Dentistry's Role in Sleep Medicine

Guest Editor

DENNIS R. BAILEY, DDS

SLEEP MEDICINE CLINICS

www.sleep.theclinics.com

March 2010 • Volume 5 • Number 1

SAUNDERS an imprint of ELSEVIER, Inc.

W.B. SAUNDERS COMPANY
A Division of Elsevier Inc.

1600 John F. Kennedy Boulevard • Suite 1800 • Philadelphia, PA 19103-2899

http://www.sleep.theclinics.com

SLEEP MEDICINE CLINICS Volume 5, Number 1
March 2010, ISSN 1556-407X, ISBN-13: 978-1-4377-1871-3

Editor: Sarah E. Barth
Developmental Editor: Donald Mumford

Sleep Medicine Clinics (ISSN 1556-407X) is published quarterly by Elsevier Inc., 360 Park Avenue South, New York, NY 10010-1710. Months of issue are March, June, September and December. Business and Editorial Offices: 1600 John F. Kennedy Blvd., Ste. 1800, Philadelphia, PA 19103-2899. Customer Service Office: 3251 Riverport Lane, Maryland Heights, MO 63043. Periodicals postage paid at New York, NY and additional mailing offices. Subscription prices are $150.00 per year (US individuals), $76.00 (US residents), $346.00 (US institutions), $185.00 (foreign individuals), $106.00 (foreign residents), and $381.00 (foreign institutions). Foreign air speed delivery is included in all *Clinics* subscription prices. All prices are subject to change without notice. **POSTMASTER:** Send change of address to *Sleep Medicine Clinics*, Elsevier Health Sciences Division, Subscription Customer Service, 3251 Riverport Lane, Maryland Heights, MO 63043 Customer Service, (orders, claims, online, change of address): **Elsevier Health Sciences Division, Subscription Customer Service, 3251 Riverport Lane, Maryland Heights, MO 63043. Tel: 1-800-654-2452 (U.S. and Canada); 314-447-8871 (outside U.S. and Canada). Fax: 314-447-8029. E-mail: journals customerservice-usa@elsevier.com (for print support); journalsonlinesupport-usa@elsevier.com (for online support).**

Reprints. For copies of 100 or more of articles in this publication, please contact the Commercial Reprints Department, Elsevier Inc., 360 Park Avenue South, New York, NY 10010-1710. Tel.: 212-633-3812; Fax: 212-462-1935; E-mail: reprints@elsevier.com.

Printed and bound by CPI Group (UK) Ltd, Croydon, CR0 4YY

Transferred to Digital Print 2011

GOAL STATEMENT

The goal of *Sleep Clinics of North America* is to keep practicing physicians up to date with current clinical practice by providing timely articles reviewing the state of the art in patient care.

ACCREDITATION

The *Sleep Clinics of North America* is planned and implemented in accordance with the Essential Areas and Policies of the Accreditation Council for Continuing Medical Education (ACCME) through the joint sponsorship of the University of Virginia School of Medicine and Elsevier. The University of Virginia School of Medicine is accredited by the ACCME to provide continuing medical education for physicians.

The University of Virginia School of Medicine designates this educational activity for a maximum of 15 *AMA PRA Category 1 Credits*™ for each issue, 60 credits per year. Physicians should only claim credit commensurate with the extent of their participation in the activity.

The American Medical Association has determined that physicians not licensed in the US who participate in this CME activity are eligible for a maximum of 15 *AMA PRA Category 1 Credits*™ for each issue, 60 credits per year.

Credit can be earned by reading the text material, taking the CME examination online at http://www.theclinics.com/home/cme, and completing the evaluation. After taking the test, you will be required to review any and all incorrect answers. Following completion of the test and evaluation, your credit will be awarded and you may print your certificate.

FACULTY DISCLOSURE/CONFLICT OF INTEREST

The University of Virginia School of Medicine, as an ACCME accredited provider, endorses and strives to comply with the Accreditation Council for Continuing Medical Education (ACCME) Standards of Commercial Support, Commonwealth of Virginia statutes, University of Virginia policies and procedures, and associated federal and private regulations and guidelines on the need for disclosure and monitoring of proprietary and financial interests that may affect the scientific integrity and balance of content delivered in continuing medical education activities under our auspices.

The University of Virginia School of Medicine requires that all CME activities accredited through this institution be developed independently and be scientifically rigorous, balanced and objective in the presentation/discussion of its content, theories and practices.

All authors/editors participating in an accredited CME activity are expected to disclose to the readers relevant financial relationships with commercial entities occurring within the past 12 months (such as grants or research support, employee, consultant, stock holder, member of speakers bureau, etc.). The University of Virginia School of Medicine will employ appropriate mechanisms to resolve potential conflicts of interest to maintain the standards of fair and balanced education to the reader. Questions about specific strategies can be directed to the Office of Continuing Medical Education, University of Virginia School of Medicine, Charlottesville, Virginia.

The faculty and staff of the University of Virginia Office of Continuing Medical Education have no financial affiliations to disclose.

The authors/editors listed below have identified no professional or financial affiliations for themselves or their spouse/partner:

David G. Austin, DDS, MS; Ronald C. Auvenshine, DDS, PhD; Dennis R. Bailey, DDS (Guest Editor); Sarah Barth (Acquisitions Editor); Cynthia Brown, MD (Test Author); R. Scott Conley, DMD; Abbey Cooper, BA, MA, CCC-SLP; Michael Friedman, MD; Christian Guilleminault, MD, DBiol; Aarnoud Hoekema, DMD, PhD; Takafumi Kato, DDS, PhD; Satish K.S. Kumar, MDSc; Gilles J. Lavigne, DMD, FRCD, PhD; Robert L. Merrill, DDS, MS; Aman A. Savani, MD; Stephen H. Sheldon, DO; Antonia Teruel, DDS, MS, PhD; and Meghan N. Wilson, MD.

The authors/editors listed below identified the following professional or financial affiliations for themselves or their spouse/partner:

Steven B. Graff-Radford, DDS is on the Speakers' Bureau for GlaxoSmithKline, Merck, and Pfizer, and is a consultant for GlaxoSmithKline, Merck, and MAP Pharmaceutical.

David C. Hatcher, DDS, MSc is a consultant for 3dMD.

Teofilo Lee-Chiong Jr, MD (Consulting Editor) is on the Advisory Board/Committee for the American College of Chest Physicians and the American Academy of Sleep Medicine.

Michael R. Littner, MD is a consultant for Balboa Sleep Disorders Laboratory; is on the Speakers' Bureau for AstraZeneca, Dey, and American Academy of Sleep Medicine (nonprofit professional organization); is an industry funded research/investigator for Schering-Plough, BioMarck, Boehringer-Ingerheim, and Novartis; and, is employed by the Department of Veterans Affairs (VA) and Sepulveda Research Corporation (nonprofit).

Disclosure of Discussion of Non-FDA Approved Uses for Pharmaceutical Products and/or Medical Devices.

The University of Virginia School of Medicine, as an ACCME provider, requires that all faculty presenters identify and disclose any off-label uses for pharmaceutical and medical device products. The University of Virginia School of Medicine recommends that each physician fully review all the available data on new products or procedures prior to clinical use.

TO ENROLL

To enroll in the Sleep Clinics of North America Continuing Medical Education program, call customer service at 1-800-654-2452 or visit us online at www.theclinics.com/home/cme. The CME program is available to subscribers for an additional fee of $99.95.

Sleep Medicine Clinics

THE CLINICS ARE NOW AVAILABLE ONLINE!

Access your subscription at:
www.theclinics.com

Contributors

CONSULTING EDITOR

TEOFILO LEE-CHIONG Jr, MD
Professor of Medicine and Chief, Division of Sleep
Medicine, National Jewish Health; Associate
Professor of Medicine, University of Colorado
Denver School of Medicine, Denver, Colorado

GUEST EDITOR

DENNIS R. BAILEY, DDS
Visiting Lecturer in Orofacial Pain and Dental Sleep
Medicine, Co-Director of Dental Sleep Medicine
Mini-Residency, UCLA School of Dentistry,
Los Angeles, California; Private Practice,
Englewood, Colorado

AUTHORS

DAVID G. AUSTIN, DDS, MS
Private Practice, Orofacial Pain, Headache, TMJ
and Sleep Disorders, Columbus, Ohio

RONALD C. AUVENSHINE, DDS, PhD
Private Practice, Temporomandibular Disorder
and Orofacial Pain; Clinical Director/Founder,
Temporomandibular Disorder/Orofacial Pain
Clinic, Veterans Affairs Hospital; Clinical Associate
Professor, Department of Restorative Dentistry
and Biomaterials, University of Texas Health
Science Center Dental Branch, Houston, Texas

DENNIS R. BAILEY, DDS
Visiting Lecturer in Orofacial Pain and Dental Sleep
Medicine, Co-Director of Dental Sleep Medicine
Mini-Residency, UCLA School of Dentistry,
Los Angeles, California; Private Practice,
Englewood, Colorado

R. SCOTT CONLEY, DMD
Clinical Associate Professor, Graduate
Orthodontic Clinical Director, Department of
Orthodontics and Pediatric Dentistry, University of
Michigan School of Dentistry, Ann Arbor, Michigan

ABBEY COOPER, MA, CCC-SLP
Front Range Speech-Language Pathology, Inc,
Englewood, Colorado

MICHAEL FRIEDMAN, MD, FACS
Professor of Otolaryngology and Chairman,
Section of Sleep Surgery - Rush University
Medical Center; Chairman of Otolaryngology -
Advocate Illinois Masonic Medical Center; Medical
Director, Advanced Center for Specialty Care,
Chicago, Illinois

STEVEN B. GRAFF-RADFORD, DDS
Director, The Program for Headache
and Orofacial Pain, The Pain Center, Cedars
Sinai Medical Center; Adjunct Associate
Professor, UCLA School of Dentistry,
Los Angeles, California

CHRISTIAN GUILLEMINAULT, MD, DBiol
Professor, Sleep Medicine Program,
Stanford University, Redwood City,
California

DAVID C. HATCHER, DDS, MSc
Clinical Professor, University of Southern Nevada, Henderson, Nevada; Adjunct Associate Clinical Professor, Arthur A. Dugoni School of Dentistry, San Francisco; Private Practice, Sacramento, California

AARNOUD HOEKEMA, DMD, PhD
Department of Oral and Maxillofacial Surgery, University Medical Center Groningen, Groningen, The Netherlands

TAKAFUMI KATO, DDS, PhD
Associate Professor, Department of Oral Anatomy and Neurobiology, Osaka University Graduate School of Dentistry, Osaka, Japan

SATISH K.S. KUMAR, MDSc
Assistant Professor of Clinical Dentistry, University of Southern California School of Dentistry, Los Angeles, California

GILLES J. LAVIGNE, DMD, FRCD, PhD
Dean and Full Professor, Faculté de Médecine Dentaire, Université de Montréal; Director of Research, Department of Surgery, Trauma Unit, Hôpital du Sacre Cœur de Montréal, Montréal, Québec, Canada

TEOFILO LEE-CHIONG Jr, MD
Professor of Medicine and Chief, Division of Sleep Medicine, National Jewish Health; Associate Professor of Medicine, University of Colorado Denver School of Medicine, Denver, Colorado

MICHAEL R. LITTNER, MD
VA GLAHS, Professor of Medicine, David Geffen School of Medicine at UCLA, Sepulveda, California

ROBERT L. MERRILL, DDS, MS
Adjunct Professor, Director, Orofacial Pain and Dental Sleep Medicine Center, UCLA School of Dentistry, Los Angeles, California

AMAN A. SAVANI, MD
Fellow, Sleep Medicine Program, Stanford University, Redwood City, California

STEPHEN H. SHELDON, DO, FAAP
Diplomate, American Board of Sleep Medicine, Diplomate in Sleep Medicine, American Board of Pediatrics, Professor of Pediatrics, Northwestern University, Feinberg School of Medicine; Director, Sleep Medicine Center, Children's Memorial Hospital, Chicago, Illinois

ANTONIA TERUEL, DDS, MS, PhD
Assistant Professor of Clinical Dentistry, University of Southern California School of Dentistry, Los Angeles, California

MEGHAN N. WILSON, MD
Research Fellow, Advocate Illinois Masonic Medical Center; Advanced Center for Specialty Care, Chicago, Illinois

Contents

The structure of the food channel is complicated by the peculiar crossing of the airway at the larynx. The oral apparatus not only prepares food but also initiates swallowing. It is designed to function in close coordination with the pharynx. The oropharyngeal system is meticulously integrated with the production of speech. One of the major reasons the upper respiratory tract of man developed as it did is partly to facilitate speech.

Orofacial Myology and Myofunctional Therapy for Sleep Related Breathing Disorders   109

Abbey Cooper

Orofacial myology or myofunctional therapy can help patients suffering from sleep breathing disorders. It aims to facilitate control of the extrinsic tongue muscles to correct, stabilize, and maintain breathing, speech, swallowing, and chewing; and to enhance the tone and mobility of orofacial structures. A speech therapist or speech-language pathologist can design orophangeal exercises to develop improved tongue posture, improved lip seal and enhanced nasal breathing.

Introduction to a Postural Education and Exercise Program in Sleep Medicine   115

David G. Austin

The 2006 American Academy of Sleep Medicine (AASM) Standards of Practice Committee supported the use of oral appliances (OAs) for patients with primary snoring and mild to moderate obstructive sleep apnea who prefer OAs to continuous positive airway pressure (CPAP) or who do not respond to CPAP. With growing public awareness and demand for alternatives to CPAP, sleep physicians are increasingly referring patients to dentists for OAs. The 2006 AASM Standards of Practice Committee noted only a 77% OA adherence after 1 year of appliance wear. Dropout rates were primarily related to OA intolerance caused by the development of temporomandibular disorders (TMDs). Many orofacial pain disorders or TMDs can be identified and managed before or in conjunction with OA therapy. With postural education and an exercise program, OA adherence can be significantly improved. It is incumbent for the sleep physician to make appropriate referrals to dentists who have advanced training in dental sleep medicine and the diagnosis and management of TMDs.

Orofacial Pain and Sleep   131

Robert L. Merrill

The relationship between orofacial pain and sleep disorders is well documented in the literature. The orofacial pain specialist is well advised to evaluate their pain patients for sleep disorders that are comorbid with orofacial pain. The interrelationship between sleep disorders and pain is complex and a two-way street. The central effects of sleep disorders on pain modulating circuitry may account for much of the association, indicating that sleep disorders should be considered in the orofacial pain population. Medications that can modulate sleep may also modulate pain where there is an overlap between the pain and sleep circuitry in which they act.

Sleep and Headache   145

Steven B. Graff-Radford, Antonia Teruel, and Satish K.S. Kumar

Sleep, shown to be associated with headaches in diverse and complex ways, has been palliative in many headaches. Sleep regulation and management of sleep disorders via multiple modalities, including continuous positive airway pressure, oral appliances, medications, surgery, behavioral sleep regulation, and psychological and cognitive behavioral management, help not only in resolving the direct consequences of poor sleeping habits and sleep disorders (eg, cardiovascular diseases and metabolic syndrome in the case of obstructive sleep apnea), but also in resolving or improving associated comorbidities, such as headaches and mood disorders. Hence, a thorough evaluation of patients with headaches and/or sleep disturbances is necessary for effective management. Dentists can play a critical role in management of these comorbid disorders of sleep and headaches.

The procedures outlined in this article are just a few of the standard methods and new advances in the treatment of obstructive sleep apnea/hypopnea syndrome (OSAHS). Thorough examination of patients' airways is necessary for identification of areas of obstruction and creation of a successful treatment plan. Multilevel therapy has been accepted as the standard for treatment because many patients have multiple levels of airway obstruction. It is important to be aware of the multiple techniques available for airway reconstruction in order to tailor therapy to meet individual patient's needs.

Obstructive sleep apnea (OSA) is common in childhood. Current epidemiologic data have shown that snoring occurs in 7% to as much as 30% of school-aged children. The most common cause of OSA in pediatric patients is hypertrophy of the tonsils or adenoids. Nonetheless, various factors are involved in upper airway obstruction during sleep in children. Craniofacial structure and function of the upper airway musculature are extensively involved in airflow dynamics. Conversely, obstructive upper airway disease can contribute to abnormalities in craniofacial structure and function. This article focuses on differences between upper airway function in children and adults, factors that predispose children to OSA, and treatment options. Bruxism, jaw clenching, and rhythmic mandibular thrusting have been associated with OSA in children, and the frequency and prevalence of these findings are discussed.

Foreword

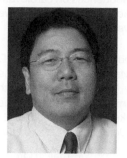

Teofilo Lee-Chiong Jr, MD
Consulting Editor

If a person snores in the forest and no one hears it, does the person make a sound? Probably no one truly knows, and no one truly cares. Until recently, snoring was, for the most part, considered simply an inescapable part of sleep, sometimes embarrassing, always a nuisance, but nonetheless harmless.

And until recently, the most common solution to snoring—a centuries-long practice that survives to this day—was banishment to another bedroom, to the far corner of the camp grounds, or to a life of nightly solitude. Other aids have been invented, mostly to allay the distress of the bed partner or roommates, rather than improve the sleep and health of the snorer. These have included chin straps of various designs and configurations, some made from cloth or leather, others of rubber or metal; chin cushions; tapes to be placed over the mouth at night, with the added benefit of abolishing speech as well, whether sleep talking or during waking; external and internal nasal dilators, including clips, braces, or strips; liniments, oils, oral sprays, and nasal decongestants; tongue retainers; sleep posture devices; pillows; background "white noise" generators; special rotating beds; magnetic strips or bands; acupuncture; hypnosis; and, if all else has failed, ear plugs. There appears to be no limit to human ingenuity, industry, aversion to snoring, and folly.

I don't need no sleep doctor/ To tell me that I snore/ My wife has told me that before/ Now I sleep outside our bedroom door/ I need help, sleep doctor, do you have/ Anything up your sleeve/ To help my poor woman/ Get some good old-fashioned sleep?/ A drug, a pill, a lotion, some magic potion/ I badly need some me-di-ca-tion./ Slept on my side, taped my mouth shut/ Stopped my boozing. I've done all that./ I'm desperate; I don't want my wife and I to fight/ So I'll sleep on the living room couch, again,/ tonight.

The early 1980s was considered by many to be a major turning point in our understanding and appreciation of the dangers of sleep-disordered breathing, including snoring. In 1981, Drs Sullivan, Issa, Eves, and Berthon-Jones, at the University of Sydney in New South Wales, Australia, described the use of a vacuum-cleaner blower motor with variable sleep control to provide continuous positive airway pressure in 5 patients with severe obstructive sleep apnea. A year earlier, at the annual meeting of the American Academy of Otolaryngology in Anaheim, California, Drs Fujita, Conway, Zorick, and Roth presented their experience with uvulopalatopharyngoplasty, described as a surgical correction of anatomic abnormalities in obstructive sleep apnea syndrome. In their paper, published a year later, they reported that, of the 12 patients who underwent this new surgical technique, relief of symptoms was seen in 9, while polysomnographic improvements in sleep patterns and nocturnal respiration were noted in 8 patients. The first description of an oral appliance for sleep-disordered breathing, the tongue-retaining device, was by Drs Cartwright and Samuelson in 1982. This device held the tongue in a forward position by negative suction and was tried on 20 male patients. The resulting reduction in obstructive and central apneic events was comparable with the efficacy rate then reported following uvulopalatopharyngoplasty or tracheostomy.

Sleep Med Clin 5 (2010) xi–xii
doi:10.1016/j.jsmc.2009.11.003

This issue of *Sleep Medicine Clinics* on dental sleep medicine comes 28 years after that first description of an oral device for sleep-disordered breathing. What a change the past 3 decades have witnessed. Currently, there are an estimated 90 oral devices for sleep-disordered breathing, and the number is increasing each year. Annually, there are several dozens of scientific papers published on the subject, and that number, too, is increasing each year. Finally, there are over 1500 dental sleep medicine specialists worldwide. Their ranks are expected to increase as well. Nevertheless, what has been the key advance in this field is the appreciation, by both patients and clinicians alike, that snoring and sleep-disordered breathing are systemic disorders with far-reaching consequences on cardiovascular, endocrine-metabolic, and neurocognitive processes as well on as overall quality of life.

Teofilo Lee-Chiong Jr, MD
Division of Sleep Medicine
National Jewish Health
University of Colorado Denver School of Medicine
1400 Jackson Street, Room J221
Denver, CO 60206, USA

E-mail address:
Lee-ChiongT@NJC.ORG

Preface

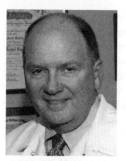

Dennis R. Bailey, DDS
Guest Editor

Dentistry has advanced in such a way that being more astute regarding medical conditions is a significant part of everyday practice. Accordingly, the role of the dentist goes beyond just the recognition of a disorder but also encompasses some degree of active participation in the patient's care. Many dentists are not sufficiently trained in the recognition of a sleep disorder, the type of referral that needs to be made, and the management of the recognized disorder. When it comes to sleep-disordered breathing one study found that less than 50% of dentists were able to identify the most common signs and symptoms.[1] This is starting to change as more courses and scientific articles in the literature read by the dentist about sleep disorders are beginning to appear.

The most common denominator associated with sleep-disordered breathing is sleep bruxism. Dentists have been actively managing this with bite splints (night guards) for decades. The recognition of bruxism as a sleep disorder and the potential for headaches and orofacial pain truly opens the door to the recognition of associated sleep disorders, especially snoring and sleep apnea. This is well documented in the article on bruxism by Drs Kato and Lavigne and is reinforced in the articles written by Dr Merrill on orofacial pain, by Drs Graff-Radford, Teruel, and Kumar on headaches, by Dr Sheldon on sleep bruxism in children, and by Dr Conley on the role of the orthodontist.

This issue brings together the comanagement and the relationship that exists between dentistry and medicine specific to the recognition and management of sleep breathing disorders. The successful completion of this issue of *Sleep Medicine Clinics* was made possible by the generous contribution of the individual authors who have shared their expertise in their respective fields. I am personally grateful for the opportunity to serve as the guest editor for this text and to those who contributed willingly to this project.

This issue demonstrates the active role of the dentist in sleep medicine and how they also need to better understand the medical side of sleep, sleep disorders, and the management of these disorders, especially sleep apnea and snoring. It also demonstrates the relationship between the various specialties in dentistry, between dentistry and medicine, their respective contribution, and how they ultimately interrelate.

Recognition of the risk for a sleep disorder and an appreciation of the craniofacial structures are brought to light by Dr Auvenshine's article on anatomy and are further reinforced in the article on the clinical screening and evaluation by the dentist. This article looks at intraoral conditions that are seen daily by the dentist that may signal that the patient is at risk for a sleep breathing disorder. In addition, the evaluation of the nasal airway is discussed along with its importance. In the article by Drs Friedman and Wilson various surgical options are discussed. Of interest are procedures designed to improve the nasal airway and other related structures that may have been impacted by growth and its impact on the craniofacial structures. In the article by Dr Conley on the role of the orthodontist the evaluation of the craniofacial structure as it relates to the airway is further developed. These articles may provide the realization that the need to evaluate the patient's growth and development is significant in

Sleep Med Clin 5 (2010) xiii–xiv
doi:10.1016/j.jsmc.2009.11.004

the potential recognition of the developing risk for a sleep breathing disorder.

The tongue and its collapse into the airway has long been a major concern as it relates to airway obstruction and the presentation of a sleep breathing disorder. In the article by Drs Savani and Guilleminault it is proposed that the collapse of the airway may be impacted by a loss of neural input and this also is applicable to the activity of the tongue. This leads to the possible contribution of orofacial and tongue exercises that are designed to improve tongue posture as described by Ms Cooper, a speech-language pathologist with advanced training in myofunctional therapy, also referred to as "orofacial myology." One study to date has described the impact this type of therapy has on sleep breathing disorders and is referenced in that article. Additionally, exercises as described by Dr Austin to improve posture and muscle tone may also have a future when it comes to improvement in breathing during sleep and during the day. Both of these areas are in need of future study to see how they may improve the treatment outcomes for snoring and sleep apnea with an oral appliance or in conjunction with surgery or continuous positive airway pressure therapy.

An area of interest among dentists who actively manage sleep apnea with an oral appliance is the use of portable monitoring to evaluate the oral appliance as a means of follow-up testing. Dr Littner provides a current view of this technology as it relates to use by the dentist for the sole purpose of determining the impact an oral appliance is having on sleep apnea. There are numerous issues to consider, study, and learn before this can be definitively implemented as a standard of care.

Imaging of the craniofacial structures and the airway now offers an added means by which sleep breathing–disordered patients may be evaluated. Dr Hatcher provides an overview of imaging from the perspective of the maxillofacial radiologist. Given the advancement of technology the dental application of this imaging that now exists may be found in dental offices and is similar to that used commonly in medicine. This imaging has the potential to evaluate patients of any age to possibly determine risk factors as they relate to the patient's craniofacial growth and their airway,

and may soon actively play a role in treatment planning.

Finally, the role of the dentist as relates to the management of sleep breathing disorders is primarily with the use of an oral appliance. The article on oral appliances reviews the use of these devices and the most current data as they relate to efficacy. This article is jointly written with Dr Hoekema, who has also published a text on oral appliances that provides a comprehensive evidence-based overview on oral appliances.[2]

It is clear that the dentist regularly encounters patients with comorbid conditions, such as headaches, orofacial pain, cardiovascular disease, hypertension, and diabetes, which may indicate the risk for a sleep breathing disorder. The risk for sleep apnea may not be the primary consideration, however, as opposed to simply being focused on the specific comorbid condition and its impact on the treatment at hand. It is hoped that over time the information and knowledge as described in this issue will be recognized by more dentists to improve the comprehensive nature of the joint effort of improved patient care by dentists and physicians. After all, as William Osler has stated: "What the brain does not know, the eye cannot see."

Dennis R. Bailey, DDS
Orofacial Pain and Dental Sleep Medicine
Dental Sleep Medicine Mini-Residency
UCLA School of Dentistry
Los Angeles, CA, USA

7901 East Belleview Avenue, Suite 200
Englewood, CO 80111, USA

E-mail address:
rmc4e@aol.com

REFERENCES

1. Levendowski DJ, Morgan T, Montague J, et al. Prevalence of probable obstructive sleep apnea risk and severity in a population of dental patients. Sleep Breath 2008;12:303–9.
2. Hoekema A. Oral-appliance therapy in obstructive sleep apnea-hypopnea syndrome: a clinical study on therapeutic outcomes. The American Academy of Dental Sleep Medicine 2008.

Oral and Nasal Airway Screening by the Dentist

Dennis R. Bailey, DDS[a,b,*]

KEYWORDS

- Oral evaluation • Nasal airway • Dentist
- Oral health • Screening

The dentist is well positioned to screen for patients at risk for a sleep disorder. When adequately trained, a dentist can use an oral appliance to treat patients diagnosed with sleep apnea. This requires some degree of awareness through training to be able to recognize the symptoms related to the more common sleep disorders. Regardless of whether the dentist intents to treat a possible sleep disorder, the dentist needs to obtain a health history to determine if the patient is at risk for some type of sleep disorder.

Because a patient's overall health may be affected by his or her oral health, the role of the dentist in managing medical conditions is expanding rapidly. This trend is evident in the literature, especially in connection with increased risk for cardiovascular disease in those individuals with periodontal disease.[1] Here, a direct link has been recognized that compels the practicing dentist for dental as well as medical reasons to be more proactive in the management of the periodontal disease process.

It has been found that the practicing dentist with some knowledge of sleep disorders is just as likely as a physician to recognize a sleep disorder in a patient.[2] The typical dentist along with the dental hygienist may see just as many patients on a daily basis as a family practitioner or an internist. A physician is more likely to uncover a sleep disorder when properly trained to obtain a sleep history and evaluate for a sleep disorder.[3] The same can be said for the dentist seeing patients on a regular basis.

SCREENING BY THE DENTIST

The dentist's first role is to screen for a sleep disorder. This can be done by adding very basic and simple questions to an already existing health questionnaire or by employing the Epworth Sleepiness Scale (ESS). The ESS is a commonly used questionnaire in sleep medicine to evaluate a patient's risk for daytime sleepiness as well as other risk factors. A more basic set of four questions, termed *STOP*, can be implemented easily by simply adding these questions to an existing form (**Box 1**).[4] The acronym STOP represents four statements that represent each of the letters. A positive response to two or more of the questions represents an increased risk for sleep apnea.

The addition of five basic questions to the health history currently in use by the dentist may also be easily implemented to detect a sleep disorder. The five questions are:

Do you have difficulty falling asleep or staying asleep?
Do you snore?
Are you frequently tired during the day?
Are you aware of or have you been told you stop breathing during sleep?
Is your sleep nonrefreshing?

Positive responses to these questions would indicate that further evaluation is needed. At this point, it would be desirable to have the patient complete the ESS. The patient should then be referred to his or her physician or to a sleep

[a] Orofacial Pain and Dental Sleep Medicine, Dental Sleep Medicine Mini-Residency, UCLA School of Dentistry, Los Angeles, CA, USA
[b] 7901 East Belleview Avenue, Suite 200, Englewood, CO 80111, USA
* 7901 East Belleview Avenue, Suite 200, Englewood, CO 80111.
E-mail address: RMC4E@aol.com

Sleep Med Clin 5 (2010) 1–8
doi:10.1016/j.jsmc.2009.10.003
1556-407X/10/$ – see front matter © 2010 Published by Elsevier Inc.

Box 1
The STOP questionnaire

S for snoring: Does the patient snore loudly?

T for tired: Does the patient often feel tired?

O for observed: Has someone observed that the patient's breathing stops during sleep?

P for pressure: Does the patient have high blood pressure?

Data from Chung F, Yegneswaran B, Pu L, et al. STOP questionnaire. Anesthesiology 2008;108: 812–21.

medicine specialist who can further evaluate the needs of the individual.

The major concern is that the dentist may not be adequately aware of symptoms or sufficiently trained in sleep medicine to recognize the possible severity of the patient's condition. Therefore, by implementing very basic questions, the possible risk may be uncovered so that the patient's problem can be adequately addressed. Unfortunately, a majority of dentists are not well versed in sleep medicine and related disorders. One study found that many dentists were not able to recognize risks of sleep apnea.[5] This is slowly changing as more articles on the topic are appearing in professional journals read by dentists and as more continuing education courses in dental schools and some predoctoral curricula are including instruction about sleep and sleep disorders.

CLINICAL RECOGNITION OF A PATIENT AT RISK FOR A SLEEP-RELATED BREATHING DISORDER

In addition to using the ESS or STOP questionnaire to gather relevant health history, the dentist needs to be acquainted with clinical observations seen daily that may indicate the risk for sleep apnea. These are findings frequently observed but which a dentist without adequate training or awareness may not associate with risk for sleep apnea. The recognition of these clinical findings should lead to a more detailed discussion about being at risk for sleep apnea or may even lead to a more extensive look at the oropharyngeal area in addition to the oral cavity.

Those who provide oral health care (ie, the dental hygienist and the dentist) should take the time to become familiar with the conditions they may encounter and to understand what those conditions may indicate. **Table 1** presents

a simplified way of correlating the clinical observations with possible risks for sleep apnea.

The dentist may uncover other sleep disorders from evidence commonly seen in practice. As an example, patients who present with orofacial pain or complaints of headaches may be at risk for insomnia. Dentists frequently treat patients for bruxism with various types of splints or appliances. The occurrence of bruxism may indicate an increased risk for restless leg syndrome or periodic limb movement disorder.[6] If a patient is found to be at risk for a sleep disorder, it is important to know what additional questions to ask to confirm this and how to properly refer the patient for more definitive care.

THE DETAILED EVALUATION

When the dentist is actively involved in the management of a sleep apnea patient, and the use of an oral appliance is called for, a more detailed evaluation is essential. This evaluation would be adjunctive to the routine clinical data that may already exist if that individual is currently a patient of record. Regardless of whether or not that data is available, the dentist needs to have some type of format for evaluating the patient so as to record data relevant to the treatment of the patient.

A more detailed evaluation is designed to look at a wide variety of factors in the oral cavity as well as the head, neck, and airway. These are areas that may be of specific concern not only dentally but also as they relate to the oropharynx and the nasal airway because conditions in these areas may affect the proposed use of an oral appliance. This examination should evaluate not only the past history, but should also review the patient's medical status and furthermore should involve a review of the findings from the sleep study. The examination format might include:

    History and chief complaints
    Review of the medical history
    Evaluation of temporomandibular joints,
        temporomandibular dysfunction, and oro-
        facial pain
    Evaluation of muscle tenderness
    Dental/oral evaluation
    Airway evaluation
    Cervical spine and postural evaluation.

The History and Chief Complaints

The history and chief complaints include information collected in a question-and-answer format about the patient's symptoms and concerns.

Table 1
Clinical findings that may indicate a risk for sleep-breathing disorders

Clinical Observation	Potential Relationship
Tongue	
Coated	Risk for gastroesophageal reflux disease or mouth breathing
Enlarged	Increased tongue activity; possible OSA
Scalloping at lateral borders (crenations)	Increased risk for sleep apnea[22]
Obstructs view of oropharynx	Mallampati score of I and II: lower risk for OSA; Mallampati score of III and IV: increased risk for OSA
Teeth and periodontal structures	
Gingival inflammation	Mouth breather; poor oral hygiene
Gingival bleeding when probed	At risk for periodontal disease
Dry mouth (xerostomia)	Mouth breather; may be medication related
Gingival recession	May be at risk for clenching
Tooth wear	May have sleep bruxism
Abfraction (cervical abrasion/wear)	Increased parafunction/clenching
Airway	
Long sloping soft palate	At risk for OSA
Enlarged/swollen/elongated uvula	At risk for OSA/snoring
Extraoral	
Chapped lips or cracking at the corners of the mouth	Inability to nose breathe
Poor lip seal; difficulty maintaining a lip seal	Chronic mouth breather
Mandibular retrognathia	Risk for OSA/snoring
Long face (doliocephalic)	Chronic mouth breathing habit
Enlarged masseter muscle	Clenching/sleep bruxism
Nose/nasal airway	
Small nostrils (nares)	Difficulty nose breathing
Alar rim collapse with forced inspiration	At risk for OSA/sleep-breathing disorder
Posture of the head/neck	
Forward head posture	Airway compromise and restriction
Loss of lordotic curve	Chronic mouth breather
Posterior rotation of the head	Tendency to mouth breathe

Abbreviation: OSA, obstructive sleep apnea.

Questions might relate to commonly found symptoms of sleep disorders, such as the presence of poor or disturbed sleep, daytime sleepiness or tiredness, snoring, observed apneas, tooth grinding (bruxism), headaches, acid reflux (gastroesophageal reflux disease), depression, mood swings or irritability, poor concentration, and low energy levels. In addition, information on history and chief complaints should summarize the findings from a sleep study if one had been done before this visit and might investigate the use of continuous positive airway pressure along with the patient's experience related to its use.

Review of the Medical History

The medical history includes a review of the current medical status of the patient along with any medications being taken. At this time, the possible health consequences of the sleep disorder and, more specifically, sleep apnea may become evident. Special emphasis should be directed toward headaches, cardiovascular disease, diabetes, asthma, allergy, neurocognitive difficulties, and any medications being used to manage these. At this time, the patient's blood pressure should also be recorded, which is a common practice in most dental practices.

Temporomandibular Joints, Temporomandibular Dysfunction, Orofacial Pain

The temporomandibular joints should be evaluated for joint sounds, joint tenderness or pain, and any dysfunction with mandibular movement. The range of motion of the mandible should be recorded as well. Many dentists do not have an adequate background in the evaluation of the patient when it comes to this area but need to become well educated and trained in it as well. It is also important to review any additional orofacial pain complaints other than those related to temporomandibular dysfunction before the initiation of any treatment.

Muscle Tenderness

Muscle tenderness in the head and neck is often a component of temporomandibular dysfunction and may be related to bruxism. Travel and Simons[7] found that muscles might have trigger points that have the potential to refer pain to a distant location. In the head and neck, the activation of these trigger points may be responsible for complaints of facial pain, headache, sinus pain, temporomandibular dysfunction, and otalgia. Some of the most commonly encountered muscles and areas of referral are:

- The masseter muscle: This may refer to the maxillary and mandibular molars, the area around the temporomandibular joints, the ear, the temples, and the face.
- The sternocleidomastoid: This may refer to the forehead, the ear, the face, the top and back of the head, and the area over the eye. Pain in this muscle may be associated with sleep-disordered breathing because it functions as a secondary muscle in respiration, elevating the rib cage and the sternum. This is a critical muscle to evaluate in the presence of frontal headaches. It has the potential to refer pain across the midline and is often described as a tight band around the head.
- The temporalis: This may refer to the side of the head and to the maxillary teeth.
- Lateral pterygoid: This is often an overlooked muscle and may refer to the face in the area of the zygomatic arch and to the temporomandibular joints.

The dentist should evaluate the patient for tenderness involving the muscles of the head and neck because these may become painful during use of an oral appliance. It is important to know in advance if there is palpable muscle tenderness so that the possibility of myofascial pain associated with the use of an oral appliance may be anticipated. It has been recommended that measuring the mandibular range of motion should be done first, since palpation may aggravate the muscles, thus limiting the movement of the mandible.[8] Many times, the patient has mostly muscle or myofascial pain that may refer to the temporomandibular joints or the surrounding areas and would then be viewed as temporomandibular joint pain or, as it is better known, temporomandibular dysfunction. It is well known that poor sleep and temporomandibular dysfunction often coexist.[9]

Dental/Oral Evaluation

All dentists are comfortable in evaluating the dental and supporting structures of the oral cavity. This evaluation is designed to look for conditions that may affect the use of the oral appliance and conditions that may be affected by the use of the oral appliance. The dentist needs to look especially for periodontal disease and, more specifically, loose teeth. The presence of dental caries also needs to be evaluated. If the patient is on medication, concern regarding xerostomia needs to be addressed as well. Certain oral and dental findings may be present that would limit the success of an oral appliance. These might include large mandibular tori, a high palatal vault associated with a narrow maxilla or posterior crossbite, and very short teeth, which might affect the secure retentive fit of the oral appliance.

In addition, the tongue should be evaluated as to its position in the mouth at rest relative to the soft palate and one's ability to view the oropharynx. Such an evaluation involves the use of the Mallampati score, which has been revised by Friedman[10] (see article by Friedman and Wilson elsewhere in this issue for discussion of this topic). The Mallampati score uses a scale from I to IV, with I being a full view of the oropharynx and IV a totally obstructed view of the oropharynx as well as of the soft palate and uvula. The more that the tongue base obstructs the view of the oropharynx and even of the soft palate, the more likely the patient is at risk for sleep apnea. One study demonstrated that, as the Mallampati score increases, so does the potential risk for obstructive sleep apnea as well as an elevated apnea-hypopnea index.[11] However, the downward slope of the soft palate should also be viewed because, if the soft palate is extended further into the oropharyngeal region, the Mallampati score may be higher than it should be to accurately reflect risk for sleep apnea. In a study using videofluorosocopy, it was found that patients with sleep apnea have longer soft palates.[12]

The lingual frenum found at the inferior surface of the tongue at the floor of the mouth should also be evaluated. If the frenum is limiting tongue mobility, the tongue may be more likely to be at a lower position and not rest in the palate as it should.

This might cause the tongue base to be further back into the oropharynx.

Airway Evaluation

From the dental perspective, the airway evaluation should be directed at the size of the uvula as it relates to its length and mass. The tonsils should be evaluated on a 0 to IV scale as is customary in medicine. As this evaluation is being done, the presence of the gag reflex needs to also be considered. Many times the patient with sleep-disordered breathing has lost the gag reflex or it has been significantly altered.

Cervical Spine and Postural Evaluation

The head posture as it relates to the cervical spine also must be evaluated. Poor posture, especially as it relates to the head and neck, may be an etiologic factor as it relates to pain, headache, temporomandibular dysfunction, and even disturbed sleep. At the same time, poor posture, especially as it relates to the head and cervical spine, may be indicative of an existing airway problem. During sleep and even during the time one is awake, the alteration in head position relative to the cervical spine may indicate the presence of airway compromise or difficulty breathing.

On clinical evaluation, a number of factors may indicate a postural problem associated with an airway problem. Addressing these findings along with the airway problems or the sleep disorder may have a positive impact on the overall treatment. The common findings associated with postural dysfunction that can be assessed on clinical evaluation are:

- Forward head posture: Here, the head is forward of the shoulders, most often visualized as the ear being forward relative to the height of the shoulder.
- Shoulder heights: When viewing the patient from the front, the shoulder heights should be even.
- Relationship of the occipital area of the skull to the cervical spine or, as it is more commonly known, posterior rotation: Here, the head appears to be rotated posteriorly

when viewed from the side and the chin may be appear to be tipped up.
- Range of motion of the head as it relates to the cervical spine: The head should freely move to the right and left such that the chin is almost over the shoulder. When the head is in flexion, the chin should nearly touch the chest and, in extension, the back of the head should be equally rotated to the posterior. All of these movements should be pain free and not feel tight or restrictive.
- Loss of the lordotic curve: When looking at the patient from the side, the cervical spine should have a slight curve, often referred to as a reverse "C" shape. If the head is forward, the neck will appear to be straight or even angled forward (forward head posture).

All of these findings can be addressed with the use of physical medicine as well as a defined exercise program. However, if the airway is compromised or obstructed, the posture of the head as it relates to the cervical spine may be more difficult to manage or correct. In these cases, head position may be compensating for the compromised or obstructed airway.

Many times, abnormal head position, poor posture, the posterior rotation of the occipital area to the first cervical vertebrae, and the loss of the lordotic curve can be visualized on a lateral head film or, as it is best know in dentistry, a cephalometric radiograph. In situations where the head is rotated to the posterior, often the chin will appear up and the occipital area will appear compressed and in close relationship to the vertebral process of the first cervical vertebrae. This is referred to as the occipital atlas space and it will appear compressed. Rocabado[13] has described and measured this on cephalometric films and has described a number of measurements that can be employed to determine if the patient has radiographic findings that would suggest postural dysfunction. The occipital atlas space is measured from the base of the occipital area to the vertebral process of the first cervical vertebrae. This distance should be 6.5 mm and the distance between the first and second vertebral process should also be 6.5 mm. When these are compressed so that these measurements are reduced, the posture of the cervical spine may be affecting the airway. In addition, the compression of the occipital atlas space may compress the greater occipital nerve, which can then lead to headaches and facial pain of cervical origin.

The hyoid, as well as the cervical spine, can be viewed. As has been described in other publications, the hyoid position is one definitive observation that indicates an increased risk for sleep apnea.[14] If the hyoid bone is more inferior and posterior as well as at an increased distance inferior to the border of the mandible, there is an increased risk for a sleep breathing disorder.

It is also possible that the posterior aspect of the airway may be affecting the airway because of some dysfunction or alteration in the posture of the cervical spine.[15] There have been reports that the posterior aspect of the airway pushed inward or an osteophyte involving the cervical vertebrae may actually impact the posterior aspect of the pharynx.[16]

THE NASAL AIRWAY EVALUATION

One of the key elements related to successful treatment involves the ability of the patient to breathe through the nose. Nasal airway screening or evaluation is not something routinely done before initiating treatment for sleep apnea or snoring. To determine the need for referral to an otorhinolaryngologist, the dentist needs to become acquainted with the process of screening for a nasal airway problem. Many people today have difficulty breathing through the nose, particularly at night. This leads to an increased tendency to be a mouth breather. The resolution of this has become a key factor in continuous positive airway pressure tolerance and effectiveness and may affect improved oxygen saturation levels during sleep.[17] The ability to breathe through the nose may be equally important when it comes to successful treatment with oral appliances and even with surgery. The reason for this is that the nose is viewed as the carburetor of the body. The nose warms the air as it flows through and humidifies it to approximately 80%.[18] This improves the lung's ability to absorb the oxygen in the inspired air. In addition, the nose and specifically the inferior turbinates filter the air. It may also be important that the patient who has difficulty nose breathing be evaluated for allergy.

To aid in the determination of nasal airway problems, it may be helpful to employ a questionnaire that determines the patient's subjective assessment of these problems. One questionnaire that is simple to use and can be combined with the ESS is the Nasal Obstruction Symptom Evaluation (NOSE) scale.[19] The scale has five questions and asks the patient to determine their perception of nasal airway problems over the last month based on a scale of 0 to 4 (no problem [0] to a severe problem [4]). It then uses a visual analog scale to determine the perception of the patient as to how difficult it is on average to nose breathe.

It is incumbent upon the dentist to be familiar with how to do a cursory nasal airway evaluation. If nasal airway obstruction or pathology appears to be present, then a referral should be made for more definitive treatment. The ultimate goal is to improve the chances that the patient is nose breathing at night, thus lessening mouth breathing, improving the sleep, and even reducing the severity of the obstructive sleep apnea.[20]

Nasal Airway Anatomy

The dentist or anyone who is screening for nasal airway problems should be acquainted with the following areas of the nose (**Fig. 1**):

- The alar rim: This is the outer area of the nose that is at times is referred to as the external nasal valve. This outer area surrounds the lateral aspect of the nose and helps form the nares (nostril).
- The turbinates: There are three paired turbinates, but the main concern here is specifically with the inferior turbinates. The inferior turbinates filter the air. The middle and superior turbinates warm and humidify the air. Enlargement of the inferior turbinates may lead to nasal airway obstruction, narrowing of the nasal valve, and difficulty breathing.
- The nasal septum: The septum divides the nose into two compartments or sides. Deviation of this can lead to airway obstruction.

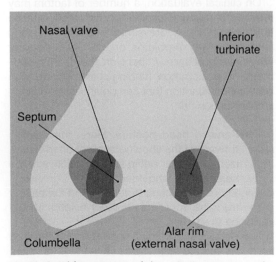

Fig. 1. Outside anatomy of the nose important to the dentist.

- The columella: This is the area at the midline of the nose located between the two nostrils that is evident externally.
- The nasal valve: This is an area that is typically viewed as long and narrow, is just inside the nose, and is formed medially by the nasal septum and laterally by the inferior turbinates. Narrowing of this area leads to increased nasal airway resistance and may tend to promote a mouth-breathing habit.

Screening by the Dentist

The screening examination for the nasal airway is done by visual observation externally and with the assistance of a nasal speculum internally. At the time of the external evaluation, the presence of a deviated septum may be evident simply by observing a bend in the nose or by the fact that the tip of the nose is not in the midline. The width of the columella can also be observed. This is a subjective observation and would be of significance if the midline tissue occupies a portion of the nostril (nares). The speculum widens the nostril, improves the view of the inferior turbinates, and enables visualization of the nasal valve. If the septum is deviated, this may also be observed.

Nasal Airway Testing

The first test is to determine if the alar rim or rims collapse during forced inspiration through the nose. If, during nasal inspiration, the alar rims collapse, this may indicate that there is a risk for increased nasal airway resistance. The collapse can usually be reduced or eliminated by placing a cotton tip applicator into the nostril where the alar rim collapses and then repeating the test. Once the collapse is reduced or eliminated, the patient should experience improvement in nasal breathing.

The second test is to determine if nasal airway dilation improves the patient's ability to nose breathe. This is referred to as the Cottle test. This is done simply by placing the fingers at the corners of the nose lateral to the alar rims and gently placing an outward (lateral) force. If this is positive and if there is alar rim collapse with inspiration, if the nasal valve or valves are constricted, or if the inferior turbinates are enlarged, then some type of nasal airway dilation may be helpful. Ultimately, surgery may prove to be beneficial.

The last test is to determine if the columella is contributing to increased nasal airway resistance. This test is done by placing the speculum into the nostrils and gently compressing the columella and asking the patient to breathe. If the patient feels his or her ability to nose breathe is improved,

then possibly some form of reduction of excess tissue making up the columella may be helpful to improve nasal breathing.

Treatment Options

Any of a variety of noninvasive treatment options can be used if any test is positive for nasal airway compromise. These options consist of:

- Nasal dilation using nasal dilator strips or other types of nasal dilators. A number of nasal dilators are available for insertion into the nose to prevent alar rim collapse and improve the caliber of the nasal valve. These have been shown to also decrease nasal airway resistance.[21]
- Nasal irrigation with a saline and sodium bicarbonate mixture. This can be helpful for reducing inflammation and removing foreign material that contributes to nasal airway obstruction. A number of over-the-counter products on the market can be used or the patient may chose to simply make their own.
- Nasal sprays. These can be prescribed to reduce inflammation. Some of these sprays are useful in cases where allergy is affecting the nasal airway. These are typically antihistamine sprays or nasal steroids.

If the patient has significant nasal airway obstruction, then a referral to an otorhinolaryngologist is indicated for a more detailed evaluation. At this time, nasal endoscopy may be indicated to more completely evaluate the nasal airway, nasopharynx, and the vocal chords; to look for nasal polyps; and to evaluate other related structures, including the tonsils and adenoids. Following this testing, more aggressive treatment may be deemed necessary. This could include surgery or long-term medication use.

Nasal airway surgical options include septoplasty, inferior turbinate reduction, removal of tonsils and adenoids, and removal of polyps. Many times, nasal airway surgery alone is not found to be curative for sleep-breathing disorders, but can be helpful with improved outcomes when the patient is using continuous positive airway pressure or an oral appliance.

SUMMARY

The evaluation process by the dentist can have many uses, including screening for sleep disorders and actively managing patients using oral appliances. As dentists become more aware of the health-related implications of conditions they observe daily, the need to be aware of sleep disorders is yet another area where additional training is necessary for optimum patient care. The first step is to become aware of conditions involving the head and neck seen every day that may indicate an increased level of risk for the patient. Being cognizant of findings in the medical history seen clinically and of the importance of the nasal airway all lead to an improved quality of life for our patients.

REFERENCES

1. Demmer RT, Desvarieux M. Periodontal infections and cardiovascular disease the heart of the matter. J Am Dent Assoc 2006;137(special suppl): 14S–20S.
2. Schwarting S, Netzer NC. Abstract from Sleep Utah 2006 (0556), Annual meeting of the APSS. Sleep apnea for the dentist—political means and practical performance. Salt Lake City, Utah, June 17–22, 2006.
3. Haponik EF, Frye AW, Richards B, et al. Sleep history is neglected diagnostic information. J Gen Intern Med 1996;11:759–61.
4. Chung F, Yegneswaran B, Pu L, et al. STOP questionnaire. Anesthesiology 2008;108:812–21.
5. Bian H. Knowledge, opinions, and clinical experience of general practice dentists toward obstructive sleep apnea and oral appliances. Sleep Breath 2004;8(2):85–90.
6. Lavigne GJ, Montplaisir JY. Restless legs syndrome and sleep bruxism: prevalence and association among Canadians. Sleep 1994;17(8):739–43.
7. Travel JG, Simons DG. Myofascial pain and dysfunction the trigger point manual. Baltimore (MD): Williams and Wilkins; 1983.
8. Wright EF. Manual of temporomandibular disorders. Ames (IA): Blackwell; 2005. p. 27.
9. Wright EF. Manual of temproromandibular disorders. Ames (IA): Blackwell; 2005. p. 14.
10. Freidman M, Tanyeri H, Lim JW, et al. Clinical predictors of obstructive sleep apnea. Laryngoscope 1999;109:1901–7.
11. Nuckton TJ, Glidden DV, Browner WS, et al. Malampati score as an independent predictor of obstructive sleep apnea. Sleep 2006;29(7):903–8.
12. Lee CH, Mo J, Lim BJ, et al. Evaluation of soft palate changes using sleep videofluroscopy in patients with obstructive sleep apnea. Arch Otolaryngol Head Neck Surg 2009;135(2):168–72.
13. Rocabado M. Biomechanical relationship of the cranial, cervical and hyoid regions. J Craniomandibular Pract 1983;1(3):61–6.
14. Hoekema A, Hovinga B, Stegenga B, et al. Craniofacial morphology and obstructive sleep apnea: a cephalometric analysis. J Oral Rehabil 2003; 30(7):690–6.
15. Finkelstein Y, Wexler D, Horowitz E, et al. Frontal and lateral cephalometry in patients with sleep-disordered breathing. Laryngoscope 2001;111:634–41.
16. Fuerderer S, Eysel-Gosepath K. Retro-pharyngeal obstruction in association with osteophytes of the cervical spine. J Bone Joint Surg Br 2004;86(6): 837–40.
17. Freidman M, Zubair S, Roee L. The role of nasal obstruction and nasal surgery in the pathogenesis and treatment of obstructive sleep apnea and snoring. Curr Opin Otolaryngol Head Neck Surg 2001;9(3):158–61.
18. Pevernagie DA, De Meyer MM, Claeys S. Sleep, breathing and the nose. Sleep Med Rev 2005;9: 437–51.
19. Stewart MG, Witsell DL, Smith TL, et al. Development and validation of the Nasal Obstruction Symptom Evaluation (NOSE) scale. Otolaryngol Head Neck Surg 2004;130:157–63.
20. McLean HA, Urton AM, Driver HS, et al. Effect of treating severe nasal obstruction on the severity of obstructive sleep apnoea. Eur Respir J 2005;25(3): 521–7.
21. Peltonen LI, Vento SI, Simola M, et al. Effects of the nasal strip and dilator on nasal breathing—a study with healthy subjects. Rhinology 2004;42(3):122–5.
22. Weiss TM, Atanasov S, Calhoun KH. The association of tongue scalloping with obstructive sleep apnea and related sleep pathology. Otolaryngol Head Neck Surg 2005;133(6):966–71.

Sleep Bruxism: A Sleep-Related Movement Disorder

Takafumi Kato, DDS, PhD[a],*,
Gilles J. Lavigne, DMD, FRCD, PhD[b,c]

KEYWORDS

- Sleep bruxism • Sleep related movement disorders
- Teeth grinding • Sleep architecture

Sleep bruxism (SB) with concomitant tooth grinding was recently reclassified as a sleep-related oromotor movement disorder falling within sleep medicine. Over several decades, however, the clinical relevance and pathophysiology of SB has been discussed by dental professionals rather than by sleep physicians, because SB has been associated with orodental consequences such as tooth wear, masticatory muscle and temporomandibular joint problems, and dental work fractures, rather than severe sleep disturbance and daytime sleepiness (rare in patients with SB). In this article, the authors review the current knowledge of SB in terms of prevalence, risk factors, diagnosis, pathophysiology, and management.

THE DEFINITION OF SLEEP BRUXISM

SB is defined as a stereotyped oromandibular activity during sleep characterized by teeth grinding and clenching. In 1990 it was classified as parasomnia in the first version of the International Classification of Sleep Disorders (ICSD-1).[1] However, in the revised version (ICSD-2) in 2005, SB was reclassified into the new category, "sleep-related movement disorders."[2] Sleep-related movement disorders are classified under simple, stereotypic, repetitive, and localized movements during sleep[3,4]; they also include periodic limb movement disorder and rhythmic movement disorder (eg, head banging).[2] On the other hand, parasomnias also include movement disorders characterized by complicated, seemingly purposeful behaviors during sleep (eg, somnambulism and rapid eye movement sleep behavior disorder [RBD]).

Sleep bruxism is regarded as primary when no clear causes are present.[2,5] SB associated with sleep disorders and neurologic diseases, drug use and medications, and can be regarded as secondary or iatrogenic. The comorbidity with SB, other medical conditions, and drugs/substances are discussed later in this article.

In dentistry, the word bruxism has been used for the diagnosis of oromandibular parafunctional activity occurring during sleeping and waking time.[6–8] This definition can include a broad spectrum of "nonfunctional" oromandibular behaviors such as clenching, bracing, tooth gnashing and grinding, nail biting, and even tongue/lip habits. Although some SB patients may be aware of bruxism during wakefulness (eg, tooth clenching), the question of whether bruxism during sleep and wakefulness shares a common physiologic alteration in oromotor controls awaits further investigation.[5,8,9]

G.J.L. holds a Canada Research Chair and his research activities are supported by the CFI, CIHR, and FRSQ. This work is supported by the Grant-in-Aid for Young Scientist (B) from the Japan Society for the Promotion of Science (No. 21791888).

[a] Department of Oral Anatomy and Neurobiology, Osaka University Graduate School of Dentistry, 1-8 Yamadaoka Suita, Osaka, 565-0871, Japan
[b] Faculté de médecine dentaire, Université de Montréal, CP6128 succursale Centre-Ville, Montréal, Québec, H3C 3J7 Canada
[c] Department of Surgery, trauma unit, Hôpital du Sacré Cœur de Montréal, Montréal, Québec, Canada
* Corresponding author.
E-mail address: takafumi@dent.osaka-u.ac.jp (T. Kato).

Sleep Med Clin 5 (2010) 9–35
doi:10.1016/j.jsmc.2009.09.003

When making a clinical diagnosis of SB followed by a management plan, clinicians need to be aware that both SB and oral parafunctions during wake time may present similar orodental problems such as orofacial pain. To avoid the confusion of the term "bruxism" and to better understand the information in the literature on bruxism, a scheme for the classification of bruxism is presented in **Fig. 1**. This article is devoted to sleep bruxism, that is, the occurrence during the sleep period of rhythmic masticatory muscle activity (RMMA) associated with occasional tooth grinding. The use of the word rhythmic refers to the fact that SB episodes tend to occur recurrently in clusters during sleep. Recording activities of the masticatory muscles with an electroencephalogram allows one to quantify data for diagnosis and to study outcomes related to various management strategies.

PREVALENCE AND RISK FACTORS

The prevalence of SB is estimated by subjective reports of tooth-grinding noise during sleep. An awareness of SB, based on sleep partner reports of tooth grinding, is reported by 5% to 8% of the adult population.[10,11] The prevalence of SB decreases from childhood (10%–20%) to old age (3%).[10–13] No gender difference is noted. The prevalence seems to decrease within a similar range in North American and European countries but might be higher in the Asian population.[10,11,14] It remains to be seen whether this difference is due to the type of questionnaire used, to a cultural awareness in relation to the sleeping environment that may increase the likelihood of tooth-grinding awareness, or to ethnicity/genetic specific factors.

Several risk factors have been reported for SB, although the causal associations between these factors and SB have not been established. SB is 1.9 times more frequent in smokers.[15,16] Caffeine and alcohol intake are reported as a risk for self-reported SB.[11,17] Drugs or substances acting on the central nervous system have been reported to increase the risk of having SB.[5,18] Adult and pediatric patients with anxiety, stress, or certain personality traits may report self-awareness or be the subject of family reports of SB more frequently than those without.[5,11,12,19–22] Familial predisposition has also been reported (see Pathophysiology section).[5]

Sleep disorders that have been reported to be concomitant with SB include obstructive sleep apnea, parasomnias, restless legs syndrome, oromandibular myoclonus, and rapid eye movement behavior disorders (RBD).[5,23,24] SB is also observed in patients with neurologic, psychiatric, and sleep disorders or following the administration or withdrawal of medication, or any combination of both.[5,8] The secondary form of SB is discussed later.

Sleep bruxism can be accompanied by a risk of secondary orodental consequences (see next section) that may include tooth destruction, dental work failure, temporomandibular joint and jaw muscle pain or jaw movement limitation, and temporal headache.[8,25–27] When tooth grinding and the habit of daytime clenching are concomitant, the odds ratio of reporting temporomandibular disorders or chronic myofascial pain in the masticatory muscles is 4 to 8, although the causal relationship remains to be proved.[5,8,28–31] A recent study reports that 43% of patients with temporomandibular disorder have 2 or more sleep disorders (eg, insomnia, sleep apnea, bruxism).[32] Most children and adult patients with SB (up to 65%) complain of headaches.[13,33–36]

CLINICAL FEATURES

Patients with SB can present the following clinical features (**Box 1**). Young SB patients do not usually complain of sleep disturbance and daytime sleepiness. However, sleep disturbance and daytime sleepiness can be reported in older SB patients or in those who have chronic head-neck pain and sleep disorders.[11,34,37] Aging and pain conditions are important factors influencing sleep organization, and the prevalence of some sleep disorders (eg, sleep apnea, periodic limb movement syndrome) is higher in the older population.[38,39]

Nonetheless, the symptom most common in SB patients is the production of an unpleasant and embarrassing noise during sleep. The noise is created by friction of the teeth related to the frequent and intense rhythmic contractions of the jaw-closing

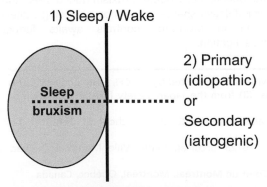

Fig. 1. Classification of bruxism. Bruxism can be classified by 2 axes: (1) sleep or waking occurrence, and (2) primary (idiopathic) or secondary (iatrogenic) type.

1) Sleep / Wake

Sleep bruxism

2) Primary (idiopathic) or Secondary (iatrogenic)

| Box 1 |
| Clinical features related to sleep bruxism |

Self-report from patient or sleep partner

- Sleep

   Sleep partner complains of grinding noise (occasionally tapping noise with oromandibular myoclonus)

- Waking in the morning

   Patient reports jaw muscle discomfort/fatigue

   Temporal headache of short duration

   Difficulty in jaw opening, jaw stiffness, temporomandibular joint noise

   Tooth hypersensitivity to cold stimuli (eg, food, beverage or air)

Clinical observations

- Visual inspection

   Tooth wear, fracture, and cervical defects

   Tongue indentation

- Digital palpation

   Masseter muscle hypertrophy during voluntary clenching (bilateral)

   Jaw muscle tenderness (masseter, temporalis) and temporomandibular joint pain

Miscellaneous

Dental restoration failure or fracture (eg, crown, denture, inlay, implant)

Occlusal trauma

Tongue biting (observed in oromandibular myoclonus)

muscles (eg, masseter and temporalis). Although the patient is usually unaware of it, a loud tooth-grinding noise often disturbs the sleep of the patient's bed partner or persons nearby.

On waking in the morning, SB patients report jaw muscle discomfort, stiffness, and fatigue.[40,41] These symptoms can be associated with a high number of jaw muscle events during sleep of the previous night. Jaw muscle symptoms can appear in the temporal regions of head (temporalis muscle area); patients may display temporal headache.

Frequent tooth grinding can be associated with secondary tooth destruction (eg, wear, noncarious cervical lesions and cracks). Tooth wear can be evident on the flat edges of anterior incisor teeth or on the flat occlusal surfaces of molar teeth.[42,43] Although tooth wear is frequent in patients with SB,[44] it cannot reliably determine the current presence of SB; wear could have happened months or

years before the time of clinical observation, and approximately 40% of normal persons can exhibit tooth wear.[45,46] Many factors contribute to tooth wear (eg, aging, diet and daytime clenching). Noncarious cervical lesions (a defect in the cervical region of the tooth) are usually associated with tooth brushing and erosion but, for reasons so far unidentified, they are more often observed in patients who are aware of tooth grinding than in those who are unaware.[47,48] The clinician needs to recognize that more cracks and failure lines may be present in the restored teeth of SB patients.[49,50] Tooth damage can be related to an unpleasant tooth sensation or pain. The morning after sleep with intense or frequent teeth grinding or clenching, patients report tooth hypersensitivity to cold liquids or air (eg, when brushing teeth). Patients may also complain of a history of acute tooth pain on chewing hard objects if they have a cracked tooth.[49]

Masseter hypertrophy can be seen in the cheek/face area between the zygomatic bone and mandibular angle when patients clench their teeth, but it does not confirm the diagnosis of SB because a habit of wake-time clenching produces the same results.[46] Tooth ridging and indentations on the buccal oral mucosa or margins of the tongue, respectively, can be observed in SB patients. Again, both masseter hypertrophy and tooth indentation can be also associated with daytime-wake time oral parafunctions such as teeth clenching, tongue pushing, and excessive swallowing.[5,51] Temporomandibular joint problems such as the limitations in jaw opening and clicking noises can be reported by SB patients.

Other conditions secondary to SB include the fracture of dental prostheses and their restoration, occlusal trauma (eg, localized bone loss around the teeth), and complaints of a metallic taste.[52]

RECOGNITION AND DIAGNOSIS
Clinical Evaluation

In ICSD-2, the following items are listed for the clinical diagnosis of SB.[2,5]

- Tooth grinding reports by parents or sleep partner (so far the most reliable)

   Plus:

- Tooth wear (again care must be taken because it may not be time related and may have other causes)
- Jaw muscle discomfort, fatigue pain, and locked jaw on waking
- Masseter muscle hypertrophy on voluntary forceful clenching

SB can be clinically recognized by interview and orofacial examination, and confirmed by electrophysiological recordings (eg, polysomnography) in the sleep laboratory or at home.[5,46,52,53] Gathering anamnestic information and clinical signs and symptoms is a starting point for a diagnosis of sleep bruxism: the information is further confirmed by sleep recording. Moreover, the information gathered from interviews about sleep habits (eg, sleep-wake pattern), sleep-related complaints (eg, daytime sleepiness and fatigue, difficulty in falling asleep, frequent awakening in night, unrefreshing sleep), signs and symptoms of sleep disorders (eg, snoring, respiratory pauses/apnea, excessive movements in sleep/periodic limb movement), and items associated with risk factors (eg, smoking, alcohol intake, medication, stress) help in managing SB and accompanying orodental problems or concomitant sleep disorders.[54] Readers can also consult the another article in this issue (by Bailey) for a better understanding of oral examination techniques and procedures.

Tooth-grinding noise

A history of tooth-grinding noise is the primary feature of SB. The grinding noise should be distinguished from other oral sounds emitted by the mouth and throat during sleep (eg, snoring, grunting, groaning, vocalization, tongue clicking, or temporomandibular joint noise) and from any squeak or clattering sounds made by the bedstead in association with body movements/sleeping position changes.[5,52] A tooth-grinding history cannot be collected in patients who sleep alone or who are edentulous. In some patients, fluctuation in grinding history can be associated with jaw muscle symptoms and with the presence of risk factors for SB (eg, stress, medication).[15,55] Because the occurrence of SB episodes and grinding noise can vary greatly over time, it is helpful to collect information about the frequency, intensity, and any temporal patterns or fluctuations in tooth grinding.[55–57]

Tooth wear

Tooth wear can be observed visually under the light after using air or cotton rolls to dry the teeth. Tooth wear does not necessarily reflect current bruxing activity.[46] The edges of worn teeth on upper and lower dentition fit together when patients slide the lower jaw laterally at an eccentric position. The severity of tooth wear can be assessed according to the previously published criteria.[42,43] Severity ranges from shiny spots on enamel, to dark yellow dentin exposure, to the reduction of crown height in a localized tooth or in a whole dentition. Severity can increase with age.[58] Attrition by dental work (eg, crown, bridge, denture) and erosion by chemicals (gastroesophageal reflux, bulimia, acid foods/beverages) should be ruled out. Wear can be very severe in SB patients in the presence of concomitant dry mouth and hyposalivation.[59] Models made from dental casts can be used to record a pattern of tooth wear and to assess time-course change. Intraoral appliances (eg, Bruxocore) are an alternative technique for indirectly assessing the mechanical impact of SB on teeth.[60,61] Patients use the appliance, which covers upper dentition, during sleep for a few weeks, and the surface area and volume of the attrition on the appliance are evaluated. When this technique is used, it is noted that jaw muscle activities during sleep are not always correlated with the degree of attrition, and that intraoral appliances can have an unpredictable influence on jaw muscle activity during sleep (see Management section).

Jaw muscle symptoms

Muscle symptoms in the face and head related to SB are distinguished from those related to other concomitant disorders. SB patients most frequently report masticatory muscle pain/discomfort on awakening in the morning, whereas myofascial pain in the jaw muscles is most likely to be reported in the evening.[62,63] Temporal headaches (mostly the tension type) on waking in the morning or in the night should be differentiated from mild generalized headache related to sleep breathing disorders (hypoventilation to hypopnea and apnea; see article in this issue by Graff-Radford).[23,64] Other orofacial symptoms related to temporomandibular disorders (eg, limited jaw opening, temporomandibular joint noise, and jaw muscle and joint pain) can be concomitant.[53] Detailed procedures for these assessments can be found in other textbooks.[53] Although several studies have suggested an association between self-reported SB and orofacial pain such as temporomandibular disorders (TMD), causation has not been established.[29,63] Polysomnographic studies were not able to prove such a link.[32,41,65] SB patients with orofacial pain have been found to exhibit significantly lower jaw motor activity than pain-free patients.[66,67] Pain sensitivity in some patients with TMD might be due to the disturbance of sleep continuity (eg, insomnia, sleep duration <6 hours or >9 hours), concomitant sleep disorders (eg, disordered breathing or limb movement), or medication, emotional disorder, persistent pain, and pain in the previous day.[32] The association between orofacial pain symptoms and SB is probably not independent of the interaction between pain and poor sleep (see the article in this issue by Merrill).[63]

Muscle hypertrophy

Masseter muscle hypertrophy can be palpated on both sides of the face. If hypertrophic, the volume of the masseter muscle increases about 2 times while the patient clenches his or her teeth, compared with the patient in a relaxed state.[5] Patients should be questioned about the presence of habitual concomitant tooth clenching during wakefulness because it can be associated with masseter muscle hypertrophy.[9] Masseter muscle hypertrophy needs to be differentiated from any swelling of parotid glands caused by tumor, inflammation, or blockage (eg, parotid-masseter syndrome).[5]

Daytime clenching

Awake bruxism, mainly characterized by tooth clenching, is thought to be a different entity from SB.[9] Awake bruxism is mainly reactive, and is induced or exaggerated by stress or anxiety.[8] It is reported by 20% of the population, more frequently among females.[9] Awake bruxism can be assessed by conscious awareness, although persons with awake bruxism are often unaware of the habit. Thus, awareness will improve after a doctor informs the patient about the habit and subsequently asks for the patient's report.[68,69] Patients with SB often report awake bruxism: mild SB patients are more frequently aware of daytime clenching and daytime stress than severe patients.[40] Awake bruxism has been reported to be associated with temporomandibular disorders (eg, jaw muscle tension/pain, joint noise, limited jaw opening capacity), tooth wear, and tongue indentation.[70,71] In addition, the coexistence of bruxism in sleep and waking may exacerbate temporomandibular disorders.[41,70,72]

Physiologic Evaluation

Jaw motor activity related to SB can be monitored at home or in sleep clinics using electrophysiological techniques. The techniques are demanding, and so far no simple system has provided a reliable proxy for valid SB diagnosis. To confirm the presence of SB in the ambulatory home setting or sleep laboratory, jaw masseter muscle electromyographic (EMG) recording of the usual polysomnographic montage with audio-video signal is strongly recommended.[4,5,23] For routine clinical purposes, the addition of one masseter EMG with audio-video will allow the frequency of RMMA episodes to be scored as described later; for research purposes burst counts and the exclusion of nonspecific oromandibular activities is mandatory.

Video monitoring

Audio-video monitoring at home can estimate jaw movements and grinding noise.[5] This technique can be useful for children or patients who refuse to sleep at the sleep laboratory with electrodes and sensors. The video camera focuses on the head/neck or upper body regions, but observation becomes difficult when the patient moves out of view. In addition, the lack of physiologic information recorded by electrodes and sensors makes it difficult to identify observed movements and sounds.[73]

Ambulatory monitoring

Ambulatory EMG recordings permit the objective measurement of jaw-closing muscle (eg, masseter) contractions during sleep. Their use in the natural sleep milieu is a major advantage. Recorded data from a single-surface EMG signal usually are stored in a portable battery-operated device. The addition of a heart rate measurement can improve the identification of SB events related to sleep arousals.[74] **Table 1** lists suggested criteria for detecting SB events using an ambulatory system.[75] However, in the absence of audio-video recording, SB episodes cannot be distinguished from oromotor events associated with swallowing, snoring, grunting, coughing, sighs, and other nonspecific jaw motor activity related to body movements, RBD, or Parkinson-related movements during sleep.[5,73] A recent study showed that 85% of body and head/neck movements were accompanied by non-SB activities in normal subjects, and that in SB patients 30% to 40% of oral and mandibular movements were not SB-related. It should be noted that in the absence of audio-video recording, confounding orofacial activities may not be properly discriminated, which can result in the overestimation of SB scoring in normals and SB patients or the misidentification of abnormal motor activities.[3,4,76]

An ambulatory EMG system can detect jaw-closing muscle bursts exceeding an EMG threshold predefined before sleep, and can quantify EMG events during sleep. Several ambulatory EMG recording systems have recently been developed to improve the reliability of recording[77] or to simplify cumbersome recording setups (Bitestrip, GrindCare).[78,79] Based on the authors' experience in a comparative sleep laboratory study, the algorithm of one of these devices does not allow the specific recognition of SB; in the other one the collection of temporalis EMG activity is a reasonable proxy that needs to be further validated in an independent sleep laboratory. Another type of ambulatory recording system has been developed to measure bite force.[80] In this system, piezoelectric film is embedded in the occlusal appliance

Table 1
Criteria for diagnosis of sleep bruxism

Ambulatory recording	
Acquisition	Sampling rate: 16.7–20 Hz (minimum)
EMG bursts	Amplitude: >10% voluntary maximum voluntary
EMG events	contraction (MVC)
	Duration: >3 s
	Interval: <5 s
	Heart rate: >5% increase
Laboratory polysomnography (audio-video plus EMG from masseter or temporalis)	
Acquisition	128 Hz (minimum) with audio-video recordings
EMG bursts	– Amplitude: >10%–20% of MVC
	– Duration:
	Phasic: 0.25–2 s
	Tonic: > 2 s
	– Interval: <3 s
Episode types	– Phasic (rhythmic): >2 phasic bursts
	– Tonic (sustained): tonic burst
	– Mixed: both phasic and tonic bursts
Polysomnographic diagnostic criteria (mild to moderate/severe case based on episode frequency estimated by EMGs)	
A: ≥4 episodes per hour of sleep for moderate/severe case Or <4 episodes per hour of sleep for low case *(mild case 2–4 episodes/h)* B: ≥25 EMG bursts per hour of sleep for moderate/severe case C: At least 2 episodes with tooth-grinding sounds at night (for both low and moderate/severe cases) Cut-off criteria: (A or B) and C	

fabricated for the patient. The diagnostic power of ambulatory systems for SB has not yet been validated in comparison with polysomnographic evaluation. With this limitation in mind, the ambulatory system can still be useful for recording jaw muscle activity in a daily life environment (eg, at home) for multiple nights in a large sample population at low cost.[5,46,81]

Polysomnographic evaluation

Compared with an ambulatory system, polysomnographic recordings are made in a controlled environment for a limited number of nights.[5] Some patients cannot sleep during the first night in unfamiliar laboratory conditions (first-night effects). Thus, in the research setting the first night is used for habituation and the data from the second night are scored for diagnosis.[5] The following biosignals are recorded in this system: a usual montage for the diagnosis of sleep disorders (eg, electroencephalograms EEGs), electro-oculograms, EMGs from submental/suprahyoid and anterior tibialis muscles, nasal air flow/pressure, thoracoabdominal movements, pulse oximetry and heart rate, and EMGs of the jaw-closing muscles (eg, masseter and temporalis) and an audio-video monitor.[73] The biosignals allow concomitant sleep disorders to be identified and permit the specific recognition of SB episodes.[5,73]

Powerful ambulatory polysomnographic systems are now available for home recording; again, simultaneous audio-video recording is recommended.[57,73,76,82]

Oromotor tasks such as swallowing, coughing, jaw opening, tooth tapping, and tooth clenching need to be recorded before sleep for further signal discrimination. In addition, other sleep disorders need to be distinguished from usual respiratory activities (exclude apnea-hypopnea and Cheyne Stokes breathing, a marker of a cardiac problem) and usual body movements (exclude periodic limb movement in sleep and RDB, a precursor of neurodegenerative disease).[4,8,52]

Scoring sleep bruxism

To begin scoring SB, jaw motor EMG episodes (single or repetitive = rhythmic) are identified in order to score bursts from at least one masseter muscle recording or, ideally, bilateral masseter plus temporalis. The EMG activity should be at least 10% to 20% of the maximum voluntary teeth clenching before sleep. All oromandibular EMG activities are scored in parallel with audio-video signals.[40] As described earlier, SB episodes should be discriminated from oromotor events associated with swallowing, snoring, grunting, coughing, sighing, and other nonspecific jaw motor contractions.

Next, EMG episodes related to SB are identified as RMMA because episodes are repeated across the sleep period. Each episode is further classified into a type: phasic (rhythmic), tonic (sustained), or mixed (a mixture of both), according to the criteria outlined in **Table 1** and **Fig. 2**.[5,83] SB episodes occurring with grinding noise are also documented. Very brief EMG bursts (duration: <0.25 second) with a brief jaw jerk or tooth-tapping movements are scored separately as myoclonic events.[84]

Diagnosis of sleep bruxism
For scoring, technicians count the number of total EMG episodes, the total number of bursts, and episodes with grinding noise. Then the frequency of bursts and episodes per hour of sleep is calculated.[84] The duration of SB episodes per hour of sleep (total duration of episodes divided by total sleep time) is a surrogate outcome variable that is also of interest.[57] Based on the diagnostic criteria, moderate to severe SB can be predicted in 83.3% of patients with SB and asymptomatic subjects can be confirmed in 81.3% of controls (sensitivity: 72%; specificity: 94%; **Table 1**) if 4 RMMA episodes per hour of sleep are scored.[83] This criterion remains constant over several years, although night-to-night variation in SB episodes (25%) and for SB episodes with tooth-grinding noise (50%) has been reported in patients with moderate to severe SB.[56] When these criteria were first proposed in 1996, patients with moderate to severe SB were clinically selected by the presence of frequent grinding noise during sleep at least 5 nights per week in the previous 6 months.[83]

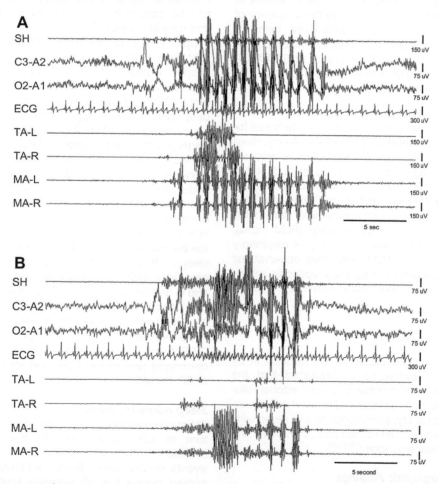

Fig. 2. Polysomnographic examples of sleep bruxism episodes. (*A*) A rhythmic type of SB episode. Phasic masseter (MA) bursts occurred rhythmically in left (L) and right (R) MA muscles. This episode is associated with grinding noise. (*B*) A mixed type of SB episode. This episode is characterized by a tonic MA burst (>2 seconds duration) followed by rhythmic MA bursts. Both episodes are associated with tachycardia on ECG and a change in brain activity on EEG (C3-A2 and O2-A1). During these episodes, EEG changes are obscured by muscle burst artifacts. SH, suprahyoid muscles; TA, anterior tibialis muscle.

When patients with a lower frequency of grinding sounds during sleep ("at least 3 nights per week") were included recently for reevaluation for RDC/SB in a study of 100 SB patients and 43 controls, a cluster of 46 SB patients did not fulfill the criteria mentioned for RDC/SB. Although they had a home history of tooth grinding, in the sleep laboratory setting they presented less than 4 episodes per hour of sleep with occasional tooth grinding.[40] These results suggest that a lower cut-off value of 2.5 RMMA episodes per hour, instead of 4.0, is clinically relevant. However, the diagnostic sensitivity and specificity of this cluster of patients with a lower frequency of SB-RMMA episodes was around 70%.[40] Moreover, the cluster of low (ie, according to frequency-based criteria rather than clinical complaint or tooth damage) SB patients formed a subgroup of patients who were different from the moderate to severe patients (again based on the frequency of EMG episodes, ie, those with more than 4.0 RMMA episodes per hour of sleep). The SB patient group with a lower EMG frequency of SB-RMMA episodes had a higher likelihood of reporting orofacial pain in morning.[40]

Supplemental sleep variables
The following sleep variables are also required for SB diagnosis: total sleep time, sleep latency, sleep stage distribution, and the frequency of arousals and awakenings. In addition, to exclude other concomitant sleep disorders and to understand the patient's sleep profile, the following also need to be documented: variables for diagnosing periodic leg movements in sleep (PLM index), sleep apnea-hypopnea index (AHI), or respiratory disturbance index (RDI), and other observations on polysomnography traces (eg, epilepsy, myoclonus) and video (eg, motor behaviors such as RBD).

PATHOPHYSIOLOGY

Although a specific cause for SB remains to be determined, studies have suggested that the occurrence of SB is subject to multifactorial influences: sleep homeostasis and arousal activity, oromotor excitability, psychological and personality traits, genetics, neurochemical activities, and oropharyngeal functions.[5,8,85,86]

Polysomnographic Findings

Sleep macrostructure
Young adult SB patients (20 to 40 years old) without concomitant medical problems (eg, no chronic pain, no sleep apnea) exhibit normal sleep architecture (eg, sleep latency, total sleep time, sleep stage distribution, sleep efficiency, number of awakenings).[8] Approximately 60% of normal subjects can exhibit RMMA in the absence of tooth grinding, at a frequency of 1.8 times per hour of sleep.[87] On the other hand, moderate to severe SB patients exhibit SB episodes 5.8 times per hour of sleep, more than 90% of which contain RMMA, occasionally associated with tooth grinding.[87,88] In SB patients, the amplitude of masseter EMG bursts is frequently as high as 30% to 40% in comparison with controls.[87] These observations suggest that RMMA in SB patients represents an extreme manifestation of a natural, physiologic oromotor activity.[8,89] As described later, 74% of RMMA episodes can be scored in a supine position and 60% of episodes are concomitant with swallowing in SB patients as well as in normal subjects.[90] Isolated or repetitive myoclonic masseter bursts can be concomitantly observed in SB patients and normal subjects.[84]

Up to 85% of SB episodes are found to occur in light non–rapid eye movement (NREM) sleep (stages 1 and 2).[27,34,83,91–96] Fewer SB-RMMA episodes are observed during rapid eye movement (REM) sleep (approximately 10%) and in deep NREM sleep (approximately 5%–10%) in young adults, in contrast to previous results.[97,98] Regarding the relationship to sleep cycles during the night, the occurrence of SB episodes is higher in the second and third NREM to REM sleep cycles compared with the first and fourth cycles (each cycle lasts between 90 and 110 minutes).[92] In addition, SB episodes are most frequently found in the ascending period within a sleep cycle (eg, the period shifting from deep NREM toward REM sleep).[92] It is known that the ascending period is correlated with an increase in sympathetic tone and in arousal activity.[99,100] Thus, the heterogenic distribution of SB episodes within the sleep cycle and across the night suggests that a normal sleep process related to endogenous ultradian (NREM and REM) or semi-circadian rhythm is an underlying physiologic condition for the genesis of SB-RMMA.

Sleep microstructures
Other observable findings in the sleep microstructure of SB patients include the association between RMMA and phasic EEG and motor events during sleep. Fewer K-complexes were scored during the 10 seconds preceding SB-RMMA episodes in SB patients (12.1%) than in normals (21.2%).[101] Unlike patients with periodic leg movements during sleep, SB patients have a smaller number of total K-complexes and K-alphas during sleep compared with normal

subjects (42.7% and 61.5% lower for K-complexes and K-alphas, respectively).[101] Sleep spindles were not associated with RMMA, and their frequency does not differ between SB patients and normal subjects.[101] Another phasic event related to SB is the microarousal (EEG arousal), characterized by a brief (more than 10 or 15 seconds) cortical, autonomic-cardiac, and motor activation.[99,100,102] Observational studies report that the changes in EEG frequency or alpha EEG waves are scored in association with SB episodes. Tachycardia (increasing up to 25% of baseline heart rate), leg jerk (>80% of episodes), and body movements (up to 24% of episodes) have also been observed in relation to SB episodes.[74,93–95,103–105] Most SB episodes result in sleep stage shifts.[92,95]

Compared with normal subjects, the frequency of microarousals (3–10 second periods of increased activity on EEG, electrocardiographic (ECG), and EMG recordings; note that in the United States the more generic but less precise word arousal is frequently used instead of microarousal) is within an upper range of the normal limit in SB patients (10 to 15 times per hour of sleep).[101,106] The association between microarousals and SB episodes is correlated with the occurrence of the cyclic alternating pattern (CAP) that is repeated every 20 to 60 seconds in clusters during NREM sleep.[93] The CAP reflects cyclic physiologic and behavioral changes in response to endogenous and environmental influences during sleep. More than 80% of SB episodes happen during CAP phase A3 (the high arousal pressure period) and more than half of SB episodes occur in a cluster within 100 seconds.[92] The frequency and duration of CAP has been shown to be similar between SB patients and normal subjects.[93] Microarousal and CAP phase A3 predominantly occur in the ascending phase of the sleep cycle in association with an increase in sympathetic balance.[100,107] The occurrence of SB episodes is thus more likely to be associated with a periodic arousal fluctuation under the influence of a subtle change in the balance of the autonomic nervous system activity during sleep.[8,85,89] However, what predisposes SB patients to be vulnerable to such powerful arousals is unknown.

Physiologic sequence

Recent studies have examined temporal relationships between SB and changes in EEG and autonomic nervous system activity to address the question, "does microarousal cause SB or does SB cause microarousal?" When sympathetic tone was assessed using heart rate frequency analysis, an increase in sympathetic tone was found to present around 4 minutes before the SB-RMMA episodes.[92] Mean heart rate subsequently starts to increase around 10 seconds before the episodes.[103] Next, a significant increase in brain alpha (fast waves) and delta (slow waves) EEG activity and an augmentation in respiratory activity occurs approximately 4 seconds before the onset of an RMMA episode, and a significant increase in heart rate occurs 1 cardiac cycle before an RMMA episode.[34,94] At the onset of RMMA, an increase in suprahyoid muscle activity and a major breathing effort precedes rhythmic jaw-closing muscle activation by 0.8 second (Fig. 3).[87,108] A clear sequence was found in 80%–90% of RMMA episodes in both SB patients and normal subjects.[87,103] These results delineate a definite physiologic sequence of autonomic/cardiac, cortical brain, and jaw motor activation in the genesis of SB-RMMA, and further demonstrate that the SB-RMMA episode is the final event during a microarousal (Fig. 4).[8,85,89]

Motor Excitability

In general, muscle tone in the limbs, upper airway, and jaw muscles decreases from wakefulness to sleep. The changes in muscle tone are attributed to the ascending or descending neural inputs, neurotransmitter release, and motoneuron excitability.[109,110] The sleep stage dependent changes in muscle tone have been reported to differ between jaw and leg muscles in humans.[111] In masticatory muscles (eg, masseter, suprahyoid), decrease in muscle tone does not differ between NREM sleep stages.[111,112] During REM sleep, masticatory muscle tone becomes minimal but does not disappear completely (eg, hypotonia). In the quiet sleep period without motor activity, masseter and suprahyoid muscle tone in SB patients does not differ from that of normal subjects during NREM and REM sleep.[112] This finding suggests that SB patients have a normal tonic motor excitability in the masticatory muscles. When microarousals were induced experimentally by sensory stimuli (auditory, vibrotactile), arousal responsiveness to stimuli did not differ between SB patients and normal subjects.[112] Nonetheless, RMMA is triggered by arousal response 7 times more frequently in SB patients than normals, and 86% of induced RMMAs involved teeth grinding.[112] SB patients may have an increased transient responsiveness of rhythmic jaw motor excitation in response to microarousal.

Most SB episodes are found to occur with leg and body movements. SB patients have been reported to exhibit increased motor activity in the body during

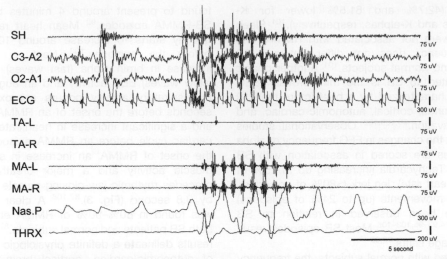

Fig. 3. An increase in respiration in association with a SB episode. A rhythmic SB episode is associated with an augmentation of nasal airway pressure (Nas.P) measured by nasal cannula (Canule). After the episode, an amplitude of respiration gradually decreased to a baseline level.

sleep.[113,114] Several studies have suggested that the degree of motor suppression or activation during sleep might differ between muscles (eg, jaw and limb muscles).[111,115,116] In addition, body movements are most likely to occur in response to the higher level of arousal response (eg, awakening).[110,117] Because arousal responsiveness is associated with an intrinsic difference in the recruitment patterns of autonomic, cortical, and motor activations,[99,110,118,119] a clarification of the thresholds (or excitability) for motor activation in jaw and body muscles would assist the understanding of increased motor activity in SB patients.[120]

Neurochemicals

The influence of neurochemicals on SB activity has been written up in case reports and in the results of clinical trials (see the Management section for more details).[18] It has been suggested that catecholamines such as dopamine, noradrenaline, and serotonin are involved in SB pathophysiology.[8,86]

One pilot imaging study has suggested that dopamine, a catecholamine, is involved in SB. In this study, researchers observed an asymmetric distribution of striatal dopamine binding sites in SB patients.[121] However, the overall density of the striatal dopamine receptors was found to be

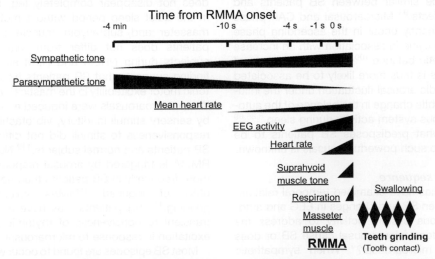

Fig. 4. Proposed sequence of physiologic changes associated to the onset or occurrence of RMMA/teeth-grinding episodes with sleep arousal.

within normal range in young adults with SB tooth grinding. A randomized experimental controlled trial using L-dopa, a catecholamine precursor, had a mild but significant suppressive effect on SB; by contrast, a moderate dopamine receptor agonist, bromocriptine, had no effect on SB episodes, and this medication failed to restore the imbalance of the striatal dopamine binding sites.[122,123] Although a case report suggested that a catecholamine-related noradrenaline β-blocker, propranolol, may reduce SB,[124] a randomized experimental controlled study failed to reproduce the results.[125] The Scandinavian group's initial supposition was of great interest, however, because an α-receptor agonist, clonidine, has been shown to decrease SB in relation to a decrease in sympathetic tone.[125]

Based on clinical observation and questionnaires, the role of serotonin is more difficult to understand: some selective serotonin reuptake inhibitors (SSRI) can exacerbate or initiate sleep bruxism (eg, fluoxetine, sertraline, citalopram), whereas a low-power study found that iatrogenic SB was suppressed by a different type of SSRI drug (eg, buspirone).[18,126,127] Other drugs related to γ-aminobutyric acid (GABA) (eg, clonazepam, diazepam, tiagabine) have suppressing effects on SB activity, but only clonazepam has been tested under a powerful methodological paradigm.[18]

This information suggests that various neurochemicals have a modulating influence on SB. Neurochemicals are known to be involved in sleep-wake regulation, autonomic functions, motor controls, and anxiety/stress conditions. In addition, these neurochemicals may interact with each other and with various endocrine functions (eg, growth hormone, corticotropin-releasing hormone, ghrelin, leptin) that regulate endogenous sleep regulations related to ultradian and circadian rhythms.[128,129] The specific roles of neurochemicals and endocrine systems during sleep and SB activity need to be investigated in a future study.

Stress and Psychological Influences

There is a common belief that psychological stress contributes to SB pathophysiology. Studies have suggested that children and adults reporting self-awareness of tooth grinding are more anxious, aggressive, and hyperactive.[11,12,19,21,22,130–134] However, the evidence is not strong.[135] Several of these studies listed had methodological limitations for interpreting the association between psychosocial factors and bruxism: some made no distinction between a daytime clenching habit and SB, and others did not perform objective physiologic recordings to validate SB diagnosis.[135] Of note, SB patients diagnosed by polysomnography showed similar reaction times and vigilance to normal controls under an attention-motor test condition.[136] However, they scored higher than normals on anxiety regarding successful test performance. A few studies suggest that SB patients are more likely to deny the impact of life events due to their coping styles or personality.[137,138] In addition, in a few case studies masseter EMG activity increased during sleep following days with emotional or physical stress,[139,140] whereas other studies did not replicate the finding.[141–143] In a study of 100 SB patients, a correlation between self-reported daytime stress and masseter muscle EMG activity during sleep was found in 8% of patients.[142] Thus, there might be a subgroup of SB patients whose psychosocial response to life events, in the form of jaw motor activity, differs from that of normal controls.

Subjective SB studies were reported to be associated with increased concentration of urinary dopamine, adrenaline, and noradrenaline during the daytime.[144,145] These results were consistent with those from a study using ambulatory EMG recording.[146] Although high urinary catecholamine is considered to be a response to sympathetic nervous activity and psychological stress, severe SB patients did not have disturbed autonomic functions and perceived less stress than mild SB patients.[92] Catecholamine concentration and sympathetic tone can be associated with other factors such as concomitant chronic orofacial pain, sleep fragmentation, and sleep-related body movements.[147–149] The significance of high catecholamine levels in SB patients clearly remains to be investigated in combination with sleep endocrinology.

To understand the relationship between SB and psychological factors, further studies are needed to clarify the roles of individual susceptibility (eg, genetic or personality traits) and the interaction of sleep and psychophysiological functions (eg, autonomic and endocrine systems) in jaw motor systems.

Genetic Factors

Some studies made using questionnaires or tooth wear examinations have suggested that there is a genetic or familial predisposition for SB. Twenty percent to 50% of SB patients may have a family member who also reports tooth grinding during childhood.[150–152] In twin studies, the report of tooth grinding is more concordant in monozygotic than in dizygotic twins.[153–155] In addition, the presence of SB in childhood persists in 86% of adults.[154] Nonetheless, a cohort study has found that self-reported tooth grinding can fluctuate over 20 years from childhood to adulthood.[156] Thus, environmental factors are also likely to be involved in the genesis of SB in addition to genetic factors. In addition, sleep parasomnias and SB have been suggested to share genetic influences.[12,153,157] Genetic influences may explain individual differences in the genesis of SB and in SB activity in response to medication, drugs, and psychological stress. The electrophysiological assessment of SB in studies conducted over several generations will be needed to determine genetic factors contributing to SB; cost is a main limiting factor for such studies.

Oropharyngeal Functions

Oropharyngeal structures play several important physiologic roles for functional and tissue integrity (eg, swallowing, respiration) during sleep.[52,59] Swallowing is a physiologic oropharyngeal motor activity that occurs 5 to 10 times per hour during sleep: a much lower rate than wakefulness (up to 60 times per hour during noneating periods).[158] The decrease in swallowing rate may be related to decreased salivary secretion and reflex sensitivity during sleep. Pharyngeal swallowing and subsequent secondary esophageal peristalsis may prevent the invasion of acid reflux to the oral cavity, pharynx, and lung in patients with gastroesophageal reflux.[159] Swallowing, therefore, plays a protective function during sleep, probably in association with saliva.[59] Swallowing occurs predominantly in light NREM sleep in relation to arousals.[89,158] Swallowing was found to occur with approximately 60% of RMMA episodes in SB patients and normal subjects.[90] Masseter EMG bursts associated with RMMA were found to occur when esophageal pH decreased in SB patients who did not suffer from sleep-related gastroesophageal reflux.[160] In children, no correlation was found between SB episodes and esophageal pH.[106] The interaction between factors such as swallowing, esophageal pH, microarousals, and salivation needs to be studied in association with autonomic and gastroenteric systems that are linked to sleep and visceral functions.[8,161,162]

During sleep, the jaw is usually open for 90% of total sleeping time because oropharyngeal muscle tone decreases.[163] The mandible and tongue collapse into the pharynx, which results in a narrowing of the upper airway during sleep.[164] The reduction in upper airway space is worst in a supine position, where obstructive sleep apnea can occur most frequently in obstructive sleep apnea syndrome (OSAS) patients.[164] Of note, 75% of RMMA episodes were found to occur in a supine position.[90] A recent study has shown that respiratory activity shows a simultaneous and significant increase on the activation of the suprahyoid muscles when RMMA episodes occur (see **Fig. 3**).[108] However, an increase in respiratory amplitude preceding RMMA episodes is more likely to be associated with an autonomic drive during the arousal response, rather than with the upper airway opening found after an obstructive apnea event. RMMA episodes rarely occur after apneic events[23] and the role of limited airway flow or upper airway resistance remains to be demonstrated, as suggested by Simmons and colleagues at the last Sleep2009 meeting in Seattle[165] (see also section on Secondary SB). Nonetheless, another study has reported that the use of an oral appliance that opens the airway reduces the frequency of RMMA episodes in SB patients who do not have sleep-disordered breathing.[166,167] It remains to be demonstrated whether arousal levels related to subclinical airflow limitation might be one of various intrinsic factors contributing to the genesis of RMMA.

Peripheral Occlusal Factors

Contrary to a common belief in dentistry, current knowledge does not support the idea that occlusal factors such as premature tooth contacts trigger SB.[8,85,86,168–170] In healthy people, an average time for tooth contacts, including meals, is 17.5 minutes per day.[171] Tooth contact is usually absent during sleep without motor activity, whereas it can occur in association with arousal, swallowing, and motor activity.[163,172] In addition, tooth contacts are found to occur in clusters approximately every 90 to 120 minutes during the night, suggesting that tooth contacts during sleep are a consequence of jaw-closing muscle activation within a sequence following microarousal.[80,172,173] In addition, edentulous patients exhibit RMMA when they sleep without their dentures.[174,175] Moreover, no correlation between dental morphology (eg, dental arch, occlusion) and SB episodes has been found in adult SB patients assessed by polysomnography.[176]

IATROGENIC AND SECONDARY BRUXISM

Various drugs and chemical substances have been reported to exacerbate SB (**Box 2**). Orofacial movements during sleep, including secondary SB, have been reported in several movement and neurologic disorders (**Box 3**).[24,177] Evidence of iatrogenic and secondary SB is scarce because

---

Box 2
Drug and chemical substances associated with sleep bruxism

Chemical substances: habitual or recreational use[5,11,15–18]

- Alcohol, caffeine, nicotine (smoking)
- Cocaine, 3,4-methylenedioxymethamphetamine (MDMA; ecstasy) (mainly for bruxism during wakefulness)

Medications[a]

- Antipsychotic drugs: haloperidol, lithium, chlorpromazine
- Antidepressive drugs: SSRI (eg, floxetine, sertraline, paroxetine, venlafaxine)
- Cardioactive drugs: Calcium blocker (eg, flunarizine)
- Psychostimulants: methylphenidate[178,179]
- Nonpsychostimulants: atomoxetine[180]

SSRI: selective serotonin reuptake inhibitors

[a] For details, see Lobbezoo et al, 2001,[181] Kato et al, 2001,[52] Winocur et al, 2003,[18] Kato et al, 2003,[24] Lavigne et al, 2005,[5] Lobbezoo et al, 2006.[181]

Box 3
Secondary sleep bruxism (eg, tooth grinding reported to be concomitant with the following medical conditions)

Movement disorders

- Hyperkinetic movement disorders: Oromandibular dystonia, Tics (Tourette syndrome), Huntington disease, Hemifacial spasms
- Hypokinetic movement disorders: Parkinson disease
- Neurologic/psychiatric disorders and other medical conditions
- Neurologic: Cerebellar hemorrhage, Olivopontocerebeller atrophy, Whipple disease, Shy-Drager syndrome, Coma, Mental retardation[a]
- Psychiatric: Anxiety disorder, Depression, Attention deficit hyperactivity disorder[a]
- Other medical conditions: Angelman syndrome[a,182] allergy[a,183]

Sleep disorders

- Insomnia
- Snoring[a], obstructive sleep apnea[a]
- NREM parasomnias: Sleep walking, night terrors, confusional awakening
- REM parasomnias: Rapid eye movement sleep behavior disorders, also named RBD
- Oromandibular myoclonus
- Sleep groaning[184]
- Sleep epilepsy[185,186]
- Enuresis[a,187,188]
- Restless legs syndrome, periodic limb movement disorders

[a] Sleep bruxism is reported in pediatric patients. For details of secondary sleep bruxism, please see Huynh and Guilleminault 2009,[189] Lavigne et al, 2005[5] and Kato et al, 2003.[24]

---

most data are derived from case reports without electrophysiological assessment of SB.

In several case reports, tooth grinding and clenching during sleep have been reported in movement disorders such as oromandibular dystonia, Parkinson disease, Huntington disease, hemifacial spasms, tic, epilepsy, and neuroleptic-induced abnormal involuntary movements. Patients with olivopontocerebellar atrophy, Whipple disease, and Shy-Drager syndrome have been reported to show SB. SB is often reported in pediatric and adult patients with psychiatric and cognitive problems.[133,190–196]

Sleep bruxism has been reported to occur in several sleep disorders.[24] Whether concomitant occurrence of SB in sleep disorders is associated with secondary influence of sleep disruption (eg, increased microarousals) or with a presence of common mechanisms for oromotor activation remains to be investigated.

In a cross-sectional epidemiologic study, snoring or OSAS was reported in more than 30% of adult subjects with signs and symptoms of SB (eg, grinding history and morning jaw muscle discomfort).[11] The odds ratio of having SB was 1.4 for snoring and 1.8 for sleep apnea. In a few polysomnographic studies, tooth grinding/RMMA events were observed in 40% to 60% of a small group of adult patients (10–20 patients) with OSAS.[197,198] However, these studies failed to show a temporal association between apneic events and EMG episodes of RMMA in patients with OSAS, suggesting that postapneic respiratory activation might be a different form of physiologic response from respiratory activation preceding RMMA.[108] Instead, tonic masseter muscle activity was frequently found at the end of apneic events, as a nonspecific oromotor activation in response to apnea-induced arousals.[177,197–201] Sensory impairment of the pharynx has been found in OSAS and snoring patients, but the influence of such changes on motor activity in response to arousals is not known (see the article in this issue by Guilleminault).[23] Further studies are needed to determine whether the concomitant occurrence of SB is associated with a degree of sleep fragmentation (eg, severity of apnea) rather than an increase in postapneic arousal responses in patients with OSAS.

The concomitant occurrence of sleep bruxism and sleep apnea or snoring has been reported in pediatric patients.[13,22,202] It has also been suggested that upper airway and face morphology contribute to the SB seen in pediatric patients.[203–206] Because upper airway morphology is a significant risk for snoring and sleep apnea in children, the occurrence of SB in children with abnormal upper airway morphology provides a future challenge to be considered in the pathophysiology and management strategies in pediatric SB patients.[189]

Parents more frequently report tooth grinding in children with common pediatric parasomnias (eg, sleep talking, sleepwalking, enuresis, night terrors) than in children without.[189] Familial predisposition and correlation with anxiety and stress have also been reported for these parasomnias.[153,207] In adults, the prevalence of SB is 1.5 to 3 times higher in patients with violent parasomnias such as REM sleep behavior disorder, sleepwalking, or night terrors.[193] Most SB episodes are associated with leg and body movements whereas periodic limb movement disorder is found in few SB patients.[24,34] Tooth grinding was reported in only 10% of patients with restless legs syndrome.[10] Oromandibular myoclonus (OMM) is characterized by repetitive or isolated tappinglike jaw movements.[84] Familial patterns can be traced for OMM.[208] Approximately 10% of SB patients can exhibit OMM, although OMM is a different entity from SB.[84,209] Patients with oromandibular myoclonus may complain of nocturnal tongue biting.

MANAGEMENT

Because researchers have yet to determine the specific causes of SB, current suggestions concentrate on managing the consequences of SB tooth grinding rather than proposing a curative treatment. The approaches proposed for managing SB range from behavioral modification and orodental appliances and splints to pharmacologic strategies (**Table 2**). It is relevant to note that not all approaches have been found to be effective, and some risks or side effects may prevent their use in some patients.[210] The clinician's choice of management option is driven by the need to protect orofacial structures from damage, to relieve any accompanying pain-related sensory complaints, and to reduce the putative risks for exacerbation, while taking into account the patient's medical history, age, and benefit-efficacy over side effect or risk ratio.[5,211–213]

Behavioral Strategies

Two major behavioral strategies for managing SB are psychological relaxation and lifestyle instruction, and approaches that include sleep hygiene and the use of biofeedback techniques.

Sleep hygiene instructions are used to guide patients toward good-quality sleep and the avoidance of several risk factors for SB (eg, stress, alcohol, smoking, and irregular life habits).[5,214,215] First, doctors or dentists explain current concepts of SB risks and pathophysiology. Then the following instructions are given: (1) avoid intense mental and physical activities during the late evening and relax before sleep; (2) avoid large meals and beverages such as coffee, tea, and alcohol, and avoid smoking in the evening; (3) install a comfortable sleep environment (eg, containing elements like a quiet room, a moderate temperature, a comfortable bed set); and (4) maintain a regular bedtime hour (if patients are engaged in shift work, the work schedule would be balanced with recovery rest periods).

For relaxation, patients learn a relaxation or meditation technique such as abdominal breathing or biofeedback practice. The patient can then practice the technique in daily life whenever he or she becomes aware of stress and tension, or before sleep. Psychologists can help patients to master these procedures. Although these instructions seem a reasonable approach to managing SB, their therapeutic effect on SB has been rarely tested. One study tested the effects of cognitive-behavioral therapy (CBT) in which patients attended a combination of stress management and nocturnal biofeedback sessions for over 12 weeks.[216] CBT reduced SB activity, as measured by abrasion on an oral device, associated symptoms, and psychological impairment. However, the effects of CBT did not differ from those observed with the use of an occlusal splint and did not last for 6 months. The approaches outlined would be appealing to patients with complaints of concomitant insomnia or sleep disturbance or whose sleep is instable. Psychological management and other strategies would also be considered for SB patients exhibiting a tendency toward maladaptive coping.[138] Because primary SB patients exhibit normal sleep structure, the efficacy of sleep hygiene, relaxation techniques, CBT, and hypnotherapy for sleep stability and SB remains to be demonstrated in a controlled study. In an open study, hypnosis reduced EMG activity and tooth grinding.[217] This result needs to be confirmed in a controlled study.

Biofeedback paradigms activated by masticatory EMG activity (eg, sound stimuli) were reported to reduce SB activity. However, the effect does not seem to persist after treatment ceases.[218,219] Because loud sound stimulation awakens patients from sleep, it is a potential cause for daytime sleepiness. In addition, sound stimuli may disturb the sleep of the patient's bed partner. Alternative stimulus modalities, such as vibration on the teeth and electrical shocks to the skin of the lip and forehead, have been tested in several studies. In a few case studies, a vibratory stimulus or an unpleasant taste stimulus applied in the mouth reduced SB activity, and the effects lasted over several months.[220,221] Non-noxious electrical stimulation to the lip at the time of tooth contact decreased the duration of SB episodes rather than the number of episodes.[222] Another study used non-noxious electrical stimulation on the skin of forehead.[78] The number of jaw motor events was decreased during a biofeedback treatment period while the signs and symptoms of temporomandibular disorders did not change. In addition, subjective sleep quality and total sleep time did not differ between the periods with and without treatment.[78] Complete polysomnographic recordings, to assess influence on sleep continuity, were rarely used in the studies employing the biofeedback paradigm.

This paradigm has transient effects during the treatment period. Thus, the efficacy of long-term use needs to be evaluated in terms of the patient's habituation to the stimulation and the accumulated influence of subtle sleep disturbance. Another question is whether sensory stimuli used in the biofeedback system suppress jaw-closing muscle activity directly by exteroceptive suppressive influence or indirectly by sleep modification and cognitive influence.

Orodental Strategies

Oral appliances such as occlusal splints and mouth guards have been used for managing SB and temporomandibular disorders in dentistry for years. However, the physiologic mechanisms underlying the action of the devices remain to be demonstrated.[223,224] Oral appliances can be fabricated in hard (acrylic resin or thermosensitive material) or soft (vinyl silicone on the occlusal surface with a hard body, or a full appliance in soft material) materials in a dental laboratory or in the clinic using special systems currently available on the market. A dentist needs to adjust such appliances to the patient's dentition.[53] Both hard acrylic occlusal splints and soft vinyl mouth guards usually cover maxillary or mandibular dentition to control the mechanical load on the teeth or dental restorations.[53,223] Based on clinical

experience, a hard occlusal splint is mainly recommended for long-term full-night use. A soft mouth guard is principally suggested for short-term use in adults, because it is less expensive. However, a soft mouth guard is the appliance of choice for pediatric SB patients with mixed dentitions because the oral device needs to be remade as teeth are replaced and grow. However, caution is needed when recommending mouth guards: they may increase SB activity in 50% of patients.[225]

Like a soft mouth guard, a hard occlusal splint does not always reduce SB activity in all subjects, and its effect on muscle activity seems to last for only a few weeks. The effect of an occlusal splint on the frequency, intensity, and duration of SB episodes has varied between or within studies (eg, decreasing or increasing effects, and no effects).[104,219,225–230] Even though an occlusal splint does not affect sleep architecture and is an effective technique to protect teeth from damage in patients with SB, the splint may disturb some physiologic orofacial activity during sleep (eg, swallowing).[227]

The choice of the best oral appliance design remains open to debate; studies comparing the effects of different designs of occlusal splint (eg, pattern of contacts between splint and dentition) on SB have failed to show any significant difference between the various models.[231] Using a cross-over design, a few studies demonstrated no difference in the effects of an occlusal splint and a palatal splint that did not cover maxillary teeth.[227,228,230] More importantly, in a study of subjects using an occlusal splint for 6 weeks, the decreasing effects, if any, lasted for only 2 weeks and did not continue after withdrawal.[219,228,232,233] These findings suggest that the occlusal splint should be used for protecting teeth from the force generated by jaw muscle contractions, rather than for controlling SB activity.[223,224,234] This concept is appropriate because the genesis of SB is regulated by the central nervous system.[8,85,86]

Although dentists have generally considered the occlusal splint to be a conservative and safe management option for SB management, a recent study has raised the possibility that it might have a harmful influence on breathing during sleep. It was found that the use of the occlusal splint in patients with obstructive sleep apnea could aggravate abnormal breathing.[235] This preliminary open study suggests that it is important for clinicians to assess a history of sleepiness and snoring in patients at risk of OSAS. It is recommended that the clinician assess sleepiness with an Epworth scale and estimate the risk of sleep breathing disorders (reports of the cessation of breathing

Table 2
Management strategies for SB

Strategies	Effects (evidence): comments
Orodental strategies	
Occlusal splint	+ or – (B): Protects tooth from grinding-related damage; short-term reduction of EMG activity but after 2–4 wk levels seems to return to baseline values; possible risk for exacerbating snoring and apnea
Mouth guard	+ or –: Short term; may increase EMG activity
NTI splint	+ (B): Short term data only; may change occlusion if used for a long term
Mandibular advancement appliance (MAA)	++ (B): Short term data only; teeth or jaw pain if not well titrated
Occlusal therapy	Questionable/Low level of evidence as a universal therapy; not reversible
Behavioral strategies	
Management of life style, stress, and sleep hygiene	+ or – (B): Lack of strong evidence/Expected to reduce SB: may help if combined with other strategies. Coping style of SB patients is considered
Biofeedback	+ (B): Reduction of EMG activity; No influences on subjective sleep quality if short-term use. Unknown influence on sleep for long-term use (may increase sleep arousal frequency and intensity)
Pharmacologic strategies	
Anxiolytic	Empiric data only
Diazepam	+ or – (B):
Clonazepam	+ (A): Risk of dependence; not for regular use—short term (1–3 nights per week)
Muscle relaxant	
Methocarbamol	+ (B) Risk of dizziness and sleepiness
Dopaminergic	
L-Dopa	+ (A)
Bromocriptine	– (A)
Pergolide	+ (one case so far)

Cardioactive	
Clonidine	++ (A): Risk of severe hypotension in the morning if given to normotensive subjects
Propranolol	– (A)
Antidepressant	
L-Tryptophan	– (A)
Amitriptyline	– (A)
Buspirone	+: reduction of SSRI-induced sleep bruxism (few cases only)
Proton-pump inhibitor	
Rabeprazole	+ (A): Reduction of SB and low esophageal pH events
Botulinum toxin	Little evidence available, small sample size controlled report

(A) and (B) correspond to the grade of evidence. Grade (A): randomized controlled trials and meta-analyses; Grade (B): other level of evidence such as well-designed controlled experimental trial and uncontrolled studies. No grade was added for case reports. For details, see text.

during sleep; hypertension, retrognathia, deep palate, large tongue, narrow dental arch) when prescribing an occlusal splint. Moreover, during the follow-up period, signs and symptoms related to sleep apnea should be reassessed. Patients need to be informed that oral splints may change the way they feel their bite during the hours following awakening, but that such effects are usually transient. It is recommended that dentists make follow-up appointments to assess oral appliance stability and oral hygiene (eg, caries or gum disease) every 6 months. Little information is available on the management of SB with occlusal splints in children. A few descriptive studies have reported that an occlusal splint prevents tooth wear in 3- to 5-year-old children.[236,237]

Apart from the occlusal splint, different types of oral devices have been tested for their efficacy in reducing SB. One oral device, the NTI (standing for Nociceptive Trigeminal Inhibitory), only covers the upper incisors, creating a one-point contact with the lower incisors. The NTI significantly reduced the frequency and intensity of SB.[238] Compared with this device, the occlusal splint has more therapeutic effects on the signs and symptoms of temporomandibular disorders, but the risk of changes in occlusion needs to be disclosed to patients if the NTI splint is used long term.[239,240] Researchers also tested the effect of another type of oral appliance on SB patients, the mandibular advancement appliance (MAA), which covers the dental arch and is made for sleep-related snoring and sleep apnea. The MAA allows a few degrees of mandibular advancement in comparison with a single arch occlusal splint.[166,167] When the jaw was placed either in an edge-to-edge tooth position or in a slightly advanced position using an MAA, the index of masticatory muscle activity was reduced significantly in comparison with an upper-maxillary or lower-mandibular occlusal splint.[167] In the first study, a thermo-molded appliance was fitted to the patient's dentition. More than 60% of patients reported discomfort or pain in the jaw and teeth when they used the oral appliances.[167] In the second study a laboratory custom-made hard appliance was used.[166] Although the mechanism for reducing SB by means of an oral appliance remains to be understood (eg, preventing airway collapse during sleep or jaw retrusion that may occlude the airway passage or the reduction of free mandibular movement due to the mechanism that advances the lower jaw), this result suggests that as long as the titration is appropriate, an MAA can be useful for managing SB in patients with sleep-disordered breathing. This possibility needs further investigation.

The belief that fine tuning the upper and lower jaw tooth contacts (ie, equilibrating tooth contacts by trimming "premature" tooth contacts on natural teeth or dental restorations) cures or relieves bruxism is not supported by controlled and bias-protected protocol.[168,241] In theory, this type of "occlusal adjustment therapy" stabilizes the forces at the temporomandibular joint or between the teeth. As described in the earlier section on Pathophysiology, current knowledge of SB does not support the concept that teeth contacts generate SB; the efficacy of occlusal adjustment is yet to be demonstrated in a controlled study.[86,170] Thus, whereas occlusal therapy is indicated for the restoration of orodental comfort when there are major prosthodontic (eg, crown, denture, bridge), restorative (eg, inlay) or orthodontic treatments, firm evidence is awaited as to its efficacy in SB management due to its irreversible nature in patients with natural dentition.[27,168,242,243]

Pharmacologic Strategies

Several drugs acting on the central nervous system have been suggested to reduce SB. However, it is unclear whether they act directly on the motor system related to SB or indirectly on the sleep arousal system. In addition, long-term efficacy has not been assessed for the drugs presented here.

In an open study, central muscle relaxants (eg, methocarbamol; 1–2 g/night) have been reported to have the effect of reducing SB.[244] Benzodiazepines (diazepam; 5 or 10 mg/night) at bedtime have been reported to reduce SB.[245] Compared with placebo, triazolam improved sleep but did not alter jaw-closing muscle activity during sleep in patients with orofacial pain.[246] In a single-blind, nonrandomized study, the acute effects of clonazepam on SB were investigated in SB patients with insomnia, restless legs syndrome, and periodic leg movements in sleep.[247,248] Clonazepam (1 mg/night) at bedtime decreased SB by approximately 30%, improved sleep quality, and reduced concomitant sleep-related movement disorders. Thus, low to modest effects can be expected when these drugs are used for a short period (eg, 1 or 2 nights). Although a long-term efficacy of clonazepam (approximately 1 mg/night for up to 3.5–8 years) has been reported for parasomnias (eg, sleepwalking, RBD) with low adverse effects,[249] further controlled trials for long-term usage are needed in SB patients not presenting other medical disorders. Patients should be informed that these drugs carry significant risks of dizziness, sleepiness, and cognitive impairment. Moreover, the risk of addiction or dependence needs to be assessed.

In a placebo-controlled study, small doses of amitriptyline (25 mg/night) or the serotonin precursor L-tryptophan failed to reduce SB activity and associated discomforts.[250–252] SSRI antidepressants should be avoided for SB management because several case reports have indicated that they may induce secondary SB.[253–258] Nonetheless, some cases with SSRI-induced SB may be resolved by a different type of SSRI drug (buspirone).[127] The influence of serotonergic drugs on SB remains unknown, and the interaction between SSRI drugs needs to be improved for an understanding of secondary SB.

In a few case reports, anticonvulsant drugs (eg, gabapentin or tiagabine) have been reported to reduce both primary and secondary self-reported bruxism.[255,259] The efficacy, role, and active mechanism of these drugs in relation to SB remains to be demonstrated.

A placebo-controlled study has reported that a catecholamine-related medication (dopamine, serotonin, adrenaline), with a major action on dopamine, L-dopa (2 doses of 100 mg/night) modestly reduced SB activity by 30%.[123] In a case study with 2 patients, the administration of the dopamine agonist bromocriptine (7.5 mg/night) resulted in a significant reduction of SB activity.[260] However, in a placebo-controlled study, bromocriptine (7.5 mg/night), in combination with domperidone (20 mg/night) for reducing nausea, failed to decrease SB.[122] A recent report presented a case in which a strong dopaminergic agonist, pergolide (0.3–0.5 mg/night) with domperidone, also reduced SB.[261] Subjects were given low doses of these medications to prevent excessive side effects such as nausea, emesis, and dizziness. The efficacy and long-term safety of dopaminergic medications requires further clarification because the side effect ratio prevents their use in most SB patients.

In 2 case reports (see earlier discussion), a reduction in SB activity in an SB patient was noted in response to the administration of the β-adrenergic receptor antagonist propranolol (2 doses of 60 mg/night). The same effect was noted in 2 secondary SB patients with antipsychotic drug exposure (up to 240 mg/d or 20 mg 3 times a day).[124,262] In a randomized experimental trial to further understand SB pathophysiology, propranolol (120 mg/night) failed to reduce SB whereas the α-receptor agonist clonidine (0.3 mg/night) decreased SB by 60%.[125] It is worth noting that clonidine acts mainly at the level of the central nervous and autonomic systems. The use of clonidine in primary SB patients is not indicated because severe hypotension in the morning was observed in 20% of patients following the administration of an intermediate dose.[125]

Compared with placebo, a proton-pump inhibitor has been reported to decrease RMMA episodes and events with decreased esophageal pH in SB patients (not patients with gastroesophageal reflux) and in controls.[160] Further study is required to assess the efficacy of this drug. The influence of visceral functions in association with autonomic nervous system activity is an area worthy of examination as regards the management of SB.

Botulinum toxin type A (BTX-A) is known to be effective for controlling involuntary orofacial movements and secondary bruxism in patients with movement disorders (eg, cranial dystonia).[263,264] One study reported a decrease in jaw muscle EMG activity during sleep after BTX–A injection.[265] However, the treatment effects of BTX-A have not yet been fully evaluated in a large sample of patients with primary SB using sleep and EMG recordings.

SUMMARY

SB is not as simple a jaw movement as chewing; it is a rhythmic movement with an intense jaw muscle contraction that can damage teeth and trigger pain or headache. When SB is clinically reported by tooth grinding, the final diagnosis is only possible with polygraphic and audio-video recordings in a home or sleep laboratory environment. The occurrence of SB is associated in some subjects with homeostatic sleep regulation (ie, biologic need for sleep over circadian rhythm) and sleep instability (eg, CAP and microarousals). Other modulating factors that need to be recognized are neurochemicals, psychological stress, and oro-esophapharyngeal functions (mucosal dryness, breathing). The contribution of child development (associated with high prevalence of tooth grinding) and aging (associated with low prevalence of tooth grinding) remains to be investigated. Concomitant sleep disorders and the use of some medication or drugs should not be overlooked. Although the complex influences of these factors can involve the genesis or exacerbation of SB, there are still discrepancies in the understanding of the relationships between sleep physiology, SB pathophysiology, and orodental consequences. Therefore, a single ideal treatment for SB has yet to be recognized. The clinician's main objective remains the prevention of damage to orofacial structures and associated orofacial sensory complaints. Thus, in managing cases of SB and related consequences, such as tooth damage or pain, and even more so if SB is secondary to medication use or a medical condition, it is necessary for the clinician to plan a multidisciplinary approach based on the best scientific evidence available.

ACKNOWLEDGMENTS

The authors thank Dr Susumu Abe for his help in preparing the manuscript and Dr Alice Petersen for English editing.

REFERENCES

1. Thorpy MJ. International classification of sleep disorders: diagnostic and coding manual. Rochester (NY): Minnesota: American Sleep Disorders Association; 1990.
2. International classification of sleep disorders: diagnostic and coding manual. 2nd edition. Westchester (IL): American Academy of Sleep Medicine; 2005.
3. Walters AS. Clinical identification of the simple sleep-related movement disorders. Chest 2007; 131:1260.
4. Walters AS, Lavigne G, Hening W, et al. The scoring of movements in sleep. J Clin Sleep Med 2007;3:155.
5. Lavigne GJ, Manzini C, Kato T. Sleep bruxism. In: Kryger MH, Roth T, Dement C, editors. Principles and practice of sleep medicine. 4th edition. Philadelphia: Elsevier Saunders; 2005. p. 946.
6. The glossary of prosthodontic terms. J Prosthet Dent 2005;94:10.
7. De Leeuw R, editor. Orofacial pain: guidelines for assessment, classification, and management. 4th edition. Chicago: Quintessence; 2008.
8. Lavigne GJ, Khoury S, Abe S, et al. Bruxism physiology and pathology: an overview for clinicians. J Oral Rehabil 2008;35:476.
9. Kato T, Dal-Fabbro C, Lavigne GJ. Current knowledge on awake and sleep bruxism: overview. Alpha Omegan 2003;96:24.
10. Lavigne GJ, Montplaisir JY. Restless legs syndrome and sleep bruxism: prevalence and association among Canadians. Sleep 1994;17:739.
11. Ohayon MM, Li KK, Guilleminault C. Risk factors for sleep bruxism in the general population. Chest 2001;119:53.
12. Laberge L, Tremblay RE, Vitaro F, et al. Development of parasomnias from childhood to early adolescence. Pediatrics 2000;106:67.
13. Ng DK, Kwok KL, Cheung JM, et al. Prevalence of sleep problems in Hong Kong primary school children: a community-based telephone survey. Chest 2005;128:1315.

14. Hicks RA, Lucero-Gorman K, Bautista J, et al. Ethnicity and bruxism. Percept Mot Skills 1999; 88:240.

15. Ahlberg J, Savolainen A, Rantala M, et al. Reported bruxism and biopsychosocial symptoms: a longitudinal study. Community Dent Oral Epidemiol 2004;32:307.

16. Lavigne GL, Lobbezoo F, Rompre PH, et al. Cigarette smoking as a risk factor or an exacerbating factor for restless legs syndrome and sleep bruxism. Sleep 1997;20:290.

17. Hojo A, Haketa T, Baba K, et al. Association between the amount of alcohol intake and masseter muscle activity levels recorded during sleep in healthy young women. Int J Prosthodont 2007;20:251.

18. Winocur E, Gavish A, Voikovitch M, et al. Drugs and bruxism: a critical review. J Orofac Pain 2003;17:99.

19. Manfredini D, Landi N, Fantoni F, et al. Anxiety symptoms in clinically diagnosed bruxers. J Oral Rehabil 2005;32:584.

20. Petit D, Touchette E, Tremblay RE, et al. Dyssomnias and parasomnias in early childhood. Pediatrics 2007;119:e1016.

21. Pingitore G, Chrobak V, Petrie J. The social and psychologic factors of bruxism. J Prosthet Dent 1991;65:443.

22. Suwa S, Takahara M, Shirakawa S, et al. Sleep bruxism and its relationship to sleep habits and lifestyle of elementary school children in Japan. Sleep Biol Rhythms 2009;7:93.

23. Kato T. Sleep bruxism and its relation to obstructive sleep apnea-hypopnea syndrome. Sleep Biol Rhythms 2004;2:1.

24. Kato T, Blanchet PJ, Montplaisir JY, et al. Sleep bruxism and other disorders with orofacial activity during sleep. In: Chokroverty S, Hening W, Walters A, editors. Sleep and movement disorders. Philadelphia: Butterworth Heinemann; 2003. p. 273.

25. Baba K, Haketa T, Sasaki Y, et al. Association between masseter muscle activity levels recorded during sleep and signs and symptoms of temporomandibular disorders in healthy young adults. J Orofac Pain 2005;19:226.

26. Lobbezoo F, Brouwers JE, Cune MS, et al. Dental implants in patients with bruxing habits. J Oral Rehabil 2006;33:152.

27. Tosun T, Karabuda C, Cuhadaroglu C. Evaluation of sleep bruxism by polysomnographic analysis in patients with dental implants. Int J Oral Maxillofac Implants 2003;18:286.

28. Casanova-Rosado JF, Medina-Solis CE, Vallejos-Sanchez AA, et al. Prevalence and associated factors for temporomandibular disorders in a group of Mexican adolescents and youth adults. Clin Oral Investig 2006;10:42.

29. Lobbezoo F, Lavigne GJ. Do bruxism and temporomandibular disorders have a cause-and-effect relationship? J Orofac Pain 1997;11:15.

30. Manfredini D, Cantini E, Romagnoli M, et al. Prevalence of bruxism in patients with different research diagnostic criteria for temporomandibular disorders (RDC/TMD) diagnoses. Cranio 2003;21:279.

31. Raphael KG, Marbach JJ, Klausner JJ, et al. Is bruxism severity a predictor of oral splint efficacy in patients with myofascial face pain? J Oral Rehabil 2003;30:17.

32. Smith MT, Wichwire EM, Grace EG, et al. Sleep disorders and their association with laboratory pain sensitivity in temporomandibular disorders. Sleep 2009;32:779.

33. Aromaa M, Sillanpaa ML, Rautava P, et al. Childhood headache at school entry: a controlled clinical study. Neurology 1998;50:1729.

34. Bader GG, Kampe T, Tagdae T, et al. Descriptive physiological data on a sleep bruxism population. Sleep 1997;20:982.

35. Camparis CM, Siqueira JT. Sleep bruxism: clinical aspects and characteristics in patients with and without chronic orofacial pain. Oral Surg Oral Med Oral Pathol Oral Radiol Endod 2006;101:188.

36. Vendrame M, Kaleyias J, Valencia I, et al. Polysomnographic findings in children with headaches. Pediatr Neurol 2008;39:6.

37. Boutros NN, Montgomery MT, Nishioka G, et al. The effects of severe bruxism on sleep architecture: a preliminary report. Clin Electroencephalogr 1993;24:59.

38. Bliwise DL. Norma aging. In: Kryger MH, Roth T, Dement WC, editors. Principles and practices of sleep medicine. 4th edition. Philadelphia: Elsevier Saunders; 2005. p. 24.

39. Lavigne GJ, McMillan D, Zucconi M. Pain and sleep. In: Kryger MH, Roth T, Dement WC, editors. Principles and practices of sleep medicine. 4th edition. Philadelphia: Elsevier Saunders; 2005. p. 1246.

40. Rompre PH, Daigle-Landry D, Guitard F, et al. Identification of a sleep bruxism subgroup with a higher risk of pain. J Dent Res 2007;86:837.

41. Rossetti LM, Pereira de Araujo Cdos R, Rossetti PH, et al. Association between rhythmic masticatory muscle activity during sleep and masticatory myofascial pain: a polysomnographic study. J Orofac Pain 2008;22:190.

42. Johansson A, Haraldson T, Omar R, et al. A system for assessing the severity and progression of occlusal tooth wear. J Oral Rehabil 1993;20:125.

43. Lobbezoo F, Naeije M. A reliability study of clinical tooth wear measurements. J Prosthet Dent 2001; 86:597.

44. Abe S, Yamaguchi T, Rompré PH, et al. Tooth wear in young subjects: a discriminator between

sleep bruxers and controls? Int J Prosthodont 2009;22:342.

45. Baba K, Haketa T, Clark GT, et al. Does tooth wear status predict ongoing sleep bruxism in 30-year-old Japanese subjects? Int J Prosthodont 2004; 17:39.

46. Koyano K, Tsukiyama Y, Ichiki R, et al. Assessment of bruxism in the clinic. J Oral Rehabil 2008;35:495.

47. Ommerborn MA, Schneider C, Giraki M, et al. In vivo evaluation of noncarious cervical lesions in sleep bruxism subjects. J Prosthet Dent 2007;98:150.

48. Rees JS, Jagger DC. Abfraction lesions: myth or reality? J Esthet Restor Dent 2003;15:263.

49. Lynch CD, McConnell RJ. The cracked tooth syndrome. J Can Dent Assoc 2002;68:470.

50. Ratcliff S, Becker IM, Quinn L. Type and incidence of cracks in posterior teeth. J Prosthet Dent 2001; 86:168.

51. Takagi I, Sakurai K. Investigation of the factors related to the formation of the buccal mucosa ridging. J Oral Rehabil 2003;30:565.

52. Kato T, Thie NM, Montplaisir JY, et al. Bruxism and orofacial movements during sleep. Dent Clin North Am 2001;45:657.

53. Okeson JP. Management of temporomandibular disorders and occlusion. 5th edition. St Louis (MO): Mosby; 2003.

54. Chervin RD. Use of clinical tools and tests in sleep medicine. In: Kryger MH, Roth T, Dement C, editors. Principles and practice of sleep medicine. 4th edition. Philadelphia: Elsevier Saunders; 2005. p. 602.

55. Egermark I, Carlsson GE, Magnusson T. A 20-year longitudinal study of subjective symptoms of temporomandibular disorders from childhood to adulthood. Acta Odontol Scand 2001;59:40.

56. Lavigne GJ, Guitard F, Rompre PH, et al. Variability in sleep bruxism activity over time. J Sleep Res 2001;10:237.

57. Van Der Zaag J, Lobbezoo F, Visscher CM, et al. Time-variant nature of sleep bruxism outcome variables using ambulatory polysomnography: implications for recognition and therapy evaluation. J Oral Rehabil 2008;35:577.

58. Van't Spijker A, Rodriguez JM, Kreulen CM, et al. Prevalence of tooth wear in adults. Int J Prosthodont 2009;22:35.

59. Thie NM, Kato T, Bader G, et al. The significance of saliva during sleep and the relevance of oromotor movements. Sleep Med Rev 2002;6:213.

60. Ommerborn MA, Giraki M, Schneider C, et al. A new analyzing method for quantification of abrasion on the Bruxcore device for sleep bruxism diagnosis. J Orofac Pain 2005;19:232.

61. Pierce CJ, Gale EN. Methodological considerations concerning the use of Bruxcore Plates to evaluate nocturnal bruxism. J Dent Res 1989;68: 1110.

62. Dao TT, Lund JP, Lavigne GJ. Comparison of pain and quality of life in bruxers and patients with myofascial pain of the masticatory muscles. J Orofac Pain 1994;8:350.

63. Svensson P, Jadidi F, Arima T, et al. Relationships between craniofacial pain and bruxism. J Oral Rehabil 2008;35:524.

64. Biondi DM. Headaches and their relationship to sleep. Dent Clin North Am 2001;45:685.

65. Camparis CM, Formigoni G, Teixeira MJ, et al. Sleep bruxism and temporomandibular disorder: clinical and polysomnographic evaluation. Arch Oral Biol 2006;51:721.

66. Arima T, Arendt-Nielsen L, Svensson P. Effect of jaw muscle pain and soreness evoked by capsaicin before sleep on orofacial motor activity during sleep. J Orofac Pain 2001;15:245.

67. Lavigne GJ, Rompre PH, Montplaisir JY, et al. Motor activity in sleep bruxism with concomitant jaw muscle pain. A retrospective pilot study. Eur J Oral Sci 1997;105:92.

68. Glaros AG, Waghela R. Psychophysiological definitions of clenching. Cranio 2006;24:252.

69. Katase-Akiyama S, Kato T, Yamashita S, et al. Specific increase in non-functional masseter bursts in subjects aware of tooth-clenching during wakefulness. J Oral Rehabil 2009;36:93.

70. Carlsson GE, Egermark I, Magnusson T. Predictors of signs and symptoms of temporomandibular disorders: a 20-year follow-up study from childhood to adulthood. Acta Odontol Scand 2002;60: 180.

71. van Selms MK, Lobbezoo F, Visscher CM, et al. Myofascial temporomandibular disorder pain, parafunctions and psychological stress. J Oral Rehabil 2008;35:45.

72. Velly AM, Gornitsky M, Philippe P. A case-control study of temporomandibular disorders: symptomatic disc displacement. J Oral Rehabil 2002;29: 408.

73. Malow BA, Aldrich MS. Polysomnography. In: Chokroverty S, Hening W, Walters A, editors. Sleep and movement disorders. Philadelphia: Butterworth Heinemann; 2003. p. 125.

74. Ikeda T, Nishigawa K, Kondo K, et al. Criteria for the detection of sleep-associated bruxism in humans. J Orofac Pain 1996;10:270.

75. Gallo LM, Lavigne G, Rompré P, et al. Reliability of scoring EMG orofacial events: polysomnography compared with ambulatory recordings. J Sleep Res 1997;6:259.

76. Dutra KM, Pereira FJ Jr, Rompre PH, et al. Orofacial activities in sleep bruxism patients and in normal subjects: a controlled polygraphic and audio-video study. J Oral Rehabil 2008;36:86.

77. Yamaguchi T, Mikami S, Okada K. Validity of a newly developed ultraminiature cordless EMG

measurement system. Oral Surg Oral Med Oral Pathol Oral Radiol Endod 2007;104:e22.

78. Jadidi F, Castrillon E, Svensson P. Effect of conditioning electrical stimuli on temporalis electromyographic activity during sleep. J Oral Rehabil 2008;35:171.

79. Shochat T, Gavish A, Arons E, et al. Validation of the BiteStrip screener for sleep bruxism. Oral Surg Oral Med Oral Pathol Oral Radiol Endod 2007;104:e32.

80. Baba K, Clark GT, Watanabe T, et al. Bruxism force detection by a piezoelectric film-based recording device in sleeping humans. J Orofac Pain 2003;17:58.

81. Nagamatsu-Sakaguchi C, Minakuchi H, Clark GT, et al. Relationship between the frequency of sleep bruxism and the prevalence of signs and symptoms of temporomandibular disorders in an adolescent population. Int J Prosthodont 2008;21:292.

82. Doering S, Boeckmann JA, Hugger S, et al. Ambulatory polysomnography for the assessment of sleep bruxism. J Oral Rehabil 2008;35:572.

83. Lavigne GJ, Rompre PH, Montplaisir JY. Sleep bruxism: validity of clinical research diagnostic criteria in a controlled polysomnographic study. J Dent Res 1996;75:546.

84. Kato T, Montplaisir JY, Blanchet PJ, et al. Idiopathic myoclonus in the oromandibular region during sleep: a possible source of confusion in sleep bruxism diagnosis. Mov Disord 1999;14:865.

85. Kato T, Thie NM, Huynh N, et al. Topical review: sleep bruxism and the role of peripheral sensory influences. J Orofac Pain 2003;17:191.

86. Lobbezoo F, Naeije M. Bruxism is mainly regulated centrally, not peripherally. J Oral Rehabil 2001;28:1085.

87. Lavigne GJ, Rompre PH, Poirier G, et al. Rhythmic masticatory muscle activity during sleep in humans. J Dent Res 2001;80:443.

88. Sjoholm T, Lehtinen II, Helenius H. Masseter muscle activity in diagnosed sleep bruxists compared with non-symptomatic controls. J Sleep Res 1995;4:48.

89. Lavigne GJ, Huynh N, Kato T, et al. Genesis of sleep bruxism: motor and autonomic-cardiac interactions. Arch Oral Biol 2007;52:381.

90. Miyawaki S, Lavigne GJ, Pierre M, et al. Association between sleep bruxism, swallowing-related laryngeal movement, and sleep positions. Sleep 2003;26:461.

91. Dettmar DM, Shaw RM, Tilley AJ. Tooth wear and bruxism: a sleep laboratory investigation. Aust Dent J 1987;32:421.

92. Huynh N, Kato T, Rompre PH, et al. Sleep bruxism is associated to micro-arousals and an increase in cardiac sympathetic activity. J Sleep Res 2006;15:339.

93. Macaluso GM, Guerra P, Di Giovanni G, et al. Sleep bruxism is a disorder related to periodic arousals during sleep. J Dent Res 1998;77:565.

94. Reding GR, Zepelin H, Robinson JE, et al. Nocturnal teeth-grinding: all-night psychophysiologic studies. J Dent Res 1968;47:786.

95. Satoh T, Harada Y. Electrophysiological study on tooth-grinding during sleep. Electroencephalogr Clin Neurophysiol 1973;35:267.

96. Wieselmann G, Permann R, Korner E, et al. Distribution of muscle activity during sleep in bruxism. Eur Neurol 1986;25(Suppl 2):111.

97. Reding GR, Rubright WC, Rechtschaffen A, et al. Sleep pattern of tooth-grinding: its relationship to dreaming. Science 1964;145:725.

98. Reding GR, Zepelin H, Robinson JEJ, et al. Sleep pattern of bruxism: a revision. In: APSS Meeting, vol. 4, p. 396, 1967.

99. Halasz P, Terzano M, Parrino L, et al. The nature of arousal in sleep. J Sleep Res 2004;13:1.

100. Terzano MG, Parrino L, Boselli M, et al. CAP components and EEG synchronization in the first 3 sleep cycles. Clin Neurophysiol 2000;111:283.

101. Lavigne GJ, Rompre PH, Guitard F, et al. Lower number of K-complexes and K-alphas in sleep bruxism: a controlled quantitative study. Clin Neurophysiol 2002;113:686.

102. EEG arousals: scoring rules and examples: a preliminary report from the Sleep Disorders Atlas Task Force of the American Sleep Disorders Association. Sleep 1992;15:173.

103. Kato T, Rompre P, Montplaisir JY, et al. Sleep bruxism: an oromotor activity secondary to micro-arousal. J Dent Res 1940;80:2001.

104. Kydd WL, Daly C. Duration of nocturnal tooth contacts during bruxing. J Prosthet Dent 1985;53:717.

105. Okeson JP, Phillips BA, Berry DT, et al. Nocturnal bruxing events: a report of normative data and cardiovascular response. J Oral Rehabil 1994;21:623.

106. Herrera M, Valencia I, Grant M, et al. Bruxism in children: effect on sleep architecture and daytime cognitive performance and behavior. Sleep 2006;29:1143.

107. Ferri R, Parrino L, Smerieri A, et al. Cyclic alternating pattern and spectral analysis of heart rate variability during normal sleep. J Sleep Res 2000;9:13.

108. Khoury S, Rouleau GA, Rompre PH, et al. A significant increase in breathing amplitude precedes sleep bruxism. Chest 2008;134:332.

109. Chase MH, Morales FR. Control of motoneurons during sleep. In: Kryger MH, Roth T, Dement C, editors. Principles and practice of sleep medicine. 4th edition. Philadelphia: Elsevier Saunders; 2005. p. 154.

110. Kato T, Montplaisir JY, Lavigne GJ. Experimentally induced arousals during sleep: a cross-modality matching paradigm. J Sleep Res 2004;13:229.

111. Okura K, Kato T, Montplaisir JY, et al. Quantitative analysis of surface EMG activity of cranial and leg muscles across sleep stages in human. Clin Neurophysiol 2006;117:269.

112. Kato T, Montplaisir JY, Guitard F, et al. Evidence that experimentally induced sleep bruxism is a consequence of transient arousal. J Dent Res 2003;82:284.

113. Bader G, Kampe T, Tagdac T. Body movement during sleep in subjects with long-standing bruxing behavior. Int J Prosthodont 2000;13:327.

114. Sjoholm TT, Polo OJ, Alihanka JM. Sleep movements in teethgrinders. J Craniomandib Disord 1992;6:184.

115. Frauscher B, Iranzo A, Hogl B, et al. Quantification of electromyographic activity during REM sleep in multiple muscles in REM sleep behavior disorder. Sleep 2008;31:724.

116. Kato T, Masuda Y, Kanayama H, et al. Muscle activities are differently modulated between masseter and neck muscle during sleep-wake cycles in guinea pigs. Neurosci Res 2007;58:265.

117. Akerstedt T, Billiard M, Bonnet M, et al. Awakening from sleep. Sleep Med Rev 2002;6:267.

118. Grosse P, Khatami R, Salih F, et al. Corticospinal excitability in human sleep as assessed by transcranial magnetic stimulation. Neurology 1988;59:2002.

119. Terzano MG, Parrino L, Rosa A, et al. CAP and arousals in the structural development of sleep: an integrative perspective. Sleep Med 2002;3:221.

120. Gastaldo E, Quatrale R, Graziani A, et al. The excitability of the trigeminal motor system in sleep bruxism: a transcranial magnetic stimulation and brainstem reflex study. J Orofac Pain 2006;20:145.

121. Lobbezoo F, Soucy JP, Montplaisir JY, et al. Striatal D2 receptor binding in sleep bruxism: a controlled study with iodine-123-iodobenzamide and single-photon-emission computed tomography. J Dent Res 1804;75:1996.

122. Lavigne GJ, Soucy JP, Lobbezoo F, et al. Double-blind, crossover, placebo-controlled trial of bromocriptine in patients with sleep bruxism. Clin Neuropharmacol 2001;24:145.

123. Lobbezoo F, Lavigne GJ, Tanguay R, et al. The effect of catecholamine precursor L-dopa on sleep bruxism: a controlled clinical trial. Mov Disord 1997;12:73.

124. Sjoholm TT, Lehtinen I, Piha SJ. The effect of propranolol on sleep bruxism: hypothetical considerations based on a case study. Clin Auton Res 1996;6:37.

125. Huynh N, Lavigne GJ, Lanfranchi PA, et al. The effect of 2 sympatholytic medications—propranolol and clonidine—on sleep bruxism: experimental randomized controlled studies. Sleep 2006;29:307.

126. Lobbezoo F, van Denderen RJ, Verheij JG, et al. Reports of SSRI-associated bruxism in the family physician's office. J Orofac Pain 2001;15:340.

127. Ranjan S, S Chandra P, Prabhu S. Antidepressant-induced bruxism: need for buspirone? Int J Neuropsychopharmacol 2006;9:485.

128. Jones BE. Basic mechanisms of sleep-wake states. In: Kryger MH, Roth T, Dement C, editors. Principles and practice of sleep medicine. 4th edition. Philadelphia: Elsevler Saunders; 2005. p. 136.

129. Van cauter E. Endorine physiology. In: Kryger MH, Roth T, Dement C, editors. Principles and practice of sleep medicine. 4th edition. Philadelphia: Elsevier Saunders; 2005. p. 266.

130. Hicks RA, Conti PA, Bragg HR. Increases in nocturnal bruxism among college students implicate stress. Med Hypotheses 1990;33:239.

131. Kampe T, Edman G, Bader G, et al. Personality traits in a group of subjects with long-standing bruxing behaviour. J Oral Rehabil 1997;24:588.

132. Kampe T, Tagdae T, Bader G, et al. Reported symptoms and clinical findings in a group of subjects with longstanding bruxing behaviour. J Oral Rehabil 1997;24:581.

133. Manfredini D, Ciapparelli A, Dell'Osso L, et al. Mood disorders in subjects with bruxing behavior. J Dent 2005;33:485.

134. Restrepo CC, Vasquez LM, Alvarez M, et al. Personality traits and temporomandibular disorders in a group of children with bruxing behaviour. J Oral Rehabil 2008;35:585.

135. Manfredini D, Lobbezoo F. Role of psychosocial factors in the etiology of bruxism. J Orofac Pain 2009;23:153.

136. Major M, Rompre PH, Guitard F, et al. A controlled daytime challenge of motor performance and vigilance in sleep bruxers. J Dent Res 1999;78:1754.

137. Ahlberg K, Ahlberg J, Kononen M, et al. Reported bruxism and stress experience in media personnel with or without irregular shift work. Acta Odontol Scand 2003;61:315.

138. Schneider C, Schaefer R, Ommerborn MA, et al. Maladaptive coping strategies in patients with bruxism compared to non-bruxing controls. Int J Behav Med 2007;14:257.

139. Funch DP, Gale EN. Factors associated with nocturnal bruxism and its treatment. J Behav Med 1980;3:385.

140. Rugh JD, Harlan J. Nocturnal bruxism and temporomandibular disorders. Adv Neurol 1988;49:329.

141. Makino M, Masaki C, Tomoeda K, et al. The relationship between sleep bruxism behavior and salivary stress biomarker level. Int J Prosthodont 2009;22:43.

142. Pierce CJ, Chrisman K, Bennett ME, et al. Stress, anticipatory stress, and psychologic measures related to sleep bruxism. J Orofac Pain 1995;9:51.

143. Watanabe T, Ichikawa K, Clark GT. Bruxism levels and daily behaviors: 3 weeks of measurement and correlation. J Orofac Pain 2003;17:65.

144. Seraidarian P, Seraidarian PI, das Neves Cavalcanti B, et al. Urinary levels of catecholamines among individuals with and without sleep bruxism. Sleep Breath 2009;13:85.

145. Vanderas AP, Menenakou M, Kouimtzis T, et al. Urinary catecholamine levels and bruxism in children. J Oral Rehabil 1999;26:103.

146. Clark GT, Rugh JD, Handelman SL. Nocturnal masseter muscle activity and urinary catecholamine levels in bruxers. J Dent Res 1980;59:1571.

147. Ahlberg K, Jahkola A, Savolainen A, et al. Associations of reported bruxism with insomnia and insufficient sleep symptoms among media personnel with or without irregular shift work. Head Face Med 2008;4:4.

148. Okura K, Lavigne GJ, Huynh N, et al. Comparison of sleep variables between chronic widespread musculoskeletal pain, insomnia, periodic leg movements syndrome and control subjects in a clinical sleep medicine practice. Sleep Med 2008;9:352.

149. Yoshihara T, Shigeta K, Hasegawa H, et al. Neuroendocrine responses to psychological stress in patients with myofascial pain. J Orofac Pain 2005; 19:202.

150. Abe K, Shimakawa M. Genetic and developmental aspects of sleeptalking and teeth-grinding. Acta Paedopsychiatr 1966;33:339.

151. Kuch EV, Till MJ, Messer LB. Bruxing and nonbruxing children: a comparison of their personality traits. Pediatr Dent 1979;1:182.

152. Reding GR, Rubright WC, Zimmerman SO. Incidence of bruxism. J Dent Res 1966;45:1198.

153. Hori A. Twin studies on parasomnias. In: Meier-Ewert K, Okawa M, editors. Sleep-wake disorders. New York: Plenum Press; 1998. p. 115.

154. Hublin C, Kaprio J, Partinen M, et al. Sleep bruxism based on self-report in a nationwide twin cohort. J Sleep Res 1998;7:61.

155. Lindqvist B. Bruxism in twins. Acta Odontol Scand 1974;32:177.

156. Carlsson GE, Egermark I, Magnusson T. Predictors of bruxism, other oral parafunctions, and tooth wear over a 20-year follow-up period. J Orofac Pain 2003;17:50.

157. Hublin C, Kaprio J, Partinen M, et al. Parasomnias: co-occurrence and genetics. Psychiatr Genet 2001;11:65.

158. Lichter I, Muir RC. The pattern of swallowing during sleep. Electroencephalogr Clin Neurophysiol 1975; 38:427.

159. Orr WC, Johnson LF, Robinson MG. Effect of sleep on swallowing, esophageal peristalsis, and acid clearance. Gastroenterology 1984;86:814.

160. Miyawaki S, Tanimoto Y, Araki Y, et al. Association between nocturnal bruxism and gastroesophageal reflux. Sleep 2003;26:888.

161. Chen CL, Orr WC. Analysis of 24-hour esophageal pH monitoring: the effect of state of consciousness. Curr Gastroenterol Rep 2008;10:258.

162. Orr WC. Gastrointestinal physiology. In: Kryger MH, Roth T, Dement C, editors. Principles and practice of sleep medicine. 4th edition. Philadelphia: Elsevier Saunders; 2005. p. 283.

163. Miyamoto K, Ozbek MM, Lowe AA, et al. Mandibular posture during sleep in healthy adults. Arch Oral Biol 1998;43:269.

164. Schwab RJ, Kuna ST, Remmers JE. Anatomy and physiology of upper airway obstruction. In: Kryger MH, Roth T, Dement C, editors. Principles and practice of sleep medicine. 4th edition. Philadelphia: Elsevier Saunders; 2005. p. 983.

165. Simmons J, Prehn R. Airway protection: the missing link between nocturnal bruxism and obstructive sleep apnea. Sleep 2009;32 (abstract supplement): A218, #0668.

166. Landry-Schonbeck A, de Grandmont P, Rompre PH, et al. Effect of an adjustable mandibular advancement appliance on sleep bruxism: a crossover sleep laboratory study. Int J Prosthodont 2009;22:251.

167. Landry ML, Rompre PH, Manzini C, et al. Reduction of sleep bruxism using a mandibular advancement device: an experimental controlled study. Int J Prosthodont 2006;19:549.

168. Ash MM. Paradigmatic shifts in occlusion and temporomandibular disorders. J Oral Rehabil 2001;28:1.

169. Manfredini D, Landi N, Romagnoli M, et al. Psychic and occlusal factors in bruxers. Aust Dent J 2004; 49:84.

170. Tsukiyama Y, Baba K, Clark GT. An evidence-based assessment of occlusal adjustment as a treatment for temporomandibular disorders. J Prosthet Dent 2001;86:57.

171. Graf H. Bruxism. Dent Clin North Am 1969;13:659.

172. Powell RN. Tooth contact during sleep: association with other events. J Dent Res 1965;44:959.

173. Powell RN, Zander HA. The frequency and distribution of tooth contact during sleep. J Dent Res 1965; 44:713.

174. Okeson JP, Phillips BA, Berry DT, et al. Nocturnal bruxing events in healthy geriatric subjects. J Oral Rehabil 1990;17:411.

175. von Gonten AS, Palik JF, Oberlander BA, et al. Nocturnal electromyographic evaluation of masseter muscle activity in the complete denture patients. J Prosthet Dent 1986;56:624.

176. Lobbezoo F, Rompre PH, Soucy JP, et al. Lack of associations between occlusal and cephalometric measures, side imbalance in striatal D2 receptor binding, and sleep-related oromotor activities. J Orofac Pain 2001;15:64.

177. Kato T, Blanchet PJ. Orofacial movement disorders in sleep. In: Lavigne GJ, Cistulli PA, Smith MT, editors. Sleep medicine for dentists: a practical overview. Hanover Park (IL): Quintessence; 2009. p. 101.

178. Gara L, Roberts W. Adverse response to methylphenidate in combination with valproic acid. J Child Adolesc Psychopharmacol 2000;10:39.

179. Mendhekar DN, Andrade C. Bruxism arising during monotherapy with methylphenidate. J Child Adolesc Psychopharmacol 2008;18:537.

180. Mendhekar D, Lohia D. Worsening of bruxism with atomoxetine: a case report. World J Biol Psychiatry 2009. DOI:10.1080/15622970802576488.

181. Lobbezoo F, Van Der Zaag J, Naeije M. Bruxism: its multiple causes and its effects on dental implants—an updated review. J Oral Rehabil 2006;33:293.

182. Bruni O, Ferri R, D'Agostino G, et al. Sleep disturbances in Angelman syndrome: a questionnaire study. Brain Dev 2004;26:233.

183. Olson RE, Laskin DM. Relationship between allergy and bruxism in patients with myofascial pain-dysfunction syndrome. J Am Dent Assoc 1980; 100:209.

184. Manconi M, Zucconi M, Carrot B, et al. Association between bruxism and nocturnal groaning. Mov Disord 2008;23:737.

185. Khatami R, Zutter D, Siegel A, et al. Sleep-wake habits and disorders in a series of 100 adult epilepsy patients—a prospective study. Seizure 2006;15:299.

186. Meletti S, Cantalupo G, Volpi L, et al. Rhythmic teeth grinding induced by temporal lobe seizures. Neurology 2004;62:2306.

187. Ghanizadeh A. Comorbidity of enuresis in children with attention-deficit/hyperactivity disorder. J Atten Disord 2009. DOI:10.1177/1087054709332411.

188. Tani K, Yoshii N, Yoshino I, et al. Electroencephalographic study of parasomnia: sleep-talking, enuresis and bruxism. Physiol Behav 1966;1:241.

189. Huynh N, Guilleminault C. Sleep bruxism in children. In: Lavigne GJ, Cistulli PA, Smith MT, editors. Sleep medicine for dentists: a practical overview. Chicago: Quintessence; 2009.

190. Bracha HS, Ralston TC, Williams AE, et al. The clenching-grinding spectrum and fear circuitry disorders: clinical insights from the neuroscience/paleoanthropology interface. CNS Spectr 2005; 10:311.

191. Ghanizadeh A. ADHD, bruxism and psychiatric disorders: does bruxism increase the chance of a comorbid psychiatric disorder in children with ADHD and their parents? Sleep Breath 2008;12: 375.

192. Lindqvist B, Heijbel J. Bruxism in children with brain damage. Acta Odontol Scand 1974;32:313.

193. Ohayon MM, Caulet M, Priest RG. Violent behavior during sleep. J Clin Psychiatry 1997;58:369.

194. Richmond G, Rugh JD, Dolfi R, et al. Survey of bruxism in an institutionalized mentally retarded population. Am J Ment Defic 1984;88:418.

195. Shur-Fen Gau S. Prevalence of sleep problems and their association with inattention/hyperactivity among children aged 6-15 in Taiwan. J Sleep Res 2006;15:403.

196. Winocur E, Hermesh H, Littner D, et al. Signs of bruxism and temporomandibular disorders among psychiatric patients. Oral Surg Oral Med Oral Pathol Oral Radiol Endod 2007;103:60.

197. Okeson JP, Phillips BA, Berry DT, et al. Nocturnal bruxing events in subjects with sleep-disordered breathing and control subjects. J Craniomandib Disord 1991;5:258.

198. Sjoholm TT, Lowe AA, Miyamoto K, et al. Sleep bruxism in patients with sleep-disordered breathing. Arch Oral Biol 2000;45:889.

199. Inoko Y, Shimizu K, Morita O, et al. Relationship between masseter muscle activity and sleep-disordered breathing. Sleep Biol Rhythms 2004;2:67.

200. Montagna P. Physiologic body jerks and movements at sleep onset and during sleep. In: Chokroverty S, Hening W, Walters A, editors. Sleep and movement disorders. Philadelphia: Butterworth Heinemann; 2003. p. 247.

201. Phillips BA, Okeson J, Paesani D, et al. Effect of sleep position on sleep apnea and parafunctional activity. Chest 1986;90:424.

202. Ng DK, Kwok KL, Poon G, et al. Habitual snoring and sleep bruxism in a paediatric outpatient population in Hong Kong. Singapore Med J 2002;43: 554.

203. DiFrancesco RC, Junqueira PA, Trezza PM, et al. Improvement of bruxism after T & A surgery. Int J Pediatr Otorhinolaryngol 2004;68:441.

204. Eftekharian A, Raad N, Gholami-Ghasri N. Bruxism and adenotonsillectomy. Int J Pediatr Otorhinolaryngol 2008;72:509.

205. Grechi TH, Trawitzki LV, de Felicio CM, et al. Bruxism in children with nasal obstruction. Int J Pediatr Otorhinolaryngol 2008;72:391.

206. Restrepo CC, Sforza C, Colombo A, et al. Palate morphology of bruxist children with mixed dentition. A pilot study. J Oral Rehabil 2008;35:353.

207. Hublin C, Kaprio J. Genetic aspects and genetic epidemiology of parasomnias. Sleep Med Rev 2003;7:413.

208. Vetrugno R, Provini F, Plazzi G, et al. Familial nocturnal facio-mandibular myoclonus mimicking sleep bruxism. Neurology 2002;58:644.

209. Loi D, Provini F, Vetrugno R, et al. Sleep-related faciomandibular myoclonus: a sleep-related movement disorder different from bruxism. Mov Disord 1819;22:2007.

210. Huynh NT, Rompre PH, Montplaisir JY, et al. Comparison of various treatments for sleep bruxism using determinants of number needed to treat and effect size. Int J Prosthodont 2006;19: 435.

211. Lobbezoo F, Blanchet PJ, Lavigne GJ. Management of movement disorders related to orofacial pain. In: Sessle B, Lavigne GJ, Lund JP, et al, editors. Orofacial pain: from basic science to clinical management. 2nd edition. Illinois: Quintessence; 2008. p. 211.

212. Lobbezoo F, van der Zaag J, van Selms MK, et al. Principles for the management of bruxism. J Oral Rehabil 2008;35:509.

213. Winocur E. Management of sleep bruxism. In: Lavigne GJ, Cistulli PA, Smith MT, editors. Sleep medicine for dentists: a practical overview. Hanover Park (IL): Quintessence; 2009.

214. Morin CM. Psychological and behavioral treatments for primary insomnia. In: Kryger MH, Roth T, Dement C, editors. Principles and practice of sleep medicine. 4th edition. Philadelphia: Elsevier Saunders; 2005. p. 726.

215. Restrepo CC, Alvarez E, Jaramillo C, et al. Effects of psychological techniques on bruxism in children with primary teeth. J Oral Rehabil 2001; 28:354.

216. Ommerborn MA, Schneider C, Giraki M, et al. Effects of an occlusal splint compared with cognitive-behavioral treatment on sleep bruxism activity. Eur J Oral Sci 2007;115:7.

217. Clarke JH, Reynolds PJ. Suggestive hypnotherapy for nocturnal bruxism: a pilot study. Am J Clin Hypn 1991;33:248.

218. Cassisi JE, McGlynn FD, Belles DR. EMG-activated feedback alarms for the treatment of nocturnal bruxism: current status and future directions. Biofeedback Self Regul 1987;12:13.

219. Pierce CJ, Gale EN. A comparison of different treatments for nocturnal bruxism. J Dent Res 1988;67: 597.

220. Nissani M. Can taste aversion prevent bruxism? Appl Psychophysiol Biofeedback 2000;25:43.

221. Watanabe T, Baba K, Yamagata K, et al. A vibratory stimulation-based inhibition system for nocturnal bruxism: a clinical report. J Prosthet Dent 2001; 85:233.

222. Nishigawa K, Kondo K, Takeuchi H, et al. Contingent electrical lip stimulation for sleep bruxism: a pilot study. J Prosthet Dent 2003;89:412.

223. Dao TT, Lavigne GJ. Oral splints: the crutches for temporomandibular disorders and bruxism? Crit Rev Oral Biol Med 1998;9:345.

224. Kato T. Peripheral sensory influences in sleep bruxism: a physiological interpretation for clinicians. In: Daniel P, editor. Bruxism: theory and practices. Hanover Park (IL): Quintessence; in press.

225. Okeson JP. The effects of hard and soft occlusal splints on nocturnal bruxism. J Am Dent Assoc 1987;114:788.

226. Clark GT, Beemsterboer PL, Solberg WK, et al. Nocturnal electromyographic evaluation of myofascial pain dysfunction in patients undergoing occlusal splint therapy. J Am Dent Assoc 1979;99:607.

227. Dube C, Rompre PH, Manzini C, et al. Quantitative polygraphic controlled study on efficacy and safety of oral splint devices in tooth-grinding subjects. J Dent Res 2004;83:398.

228. Harada T, Ichiki R, Tsukiyama Y, et al. The effect of oral splint devices on sleep bruxism: a 6-week observation with an ambulatory electromyographic recording device. J Oral Rehabil 2006;33:482.

229. Okkerse W, Brebels A, De Deyn PP, et al. Influence of a bite-plane according to Jeanmonod, on bruxism activity during sleep. J Oral Rehabil 2002;29:980.

230. van der Zaag J, Lobbezoo F, Wicks DJ, et al. Controlled assessment of the efficacy of occlusal stabilization splints on sleep bruxism. J Orofac Pain 2005;19:151.

231. Rugh JD, Graham GS, Smith JC, et al. Effects of canine versus molar occlusal splint guidance on nocturnal bruxism and craniomandibular symptomatology. J Craniomandib Disord 1989;3:203.

232. Rugh JD, Solberg WK. Electromyographic studies of bruxist behavior before and during treatment. J Calif Dent Assoc 1975;3:56.

233. Solberg WK, Clark GT, Rugh JD. Nocturnal electromyographic evaluation of bruxism patients undergoing short term splint therapy. J Oral Rehabil 1975;2:215.

234. Macedo CR, Silva AB, Machado MA, et al. Occlusal splints for treating sleep bruxism (tooth grinding). Cochrane Database Syst Rev 2007;4: CD005514.

235. Gagnon Y, Mayer P, Morisson F, et al. Aggravation of respiratory disturbances by the use of an occlusal splint in apneic patients: a pilot study. Int J Prosthodont 2004;17:447.

236. Hachmann A, Martins EA, Araujo FB, et al. Efficacy of the nocturnal bite plate in the control of bruxism for 3 to 5 year old children. J Clin Pediatr Dent 1999;24:9.

237. Jones CM. Chronic headache and nocturnal bruxism in a 5-year-old child treated with an occlusal splint. Int J Paediatr Dent 1993;3:95.

238. Baad-Hansen L, Jadidi F, Castrillon E, et al. Effect of a nociceptive trigeminal inhibitory splint on electromyographic activity in jaw closing muscles during sleep. J Oral Rehabil 2007;34:105.

239. Magnusson T, Adiels AM, Nilsson HL, et al. Treatment effect on signs and symptoms of temporomandibular disorders—comparison between stabilisation splint and a new type of splint (NTI). A pilot study. Swed Dent J 2004;28:11.

240. Stapelmann H, Türp JC. The NTI-tss device for the therapy of bruxism, temporomandibular disorders, and headache - where do we stand? A qualitative systematic review of the literature. BMC Oral Health 2008;8:22. DOI:10.1186/1472-6831-8-22.

241. Yustin D, Neff P, Rieger MR, et al. Characterization of 86 bruxing patients with long term study of their management with occlusal devices and other forms of therapy. J Orofac Pain 1993;7:54.

242. Ash MMJ. Philosophy of occlusion: past and present. Dent Clin North Am 1995;39:233.

243. De Boever JA, Carlsson GE, Klineberg IJ. Need for occlusal therapy and prosthodontic treatment in the management of temporomandibular disorders. Part II: tooth loss and prosthodontic treatment. J Oral Rehabil 2000;27:647.

244. Chasins AI. Methocarbamol (Robaxin) as an adjunct in the treatment of bruxism. J Dent Med 1959;14:166.

245. Montgomery MT, Nishioka GJ, Rugh JD, et al. Effect of diazepam on nocturnal masticatory muscle activity (abstract). J Dent Res 1986;65:96.

246. DeNucci DJ, Sobiski C, Dionne RA. Triazolam improves sleep but fails to alter pain in TMD patients. J Orofac Pain 1998;12:116.

247. Saletu A, Parapatics S, Anderer P, et al. Controlled clinical, polysomnographic and psychometric studies on differences between sleep bruxers and controls and acute effects of clonazepam as compared with placebo. Eur Arch Psychiatry Clin Neurosci 2009. DOI:10.1007/s00406-009-0034-0.

248. Saletu A, Parapatics S, Saletu B, et al. On the pharmacotherapy of sleep bruxism: placebo-controlled polysomnographic and psychometric studies with clonazepam. Neuropsychobiology 2005;51:214.

249. Schenck CH, Mahowald MW. Long-term, nightly benzodiazepine treatment of injurious parasomnias and other disorders of disrupted nocturnal sleep in 170 adults. Am J Med 1996;100:333.

250. Etzel KR, Stockstill JW, Rugh JD, et al. Tryptophan supplementation for nocturnal bruxism: report of negative results. J Craniomandib Disord 1991;5:115.

251. Mohamed SE, Christensen LV, Penchas J. A randomized double-blind clinical trial of the effect of amitriptyline on nocturnal masseteric motor activity (sleep bruxism). Cranio 1997;15:326.

252. Raigrodski AJ, Mohamed SE, Gardiner DM. The effect of amitriptyline on pain intensity and perception of stress in bruxers. J Prosthodont 2001;10:73.

253. Alonso-Navarro H, Martin-Prieto M, Ruiz-Ezquerro JJ, et al. Bruxism possibly induced by venlafaxine. Clin Neuropharmacol 2009;32:111.

254. Bostwick JM, Jaffee MS. Buspirone as an antidote to SSRI-induced bruxism in 4 cases. J Clin Psychiatry 1999;60:857.

255. Brown ES, Hong SC. Antidepressant-induced bruxism successfully treated with gabapentin. J Am Dent Assoc 1999;130:1467.

256. Ellison JM, Stanziani P. SSRI-associated nocturnal bruxism in four patients. J Clin Psychiatry 1993; 54:432.

257. Romanelli F, Adler DA, Bungay KM. Possible paroxetine-induced bruxism. Ann Pharmacother 1996; 30:1246.

258. Stein DJ, Van Greunen G, Niehaus D. Can bruxism respond to serotonin reuptake inhibitors? J Clin Psychiatry 1998;59:133.

259. Kast RE. Tiagabine may reduce bruxism and associated temporomandibular joint pain. Anesth Prog 2005;52:102.

260. Lobbezoo F, Soucy JP, Hartman NG, et al. Effects of the D2 receptor agonist bromocriptine on sleep bruxism: report of two single-patient clinical trials. J Dent Res 1997;76:1610.

261. Van der Zaag J, Lobbezoo F, Van der Avoort PG, et al. Effects of pergolide on severe sleep bruxism in a patient experiencing oral implant failure. J Oral Rehabil 2007;34:317.

262. Amir I, Hermesh H, Gavish A. Bruxism secondary to antipsychotic drug exposure: a positive response to propranolol. Clin Neuropharmacol 1997;20:86.

263. Tan EK, Jankovic J. Treating severe bruxism with botulinum toxin. J Am Dent Assoc 2000;131: 211.

264. Tan EK, Jankovic J, Ondo W. Bruxism in Huntington's disease. Mov Disord 2000;15:171.

265. Lee SJ, McCall WD Jr, Kim YK, et al. Effect of botulinum toxin injection on nocturnal bruxism: a randomized controlled trial. Am J Phys Med Rehabil 2009. DOI:10.1097/PHM.0b013e3181bc0c78.

Neurologic Basis of Sleep Breathing Disorders

Aman A. Savani, MD, Christian Guilleminault, MD, DBiol*

KEYWORDS
- Obstructive sleep apnea syndrome • Neurologic basis
- Upper airway • Anatomic abnormalities

Obstructive sleep apnea syndrome (OSAS) is a disorder resulting from partial or complete repetitive collapse of the pharynx occurring while an individual is sleeping. It is a common problem affecting about 2% to 4% of the adult population in the United States.[1] The diagnosis is made when 5 or more such events, lasting a minimum of 10 seconds per hour of sleep, are observed on a polysomnogram. Patients suffering from sleep apnea are variably symptomatic from the disease. Snoring is a commonly reported symptom of OSAS, but it is neither necessary nor sufficient for diagnosis. Waking up gasping, choking, drooling, or with a dry mouth and bruxism are also commonly associated nocturnal symptoms of OSAS. Disturbed nighttime sleep can be associated with excessive daytime sleepiness, impaired concentration, cognitive deficits, increased irritability, depression, and anxiety.

There are several risk factors for the disease, including increasing age, obesity, postmenopausal state, and positive family history.[2] There are also several anatomic factors that are associated with obstructive sleep apnea, including neck circumference of 17 in or more, turbinate hypertrophy, narrow mandible and maxilla, retrognathia, and dental malocclusion. One study showed that the single most important cephalometric variable in predicting the severity of sleep apnea is the horizontal dimension of the maxilla.[3] The role of gender in the development of sleep-disordered breathing has also been evaluated. Men may have inherent structural and functional differences in their airways making them more vulnerable to collapse and obstruction.[4] Based on these observations, obstructive sleep apnea is often approached as a purely mechanical problem or a structural disorder that leads to increased respiratory effect and sleep fragmentation.

The evolution of the field of sleep medicine into a multidisciplinary specialty has enhanced the understanding of this prevalent disorder. Specifically, advances in neuroscience are increasing the understanding of OSAS as a more complex problem with sensory impairment, motor dysfunction, and altered cortical processing, all playing a role in the underlying pathogenesis of the disease in addition to the observed structural abnormalities. One particular study suggested that two-thirds of OSAS cases are attributable to neurologic factors.[5] This article reviews the evidence supporting a neurologic basis for obstructive sleep apnea. A review of the normal upper airway anatomy will precede the discussion of sensory impairment, abnormal cortical processing, motor dysfunction, and histopathologic derangements associated with OSAS.

UPPER AIRWAY ANATOMY

The upper airway is separated into 3 regions: the nasophayrnx, the oropharynx, and the hypopharynx. The nasopharynx is the path from the nasal turbinates to the hard palate. The oropharynx is further subdivided into the retropalatal region, which extends from the hard palate to the caudal border of the soft palate, and the retroglossal region, which extends from the caudal border of the soft palate to the base of the

Sleep Medicine Program, Stanford University, 450 Broadway Street, M/C 5704, Redwood City, CA 94063, USA
* Corresponding author.
E-mail address: cguil@stanford.edu (C. Guilleminault).

Sleep Med Clin 5 (2010) 37–44
doi:10.1016/j.jsmc.2009.09.005

sleep.theclinics.com

epiglottis. The hypopharynx is defined as the region from the base of the tongue to the larynx. The soft palate and the tongue form the anterior wall of the oropharynx, whereas the posterior wall is composed of superior, middle, and inferior constrictor muscles. The lateral walls are formed by several structures, including the hypoglossus, styloglossus, stylohyoid, stylopharyngeus, palatoglossus, palatopharyngeus, and pharyngeal constrictors. The pharyngeal airway is largely unsupported by bony structures, and so it is susceptible to collapse under the negative pressures generated during inspiration. Obesity influences airway collapsibility by increasing the amount of soft tissue surrounding the pharyngeal airway.[6] Body position can also affect airway collapsibility. It has been frequently observed that obstructive breathing events occur more frequently in the supine position. Without changing the cross sectional area, the upper airway assumes a more elliptical shape when supine as opposed to a more circular shape when in the lateral recumbent position. Thus, the closer opposition of the pharyngeal walls in the supine position may make the upper airway more susceptible to collapse.[7] In OSAS, the muscles surrounding the pharyngeal airway can influence its patency by actively dilating and opening the airway or stiffening to reduce susceptibility to negative pressure collapse. The most active and relevant of these muscles is an extrinsic tongue muscle, the genioglossus.

The genioglossus is the largest of the upper airway dilator muscles and is often modified in sleep apnea surgery. Anterior movement of the tongue and widening of the oropharyngeal airway is facilitated by contraction of this muscle. The genioglossus is innervated by the medial branch of the hypoglossal nerve and receives input from the pre-Botzinger complex and the neurons that regulate sleep-wake states.[8] Evidence from single motor unit recordings indicates that the genioglossus consists of motor units with a variety of firing patterns. The activity of individual units can be divided into 6 classes based on their discharge patterns. One study showed that 29% of sampled units discharged tonically without phasic respiratory control, 16% increased their firing during expiration, and 50% increased firing during inspiration. Adjacent units had differing respiratory and tonic drives, suggesting a complex interaction of tonic and phasic activities at the hypoglossal motor nucleus.[9] Wilkinson and colleagues[10] studied sampled motor units from healthy patients at the onset of sleep and found that 50% of the units ceased activity entirely. The different units probably have different functional roles. Inspiratory

motor units may be phasically active to compensate for negative pressures generated during inspiration while inspiratory/expiratory units tonically discharge to maintain tongue position.[11] The genioglossus also receives input from the negative pressure receptors in the upper airway. Consequently, genioglossus activity is increased during inspiration to prevent negative pressure collapse. It also remains active during expiration, although to a lesser degree. Thus, genioglossus activity is increased in response to respiratory drive through its connection to respiratory rhythm–generating neurons and in response to negative airway pressure. This has been demonstrated through the application of brief negative pressure pulses to the upper airway. However, the genioglossus reflex to negative pressure seems to be inhibited during rapid eye movement sleep, and this probably explains why the upper airway is more susceptible to collapse during this stage of sleep.[12] It has also been shown that increased genioglossus muscle tone is associated with spontaneous periods of stable flow limited breathing in patients with obstructive sleep apnea.[13] The mechanism behind this observation could be the long-term facilitation of genioglossus activity due to repeated hypoxia. A study of anesthetized, spontaneously breathing rats showed that increases in peak genioglossus activity after 8 hypoxic episodes measured by electromyography 1 hour after the last episode demonstrated a long-term facilitatory change.[14]

The stiffness and position of the palate, tongue, and pharynx and the shape of the uvula are determined by the palatal muscles (tensor palatine, levator veli palatine, palatoglossus, palatopharyngeus, and musculus uvulae). These muscles are important to maintain upper airway patency. McWhorter and colleagues[15] showed that in cats, stimulation of the tensor veli palatini decreases upper airway collapsibility. The pharyngeal branch of the vagus nerve innervates all these muscles with the exception of the tensor veli palatini, which is innervated by the trigeminal nerve. Another study showed that vagal nerve stimulation in patients suffering from epilepsy can adversely affect respiration during sleep.[16]

There are 3 pharyngeal constrictor muscles: superior, middle, and inferior. These muscles are innervated by the vagus nerve and may play a role in stiffening the posterior pharyngeal wall. Kuna[17] showed that activation of the pharyngeal constrictor muscles constricts the airway at relatively high airway volumes but dilates the airway at relatively low volumes. This suggests that the pharyngeal constrictor muscle activation at the end of an apneic episode, when airway volumes are low, could help restore airway patency in individuals with obstructive sleep apnea. However, there is little evidence supporting the role of these muscles in apnea pathogenesis.

The hyoid arch and its muscle attachments, including the geniohyoid, mylohyoid, sternohyoid, stylohyoid, and thyrohyoid muscles, strongly influence hypopharyngeal airway patency and resistance. These muscles are innervated by the hypoglossal nerve (geniohyoid and thyrohyoid muscles), the trigeminal nerve (mylohyoid muscle), facial nerve (stylohyoid muscle), and ansa cervicalis (sternohyoid muscle). The geniohyoid and mylohyoid muscles act to pull the hyoid bone forward and upward, whereas the sternohyoid and thyrohyoid muscles pull the bone caudally. Tandem activation of both muscle groups results in ventral/caudal movement of the hyoid, facilitating airway dilation.[18]

SENSORY DYSFUNCTION

There are different types of sensory receptors in the upper airway, and they respond to various stimuli, including pressure, cold, heat, irritants, and respiratory muscle drive. Among the various types of receptors, mechanoreceptors have been well studied.

The upper airway reflex opposes the negative pressure collapsing forces generated during inhalation. This process is accomplished through the activation of pharyngeal dilator muscles, which can increase airway patency. The sensory input for this reflex comes from the mechanosensory receptors of the upper airway through the central respiratory centers. This represents a true reflex, as increase in pharyngeal dilator activity can be demonstrated with a shorter latency than would be expected with voluntary activation.[19]

Proprioceptive feedback from thoracic and upper airway receptors can alter motor output to the pharyngeal muscles. Studies in animal models have shown that negative pressure generation in the upper airway can increase activity in the genioglossus. This response can be blocked by transecting the superior laryngeal nerve or by applying topical anesthesia. In animal models, the diversion of tidal volume away from mechanosensory receptors in the upper airway through a tracheostomy tube also induced pharyngeal closure, which was reversible on restoration of normal flow.[20] Because topical anesthesia can block this response, it is believed that the receptors mediating this reflex are located superficially in the airway wall. Most of these receptors appear to be located in the upper trachea and transmit information through the superior laryngeal nerve as well as the glossopharyngeal and trigeminal nerves.

During apneas and hypopneas, receptors distal to the obstruction sense and transmit information about the resultant pressure changes. Abnormalities in the sensory component of the airway reflex, which contribute to obstructive sleep apnea, can be primary, secondary, or both.[21] In certain individuals, primary sensory deficits are thought to be a preexisting factor that increases the threshold for the negative pressure reflex, making the airway more collapsible. Secondary deficits are thought to be the result of accumulated damage due to local trauma in the setting of snoring and obstructive sleep apnea, creating a vicious cycle that perpetuates the disease.

Snoring is a common symptom associated with obstructive sleep apnea. Snoring is a manifestation of airway resistance that creates turbulent flow and vibrates distensible tissues. Repetitive snoring and upper airway occlusion have been shown to lead to edema of the upper airway soft tissue structures, which further narrows the airway and increases resistance to normal airflow. Snoring also causes damage to mechanosensory receptors. Occupational and environmental health studies have shown that repetitive use of vibrating tools can lead to localized nerve lesions. In the vibration-induced white finger syndrome, 3 characteristic pathologic changes were found. First, the muscular layer of arteries showed thickening with significant hypertrophy of muscle cells. Second, a demyelinating peripheral neuropathy was noted with marked loss of nerve fibers. Third, there was an increase in connective tissue and collagen.[22,23] Continuous snoring produces low-frequency vibration, and this vibration from long-term snoring presents repetitive trauma to the palate and other upper airway structures. A recent study showed that the mechanical stimulus of vibration triggered an early proinflammatory process in the upper airway of rats; there was significant overexpression of tumor necrosis factor alpha and macrophage inflammatory protein-2.[24] This inflammation appeared to be related to contractile dysfunction, loss of sensory afferents, and impaired vascular reactivity in pharyngeal structures, which further compromised the negative pressure reflex and increased the likelihood of partial or complete closure of the airway.[25]

The importance of sensory feedback in the upper airway reflex has been demonstrated in studies of sleep and awake patients in whom the selective anesthetization of various upper airway structures with topical lidocaine resulted in diminished upper airway patency. Similar studies of snorers have shown increase in the frequency of abnormal breathing events (hypopneas and sometimes even apneas) with application of topical lidocaine and bupivacaine to the oropharynx.[26] These findings suggest that the receptors sensitive to airflow may be important in maintaining breathing rhythmicity during sleep.[27] Other studies performed to support this theory have shown reduced temperature thresholds for sensations of heat and cold on the tonsillar pillars and exaggerated vasodilation and vascular reactivity in snorers when compared with control subjects. There is also evidence that 2-point discrimination, vibratory sensation, and mucosal sensory function at multiple points in the upper airway are impaired in patients with snoring and obstructive sleep apnea.[28,29] Two-point palatal discrimination has also been evaluated in normal subjects compared with individuals with upper airway resistance syndrome (UARS) and individuals with obstructive sleep apnea. Patients with OSAS had clear impairment of their palatal sensory response with a decrement in 2-point discrimination when compared with patients with UARS, suggesting that they are less capable of transmitting sensory inputs.[30] Upper airway sensory impairment also contributes to altered swallowing function in patients with OSAS, as measured by prolongation of the respiratory cycle after swallowing.[31] There is also evidence that a prior history of sleep apnea increases the arousal threshold to upper airway occlusion and prolongs the duration of apneic events.[32]

It is not clear whether upper airway sensory dysfunction represents a cause or an effect of obstructive sleep apnea. However, these findings underscore the importance of recognizing the disease early to avoid further damage and perpetuation of the disorder.

IMPAIRED CORTICAL PROCESSING

One of the principal features of obstructive sleep apnea is the presence of electroencephalography (EEG) arousals associated with hypopneas, apneas, and increased respiratory effort. The EEG arousal can be considered an important part of the neural mechanism required to abort an abnormal breathing event and restore normal airway patency. However, EEG arousals are state changes that result in sleep fragmentation. In obstructive sleep apnea, cortical arousability is diminished, suggesting that arousal thresholds are blunted. This would increase the duration of apneas and the likelihood of additional events.

Neurogenic activity can be recorded in the somatosensory area of the cortex in relation to respiratory occlusion. The respiratory-related evoked potential (RREP) is a cortical response to the rapid application of resistive loads to breathing.[33] During wakefulness, RREPs are formed of early and late components. P1 and Nf are the early positive and negative responses occurring 40 and 80 seconds after the inspiratory resistive load is applied, as recorded in the parietal and frontal scalp regions, respectively. The potentials are present bilaterally but diminished over midline sites.[34] Additional components of the RREP during wakefulness include N1 and P300 components, which are thought to be related to attention and perception of respiratory sensitivity and effort.[35]

Patients with obstructive sleep apnea have a significantly increased inspiratory effort–related arousal threshold when compared with control subjects. Thus, more stimulus is required to produce an arousal during an obstructive breathing event. This abnormality could be attributed to differences in afferent processing caused by focal neuropathic lesions. Studies of RREPs in both asleep and awake subjects have been performed in patients with OSAS to further investigate this finding. During wakefulness it appears that the cortical processing of airway occlusion–related afferents is abnormal in untreated patients with obstructive sleep apnea. Specifically, N1 latencies and P2 and N2 were significantly delayed despite there being no significant differences in P1 latencies.[36] However, this finding has been disputed by some studies. Gora and colleagues[37] found that the RREP waveform is broadly similar in patients with obstructive sleep apnea while awake but differed significantly during stage 2 non-rapid eye movement (NREM) sleep. Specifically, fewer K-complexes were elicited in response to occlusion stimuli in the OSAS group. To determine whether these observations reflect a sleep-specific dampening of inspiratory effort–related stimuli, Afifi and colleagues[38] studied respiratory- and auditory-evoked potentials in NREM sleep and wakefulness in patients with OSAS and in control subjects. The amplitude of the N550 potential and the proportion of elicited K-complexes did not differ between the 2 groups in response to auditory stimuli presented during stage 2 NREM sleep. However, in response to respiratory stimuli presented during stage 2 sleep, the N550 amplitude and K-complex elicitation rate was significantly reduced in patients with OSAS when compared with controls. These results confirm a sleep-specific blunted cortical response to inspiratory occlusions. The sleep-related differences in patients with OSAS specific to the processing of inspiratory stimuli is highlighted by the absence of a significant difference between the 2 groups in response to auditory stimuli.

The question that follows is whether or not the changes in cortical processing are reversible with continuous positive airway pressure (CPAP) treatment. Sangal and Sanga[39] performed auditory and visual P300 testing in patients with severe obstructive sleep apnea (defined as a respiratory disturbance index>40) before and after CPAP therapy for 2 to 4 months. Though there was significant symptomatic improvement with therapy, there was no significant change in the P300 latencies. Patients with severe obstructive sleep apnea had prolonged P300 latencies before and after treatment. These results suggest that the changes in cortical processing associated with severe sleep apnea are irreversible and reinforce the importance of early diagnosis and treatment of this disorder.

MOTOR DEFICITS

Airway patency during wakefulness and sleep is determined by pharyngeal motor control, which requires an intact neural response. This explains the observation that not all patients with predisposing anatomic features have obstructive sleep apnea and not all patients with obstructive sleep apnea have obvious anatomic abnormalities. Patients with obstructive sleep apnea are able to maintain sufficient airway patency during wakefulness, suggesting that a compensatory mechanism must be functioning to prevent collapse. Failure of these mechanisms compromises airway patency and leads to collapse under negative inspiratory pressure and obstruction.

Pharyngeal dilator muscle activity is influenced by inputs from the central respiratory center in the medulla, by mechanoreceptor feedback from the pharynx itself, by vagal input from the lungs, and by the drive for wakefulness.[13] These muscles function to keep the airway open against the negative pressures generated during inhalation. The action of the genioglossus, palatopharyngeus, levator veli palatini, and tensor veli palatini represents the final common pathway of the negative pressure airway reflex. Dysfunction in the genioglossus and tensor palatine has been well described in patients with obstructive sleep apnea.

Impaired electromyographic activation of the levator veli palatini and palatoglossus in response to negative pressure pulses was described in awake patients with OSAS compared with control participants. Patients showed improved responses with long-term nightly CPAP therapy.[40]

Unlike the palatal muscles, the genioglossus seems to be more active during wakefulness in sleep apnea patients compared with control participants and has a well-preserved response to negative pressure, possibly representing a compensatory mechanism for a more collapsible airway.[41,42] Single motor unit recordings from the genioglossus of awake patients with severe OSAS showed larger area and longer duration action potentials with earlier recruitment and higher discharge frequencies. Patients with obstructive sleep apnea also have a greater reduction in genioglossus muscle tone at sleep onset compared with control participants, even when airway resistance is controlled for by application of CPAP.[43] These findings suggest that neurogenic changes occur in patients with severe obstructive sleep apnea with possibly altered output from the hypoglossal nucleus.[44]

HISTOPATHOLOGIC CORRELATES

Several studies have demonstrated other pathologic changes associated with OSAS. There is evidence that motor neuron lesions and damage to airway musculature can lead to weakness of the pharyngeal muscles, making the airway more susceptible to collapse. Muscle biopsies of the palatopharyngeal muscle performed during uvulopalatopharyngoplasty on patients with obstructive sleep apnea showed atrophy with a fascicular distribution, increased number of angulated atrophic fibers, and abnormal distribution of fiber types in many muscle fascicles.[45] There is also evidence of hypertrophy of the salivary glands, congestion and dilation of the thin-walled vessels, and lymphocytic infiltrates reflective of inflammatory changes.[46] Vasodilation in response to electrical stimulation is also exaggerated in habitual snorers and patients with mild OSAS in comparison with normal subjects.[47] In apneics and snorers, light microscopy has revealed mucous gland hypertrophy with ductal dilation and focal squamous metaplasia, disruption of muscle bundles by infiltrating mucous glands, focal atrophy of muscle fibers, and significant edema of the lamina propria. Electron microscopy of pharyngeal tissues in severe apneics has shown focal degeneration of myelinated nerve fibers and axons.[48] Confirmatory digital analysis of uvular specimens from patients with obstructive sleep apnea has demonstrated an increase in the total muscle bulk of the palatine muscles when compared with patients who snore but do not meet the diagnostic criteria for OSAS. This finding suggests that muscular hypertrophy may also underlie the pathophysiology of the disease.[49] Biopsies of palatopharyngeal muscle from subjects with habitual snoring and different degrees of upper airway obstruction showed numerous morphologic abnormalities, including neurogenic signs (eg, type grouping). The extent of the abnormality was significantly increased in these patients compared with control subjects and correlated to the severity of obstructive sleep apnea but not to oxygen desaturation. Analyses of the individual fiber-size spectra have demonstrated a significantly increased number of hypertrophied and/or atrophied fibers in these patients when compared with control participants.[50]

The genioglossus is a well-studied muscle in patients with obstructive sleep apnea. Biopsies of this muscle in patients with OSAS have shown an increase in the percentage of type II (fast-twitch) fibers when compared with control subjects. Analysis of these muscle fibers also demonstrated increased fatigability compared with control subjects.[51] These changes are present to a greater extent in obese patients with OSAS, potentially making the airway in this group of patients even more collapsible.[52]

These studies support the hypothesis that upper airway efferent nerve lesions are present in patients with OSAS. However, it is still unclear whether these lesions represent a cause or an effect of obstructive sleep apnea.

REVERSAL OF NEUROLOGIC LESIONS WITH TREATMENT

There is a growing body of evidence suggesting that upper airway neurologic lesions are associated with obstructive sleep apnea. Nasal CPAP therapy is recognized as an effective means of treating sleep-related obstructive breathing events. Studies have shown improvement of the symptoms associated with obstructive sleep apnea, including excessive daytime sleepiness, snoring, and cognitive impairment. However, improvement in the associated neurologic lesions has not been demonstrated as consistently with the use of CPAP therapy. Carrera and colleagues[51] showed that pathologic and physiologic alterations in the genioglossus of patients with OSAS improved after treatment with CPAP. Guilleminault and colleagues[53] evaluated healthy, nonobese subjects over a period of 5 years. Despite compliance with CPAP therapy and maintenance of body mass index, pressure had to be increased by at least 2 cm of H_2O in two-thirds of the subjects in the study. Additionally, abnormal 2-point palatal discrimination during wakefulness was present at the conclusion of the study when compared with control subjects. Both these observations suggest that the neurologic lesions persist despite otherwise effective treatment with CPAP.

However, as with larger muscle groups that are weakened by underlying neurologic lesions, the muscles of the pharyngeal airway may be amenable to rehabilitation with physical therapy. A recent study evaluated the effectiveness of a set of oropharyngeal exercises involving the tongue, soft palate, and lateral pharyngeal wall versus sham therapy in patients with moderate obstructive sleep apnea. After 3 months of daily exercise for approximately 30 minutes, reduction in OSAS severity and symptoms was noted in the treatment group, suggesting some degree of improvement in the targeted muscles.[54]

SUMMARY

There is good evidence that OSAS is associated with local neurologic impairment and that some of the impairment may persist despite adequate treatment. The number of local neurogenic lesions is not well evaluated in the workup of a patient with OSAS, despite the fact that such lesions may greatly affect the long-term results of therapeutic efforts. Development of specific tools to explore the severity and extension of the neurogenic impairment should be a clinical goal. Furthermore, the development of guidelines to recognize, diagnose, and treat individuals with known risk factors for collapsible airways should be a priority. Specifically, opening the upper airway in young individuals with high-risk anatomic features should be a primary goal to prevent the development, progression, and irreversible sequelae of associated neurologic lesions. Dentists and orthodontists should clearly incorporate an assessment of the upper airway in their general evaluation of the oral and dental development of young individuals and in the routine dental examination of adults.

REFERENCES

1. Young T, Palta M, Dempsey J, et al. The occurrence of sleep disordered breathing among middle-aged adults. N Engl J Med 1993;328:1230–5.
2. Young T, Peppard PE, Gottlieb DJ. Epidemiology of obstructive sleep apnea: a population health perspective. Am J Respir Crit Care Med 2002; 165(9):1217–39.
3. Dempsey JA, Skatrud JB, Jacques AJ, et al. Anatomic determinants of sleep-disordered breathing across the spectrum of clinical and nonclinical male subjects. Chest 2002;122(3): 840–51.
4. Mohsenin V. Gender differences in the expression of sleep-disordered breathing: role of upper airway dimensions. Chest 2001;120(5):1442–7.

5. Younes M. Role of respiratory control mechanisms in the pathogenesis of obstructive sleep disorders. J Appl Phys 2008;105:1389–405.

6. Kryger MH, Roth T, Dement WC. Principles and practice of sleep medicine. Elsevier Saunders; 2005. p. 983–8.

7. Walsh JH, Leigh MS, Paduch A, et al. Effect of posture on pharyngeal shape and size in adults with and without obstructive sleep apnea. Sleep 2008;31(11):1543–9.

8. Phillipson EA. Regulation of breathing during sleep. Am Rev Respir Dis 1977;115:217–24.

9. Sabiosky JP, Butler JE, Fogel RB, et al. Tonic and phasic respiratory drives to human genioglossus motoneurons during breathing. J Neurophysiol 2006;95(4):2213–21.

10. Wilkinson V, Malhotra A, Nicholas CL, et al. Discharge patterns of human genioglossus motor units during sleep onset. Sleep 2008;31(4):525–33.

11. Tsuiki S, Ono T, Ishiwata Y, et al. Functional divergence of human genioglossus motor units with respiratory-related activity. Eur Respir J 2000;15(5):906–10.

12. Shea SA, Edwards JK, White DP. Effect of wake-sleep transitions and rapid eye movement sleep on pharyngeal muscle response to negative pressure in humans. J Physiol 1999;520:897–908.

13. Jordan AS, White DP, Wellman A, et al. Airway dilator muscle activity and lung volume during stable breathing in obstructive sleep apnea. Sleep 2009; 32(3):361–8.

14. Ryan S, Nolan P. Episodic hypoxia induces long-term facilitation of upper airway muscle activity in spontaneously breathing anaesthetized rats. J Physiol 2009;587(Pt 13):3329–42.

15. McWhorter AJ, Rowley JA, Eisele DW. The effect of tensor veli palitini stimulation on upper airway patency. Arch Otolaryngol Head Neck Surg 1999; 125(9):937–40.

16. Marzec M, Edwards J, Sagher O, et al. Effects of vagus nerve stimulation on sleep related breathing disorders in epilepsy patients. Epilepsia 2003; 44(7):930–5.

17. Kuna ST. Respiratory-related activation and mechanical effects of the pharyngeal constrictor muscles. Respir Physiol 2000;119(2–3):155–61.

18. Van de Graaff WB, Gottfried SB, Mitra J, et al. Respiratory function of the hyoid muscles and the hyoid arch. J Appl Physiol 1984;57(1):197–204.

19. Horner RL, Innes JA, Murphy K, et al. Evidence for reflex upper airway dilator muscle activation by sudden negative airway pressure in man. J Physiol 1991;436:15–29.

20. Abu-Osba YK, Mathew OP, Thach BT. An animal model for airway sensory deprivation producing obstructive sleep apnea with postmortem findings of sudden infant death syndrome. Pediatrics 1981; 68:796–801.

21. Broderick M, Guilleminault C. Neurological aspects of obstructive sleep apnea. Ann N Y Acad Sci 2008;1142:44–57.

22. Sauni R, Pääkkönen R, Virtema P. Vibration-induced white finger syndrome and carpal tunnel syndrome among Finnish metal workers. Int Arch Occup Environ Health 2009;82(4):445–53.

23. Takeuchi T, Futatsuka M, Imanishi H, et al. Pathological changes observed in the finger biopsy of patients with vibration-induced white finger. Scand J Work Environ Health 1986;12:280–3.

24. Almendros I, Acerbi I, Puig F. Upper-airway inflammation triggered by vibration in a rat model of snoring. Sleep 2007;30(2):225–7.

25. Ramar K, Guilleminault C. Neurologic aspects of sleep apnea: is obstructive sleep apnea a neurologic disorder? Semin Neurol 2009;(4):368–71.

26. Chadwick GA, Crowley P, Fitzgerald MX, et al. Obstructive sleep apnea following topical oropharyngeal anesthesia in loud snorers. Am Rev Respir Dis 1991;143(4):810–3.

27. White DP, Cadieux RJ, Lombard RM, et al. The effects of nasal anesthesia on breathing during sleep. Am Rev Respir Dis 1985;132(5):972–5.

28. Kimoff RJ, Sfozra E, Champagne V, et al. Upper airway sensation in snoring and obstructive sleep apnea. Am J Respir Crit Care Med 2001;164(2):250–5.

29. Nguyen AT, Jobin V, Payne R, et al. Laryngeal and velopharyngeal sensory impairment in obstructive sleep apnea. Sleep 2005;28(5):585–93.

30. Guilleminault C, Li K, Poyares D. Two-point palatal discrimination in patients with upper airway resistance syndrome, obstructive sleep apnea syndrome, and normal control subjects. Chest 2002;122(3):866–70.

31. Jobin V, Champagne V, Beauregard J, et al. Swallowing function and upper airway sensation in obstructive sleep apnea. J Appl Physiol 2007; 102(4):1587–94.

32. Berry RB, Kouchi KG, Der DE, et al. Sleep apnea impairs the arousal response to airway occlusion. Chest 1996;109(6):1490–6.

33. Davenport PW, Friedman WA, Thompson FJ. Respiratory-related evoked potentials evoked by inspiratory occlusion in humans. J Appl Physiol 1986; 60(6):1843–8.

34. Davenport PW, Colrain IM, Hill PM. Scalp topography of the short-latency components of the respiratory-related evoked potential in children. J Appl Physiol 1996;80(5):1785–91.

35. Webster KE, Colrain IM. The relationship between respiratory-related evoked potentials and the perception of inspiratory resistive loads. Psychophysiology 2000;37(6):831–41.

36. Donzel-Raynaud C, Redolfi S, Arnulf I, et al. Abnormal respiratory-related evoked potentials in untreated awake patients with severe obstructive

sleep apnoea syndrome. Clin Physiol Funct Imaging 2009;29(1):10–7.

37. Gora J, Trinder J, Pierce R, et al. Evidence of a sleep specific blunted cortical response to inspiratory occlusions in mild obstructive sleep apnea syndrome. Am J Respir Crit Care Med 2002; 166(9):1225–34.

38. Afifi L, Guilleminault C, Colrain IM. Sleep and respiratory stimulus specific dampening of cortical responsiveness in OSAS. Respir Physiolo Neurobiol 2003;136(2–3):221–34.

39. Sangal RB, Sanga JM. Abnormal visual P300 latency in obstructive sleep apnea does not change acutely upon treatment with CPAP. Sleep 1997; 20(9):702–4.

40. Mortimore IL, Douglas NJ. Palatal muscle EMG response to negative pressure in awake sleep apneic and control subjects. Am J Respir Crit Care Med 1997;156:867–73.

41. Fogel RB, Malhotra A, Pillar G, et al. Genioglossal activation in patients with obstructive sleep apnea versus control subjects: mechanisms of muscle control. Am J Respir Crit Care Med 2001;164(11):2025–30.

42. Berry RB, White DP, Roper J, et al. Awake negative pressure reflex response of the genioglossus in OSAS patients and normal subjects. J Appl Physiol 2003;94(5):1875–82.

43. Fogel RB, Trinder J, White DP, et al. The effect of sleep onset on upper airway muscle activity in patients with sleep apnoea versus controls. J Physiol 2005;564:549–62.

44. Sabiosky JP, Butler JE, McKenzie DK, et al. Neural drive to human genioglossus in obstructive sleep apnoea. J Physiol 2007;585(1):135–46.

45. Edstrom L, Larsson J, Larsson L. Neurogenic effects on the palatopharyngeal muscle in patients with obstructive sleep apnoea: a muscle biopsy study. J Neurol Neurosurg Psychiatr 1992;55(10):916–20.

46. Namyslowski G, Scierski W, Zembala-Nosynska E, et al. [Histopathologic changes of the soft palate in snoring and obstructive sleep apnea syndrome patients]. Otolaryngol Pol 2005;59(1):13–9 [in Polish].

47. Friberg D, Gazelius B. Evaluation of the vascular reaction in pharyngeal mucosas. Acta Otolaryngol 1998;118(3):413–8.

48. Woodson BT, Garancis JC, Toohill RJ. Histopathological changes in snoring and obstructive sleep apnea syndrome. Laryngoscope 1991;101: 1318–22.

49. Bassiouny A, Mashaly M, Nasr S, et al. Quantitative analysis of uvular muscles in cases of simple snoring and obstructive sleep apnea: an image analysis study. Eur Arch Otorhinolaryngol 2008; 265(5):581–6.

50. Friberg D, Ansved T, Borg K, et al. Histological indications of a progressive snorer's disease in an upper airway muscle. Am J Respir Crit Care Med 1998;157(2):586–93.

51. Carrera M, Barbe F, Sauleda J, et al. Patients with obstructive sleep apnea exhibit genioglossus dysfunction that is normalized after treatment with continuous positive airway pressure. Am J Respir Crit Care Med 1999;159(6):1960–6.

52. Carrera M, Barbe F, Sauleda J, et al. Effects of obesity upon genioglossus structure and function in obstructive sleep apnoea. Eur Respir J 2004; 23(3):425–9.

53. Guilleminault CG, Huang YS, Kirisoglu C, et al. Is obstructive sleep apnea syndrome a neurological disorder? A continuous positive pressure follow-up study. Ann Neurol 2005;58(6):880–7.

54. Guimaraes KC, Drager LF, Genta PR. Effects of oropharyngeal exercises on patients with moderate obstructive sleep apnea syndrome. Am J Respir Crit Care Med 2009;179(10):962–6.

Anatomy of the Airway: An Overview

Ronald C. Auvenshine, DDS, PhD[a,b,c,]*

KEYWORDS

• Airway • Larynx • Pharynx • Anatomy

The adult human supralaryngeal vocal tract must be viewed from a phylogenetic and a growth and development perspective. As man has assumed an upright position, variations have evolved that make the anatomy of humans different from the anatomy of close ancestors and other mammals. The face, eyes, maxilla, and mandible have migrated inferiorly and posteriorly, creating a short face or splanchnocranium. The splanchnocranium is composed of the mandible, palate, ethmoid, maxilla, and sphenoid bones, as well as a narrow supralaryngeal vocal tract and a more posterior oropharyngeal tongue, along with a descended larynx and shortened soft palate with the loss of an epiglottic–soft palate lockup. These anatomic features have allowed man the ability to speak and to develop language (**Box 1**).[1]

EMBRYOLOGIC DEVELOPMENT OF THE SUPRALARYNGEAL VOCAL TRACT

The head and neck are formed by pharyngeal (branchial) arches. These arches appear in the fourth and fifth weeks of development and contribute to the characteristic external appearance of the embryo. In humans, there are 5 pairs of arches. These arches correspond in numbers I, II, III, IV, and VI. The pharyngeal arches consist of bars of mesenchymal tissue separated by pharyngeal pouches or clefts. Each arch has its own outer covering of ectoderm, an inner covering of endoderm, and a core of mesenchyme derived from paraxial and lateral plate mesoderm cells

and neural crest cells. Each arch contains its own artery, cranial nerve, muscle component, and cartilage bar or skeletal element (**Fig. 1**, **Table 1**). During the fourth and fifth weeks of development, outpocketings appear in the lateral wall of the pharyngeal gut. These outpocketings are referred to as pharyngeal pouches. The pouches penetrate the surrounding mesenchyme but do not establish open communication with the external clefts (**Fig. 2**).

Each of the pharyngeal pouches gives rise to an adult structure. The first pouch becomes the tympanic cavity and auditory (eustachian) tube. The second pouch gives rise to the palatine tonsils. The third pouch forms the thymus gland and inferior parathyroid glands, and the fourth pouch forms the superior parathyroid glands. The thymus and parathyroid glands migrate to their final position. The thyroid gland forms as a midline, ventral, endodermal invagination in the floor of the pharynx. Its point of invagination is marked in the adult by the foramen cecum on the upper surface of the tongue. This primordium of the thyroid gland elongates after its evagination, detaches from the pharyngeal endoderm, and finally migrates to its definitive location just inferior and ventral to the larynx.[2]

The tongue appears in embryos at approximately 4 weeks. It is formed by 2 lateral lingual swellings and 1 medial swelling (the tuberculum impar). These 3 swellings develop from the first pharyngeal arch. A second medial swelling, the copula, is formed by mesoderm of the second,

[a] Private practice, Temporomandibular Disorder and Orofacial Pain, 7505 South Main, Suite 210, Houston, TX 77030, USA
[b] Temporomandibular Disorder/Orofacial Pain Clinic, Veterans Affairs Hospital, 2002 Holcombe Boulevard, Houston, TX 77030-4298, USA
[c] Department of Restorative Dentistry and Biomaterials, University of Texas Health Science Center Dental Branch, 6516 John Freeman Street, Houston, TX 77030, USA
* Temporomandibular Disorder/Orofacial Pain Clinic, Veterans Affairs Hospital, 2002 Holcombe Boulevard, Houston, TX 77030-4298.
E-mail address: auvenshine244@pol.net

Sleep Med Clin 5 (2010) 45–57
doi:10.1016/j.jsmc.2009.09.001

third, and fourth arches. The third medial swelling that is formed by the posterior part of the fourth arch marks the development of the epiglottis. Immediately behind this swelling is the laryngeal orifice. The laryngeal orifice is completed posteriorly by the arytenoid swellings (**Fig. 3**).[2]

The lateral lingual swellings increase in size and begin to overgrow the tuberculum impar. As a result, the anterior two-thirds of the tongue, or body of the tongue, is composed of the merging 2 lateral lingual swellings and the disappearance of the tuberculum impar. The mucosa covering the tongue originates from the first pharyngeal arch; therefore, the sensory innervation is from the mandibular branch of the trigeminal nerve. The sulcus terminalis separates the posterior one-third of the tongue from the anterior two-thirds of the tongue. Because the posterior

one-third of the tongue originates from the second and third arches and part of the fourth pharyngeal arch, the sensory innervation is supplied by the glossopharyngeal nerve and pharyngeal plexus.

The epiglottis and extreme posterior part of the tongue are innervated by the superior laryngeal nerve in keeping with their development from the fourth pharyngeal arch. The muscles of the tongue develop from myoblasts originating in occipital somites. Therefore, the tongue musculature is innervated by the hypoglossal nerve. The chorda tympani branch of the facial nerve provides special sensory innervation (taste) to the body of the tongue.[3]

The hard palate is made up of fusion of the primary palate, which is derived from the intermaxillary segment and the 2 shelflike outgrowths of the maxillary processes (palatine shelves). These palatal shelves appear in the sixth week of development and are positioned on each side below the developing tongue. Between the seventh and eighth week of development, the tongue moves inferiorly between the 2 shelves, allowing the lateral shelves to fuse, forming the secondary palate (**Fig. 4**). The most reliable explanation for the mechanism by which the tongue drops between the palatine shelves is that the mouth first opens in the human embryo at seven and a half weeks.[4,5] The movement provided by mouth opening is necessary for the development of the temporomandibular joint.[6] The process by which a joint space is created is called cavitation.[7]

GROWTH AND DEVELOPMENT

According to Enlow, "morphogenesis works constantly toward a state of composite, architectonic balance among all the separate growing

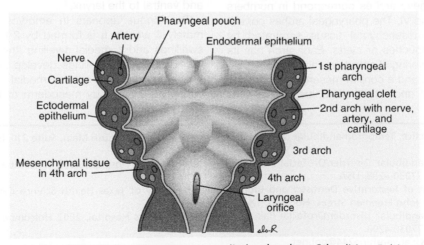

Fig. 1. Pharyngeal arches. (*From* Sadler TW. Langman's medical embryology. 8th edition. Baltimore (MD): Lippincott Williams & Wilkins; 2000. p. 351; with permission.)

Table 1
Derivatives of the pharyngeal arches and their innervation

Pharyngeal Arch	Nerve	Muscles	Skeleton
1 Mandibular	V. Trigeminal mandibular division	Mastication (temporal, masseter, medial, lateral pterygoids); mylohyoid; anterior; tensor palatine; tensor tympani	Quadrate cartilage; incus; Meckel cartilage; malleus; anterior ligament of melleus; sphenomandibular ligament; portion of mandible
2 Hyoid	VII. Facial	Facial expression (buccinator, auricularis, frontalis, platysma, orbicularis oris, orbicularis oculi); posterior belly of digastric; stylohyoid; stapedius	Stapes; styloid process; stylohyoid ligament; lesser horn and upper portion of body of hyoid bone
3	IX. Glossopharyngeal	Stylopharyngeus	Greater horn and lower portion of body of hyoid bone
4–6	X. Vagus Superior laryngeal branch (nerve to fourth arch) Recurrent laryngeal branch (nerve to sixth arch)	Cricothyroid; levator palatini; constrictors of pharynx Intrinsic muscles of larynx	Laryngeal cartilages (thyroid, cricoid, arytenoids, corniculate, cuneiform)

Data from Sadler TW. Langman's medical embryology. 8th edition. Baltimore (MD): Lippincott Williams & Wilkins; 2000. p. 348.

parts. This means that the various parts developmentally merge into a functional whole, with each part complimenting the others as they all grow and function together. During development, balance is continuously transient and can never actually be achieved because growth itself constantly creates ongoing, normal, regional imbalances."[8]

Enlow and Hans[8] state, "The facial and pharyngeal airway is a space determined by the multitude of separate parts comprising its enclosing walls. The configuration and dimensions of the airway are thus a product of the composite growth and development of the many hard and soft tissues along its pathway from the nares to the glottis. Although determined by surrounding parts, both parts in turn are dependent on the airway for maintenance of their own functional and anatomic positions. If there develops any regional childhood variations along the course of the airway that significantly alters its configuration or size, then growth proceeds along a different course, leading to variation in overall facial asymmetry that may exceed the bounds of normal pattern. The airway functions, in a real sense, as a keystone for the face."[9]

According to Enlow, the major but mutually interrelated form/functional components involved in the development are the brain and brain cranium, airway, and oral region. Each has its own separate timetable of development even though all are interrelated as a whole.

During later childhood and into adolescents, vertical nasal enlargement keeps pace with the growing body and lung size. Dental and other oral components approach adult sizes and configuration. The mandibular arch is lowered by the increasing vertical ramus length. Overall, the early wide face of the infant has become altered and in proportion by later vertical changes, leading more to the adult configuration of an elongated face (**Fig. 5**).

DIFFERENCES BETWEEN INFANT AND ADULT LARYNX

The infant larynx is more inferior. The cricoid cartilage is approximate to C3 and C4 but not C6. The epiglottis is longer, stiffer, and further away from the anterior pharyngeal wall. The narrowest portion is the cricoid cartilage, not the vocal cords. The tongue is relatively larger compared with that

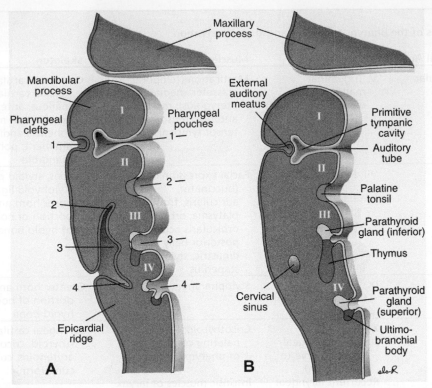

Fig. 2. Pharyngeal pouches (*A, B*). (*From* Sadler TW. Langman's medical embryology. 8th edition. Baltimore (MD): Lippincott Williams & Wilkins; 2000. p. 355; with permission.)

of the adult. Other differences include a more rostral larynx, angled vocal cords, differently shaped epiglottis, and funnel-shaped larynx, the narrowest part of which is the cricoid cartilage, not the vocal cords.[10]

KLINORYNCHY

Klinorynchy is described as the posterior migration of the facial skeleton under the brain case.[1]

According to Barsh's[9] studies, the maxilla and other facial bones, along with the mandible, moved posteriorly and rotated downwardly. This posterior migration caused the pharynx to become compressed. To preserve the pharynx for respiration and deglutition, the mandible and maxilla, along with the ethmoid and palate, became shortened.[9] Evidence of this change is seen within the teeth also. The narrowing of the dental arches in the maxilla and the mandible has been proved by

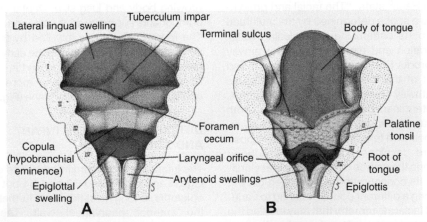

Fig. 3. Development of the tongue (*A, B*). (*From* Sadler TW. Langman's medical embryology. 8th edition. Baltimore (MD): Lippincott Williams & Wilkins; 2000. p. 363; with permission.)

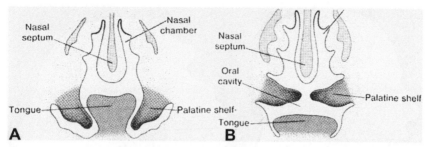

Fig. 4. (*A*) Frontal section through head at 6.5 weeks. Tongue is between palatine shelves. (*B*) Frontal section through head at 7.5 weeks. Tongue is below palatine shelves. (*From* Sadler TW. Langman's medical embryology. 8th edition. Baltimore (MD): Lippincott Williams & Wilkins; 2000. p. 371–72; with permission.)

the fact that man is the only primate with impacted third molars. The narrowing of the dental arches anterior-posteriorly with expansion laterally has resulted in the shortening of the oral cavity and has contributed to the narrowing of the pharynx. Crelin[11] notes that man is the only animal whose tongue resides partially in the pharynx. In all other animals, the tongue resides exclusively in the oral cavity. The human oral cavity is smaller than that of similar-sized primates, yet the tongue remains approximately the same volume. Therefore, according to Negus, the tongue is oversized and has pushed the larynx inferiorly. The tongue now protrudes into the oropharynx. Although in most animals the tongue is flat, the tongue of man is curvilinear and folds posteriorly and inferiorly (**Fig. 6**).[9,12]

Throughout the animal kingdom, there seems to be an overlap that exists between the soft palate and epiglottis. This is referred to as lockup. Man is the only animal that, in the adult form, has lost this epiglottic–soft palate lockup. This is because of laryngeal descent and shortening of the soft palate.[1]

The anatomy of human newborns and infants closely approximates the anatomy of the upper respiratory tract of primates. The close approximation and locking of the uvula and epiglottis allow for simultaneous suckling of milk and breathing (**Fig. 7**). However, the notion that infants can breath air and swallow liquid simultaneously has been challenged by several research studies.[10] Sensation of nasal airflow has been documented during nonfeeding and feeding swallows in term and preterm infants. However, the differences in relationship between anatomic structures and swallowing physiology suggest that the infant swallow must be viewed as distinct and not as a miniature adult swallow.

At approximately 18 months of development, the human infant experiences an anatomic change in the supralaryngeal vocal tract. The laryngeal complex migrates from its original subcranial

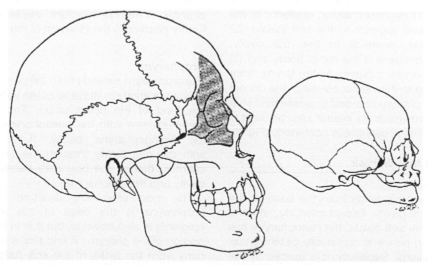

Fig. 5. Facial growth. (*From* Enlow DH, Hans MG. Essentials of facial growth. 2nd edition. Ann Arbor (MI): Needham Press; 2008. p. 30; with permission.)

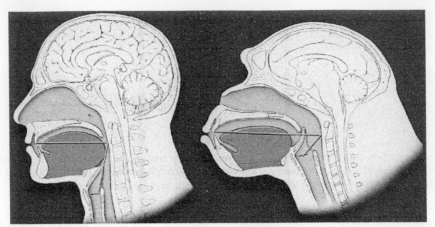

Fig. 6. Oropharyngeal tongue and oropharynx of human compared with oral tongue and palate lockup of chimpanzee. (*From* Davidson TM. The great leap forward; the anatomic basis for the acquisition of speech and obstructive sleep apnea. Sleep Med 2003;4:192; with permission.)

position to a more descended position. This leads to a gradual separation of the uvula from the epiglottis, and the interdigitation or lock is lost. In the mature human, however, the anterior wall of the respiratory tube is breached throughout the extended length of the newly developed oropharynx. The development of a wide, soft-walled oropharyngeal structure has an advantage in providing a resonating chamber in which the basis of human speech can be generated.

STRUCTURAL OVERVIEW OF THE PHARYNX

The pharynx is a fibromuscular, funnel-shaped tube, which is approximately 15 cm long. It serves as a common passageway for air and food. It extends from the base of the skull superiorly to the esophagus inferiorly.[13] The pharynx is divided into 3 parts: (1) the nasopharynx, posterior to the nasal cavity and superior to the soft palate, (2) the oropharynx, posterior to the oral cavity, between the palate and the hyoid bone, and (3) the laryngopharynx, posterior to the larynx, from the hyoid bone to the inferior border of the cricoid cartilage. The pharynx is widest opposite the hyoid bone and narrowest at its inferior end, where it is continuous with the esophagus posteriorly (**Fig. 8**).

Divisions of the Pharynx

Nasopharynx
The nasopharynx extends from the base of the skull to the soft palate. Except inferiorly, where it is bound by the soft palate, the nasopharynx has rigid walls and hence is continually patent under normal conditions. Superiorly, it is formed by the body of the sphenoid bone and the basilar part of the occipital bone. The body wall extends as

far as the pharyngeal tubercle. Below this, the wall is formed by the pharyngobasilar fascia that overlies the anterior arch of the atlas. The cervical vertebrae form the posterior boundary of the nasopharynx. Inferiorly, the nasopharynx is continuous with the oropharynx. Pharyngeal openings of the eustachian tube are situated on the lateral walls of the nasopharynx, just posterior to the inferior turbinate. The posterior wall contains a condensation of lymphoid tissue, the pharyngeal tonsils. Just posterior to the auditory tube is an elevation, which separates the tube from the fairly deep fossa, the pharyngeal recess.

The soft palate can be considered as a partial floor for the anterior part of the nasopharynx. This flexible structure is attached to the posterior part of the hard palate and laterally to the walls of the pharynx. It extends into the cavity of the pharynx. A midline structure, the uvula, projects further posteriorly than the rest of the soft palate.[14]

Oropharynx
The oropharynx extends from the plane of the hard palate superiorly to the level of the valleculae (also the level of the hyoid bone). The oropharynx communicates with the nasopharynx above and the laryngopharynx below. It is continuous with the oral cavity through the oropharyngeal isthmus, that is, the boundary between the oral cavity and the oropharynx.

The most prominent structure seen in the oropharynx is the base of the tongue. The epiglottis is also obvious, but it is in the laryngeal portion of the pharynx. A fold tissue extends inferiorly from the sides of the soft palate to blend with the sides of the walls of the pharynx. This fold covers the palatopharyngeus muscle and

A

B

C

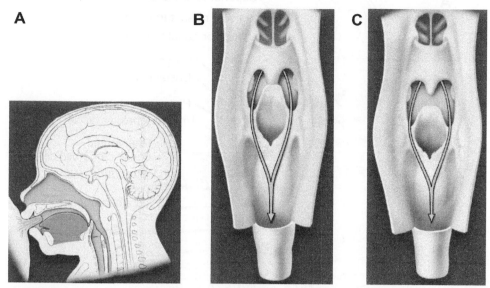

Fig. 7. (*A*) Infant epiglottic–soft palate lockup. (*B*) Epiglottic–soft palate lockup as viewed from the posterior pharynx. In human infants, the epiglottis overlaps the soft palate and food is diverted laterally around the epiglottis. Swallowing and respiration can occur simultaneously. (*C*) In human adults, the larynx is descended, the soft palate is shortened, and the epiglottic–soft palate lockup is lost. (*From* Davidson TM. The great leap forward: the anatomic basis for the acquisition of speech and obstructive sleep apnea. Sleep Med 2003;4: 189; with permission.)

takes the same name. Another pair of folds, palatoglossal, is located anterior to the palatopharyngeal folds and contains muscles of the same name. These 2 folds form an arch, which is clinically referred to as the palatine arch. Two important structures, the palatine tonsils, are located in the tonsilar fossa between the palatoglossus and palatopharyngeous muscle. Blood supply to the palatine tonsil is contributed by branches of the ascending pharyngeal branch of the external carotid artery from the lesser palatine branches of the maxillary artery and from the dorsal lingual artery and also by the ascending palatine and tonsilar branches of the facial artery.[14]

Laryngopharynx

The laryngopharynx is a region of the pharynx that lies behind the larynx and is continuous with the oropharynx above and the esophagus below. This part of the pharynx decreases rapidly in size from superior to inferior. The opening of the larynx is bounded anteriorly and superiorly by the upper portion of the epiglottis, laterally by the aryepiglottic folds and posteriorly by the elevation of the arytenoid cartilages. Below the opening of the larynx, the anterior wall of the laryngopharynx is formed by the posterior surfaces of the arytenoid cartilages and the posterior plate of the cricoid cartilage. The pyriform recess is situated on each side of the larynx. It is bounded laterally by the

thyroid cartilage. The pyriform recess extends from the lateral pharyngoepiglottic fold to the upper portion of the esophagus. The superior laryngeal nerve lies deep to the mucosal fold in the lateral wall of the pyriform recess.

The pyriform recess is a fairly deep hollow between the arytenoid cartilages and aryepiglottic folds medially. The recess is situated on each side of the larynx.

The Pharyngeal Wall

The pharyngeal wall is composed of 4 layers: (1) a mucosa that is composed of ciliated columnar epithelium in the nasopharynx and stratified columnar epithelium in the oropharynx and laryngopharynx, (2) a fibrous layer, which forms the pharyngobasilar fascia and is attached superiorly to the skull, (3) a muscular layer composed of inner longitudinal and outer circular parts, and (4) a loose connective tissue layer that forms the buccopharyngeal fascia. The buccopharyngeal fascia is continuous with the epimysium (deep surface) of the pharyngeal muscles, and it contains the pharyngeal plexus of nerves and veins.

Pharyngeal Musculature

The muscles of the pharynx are

1. Superior constrictor
2. Middle constrictor

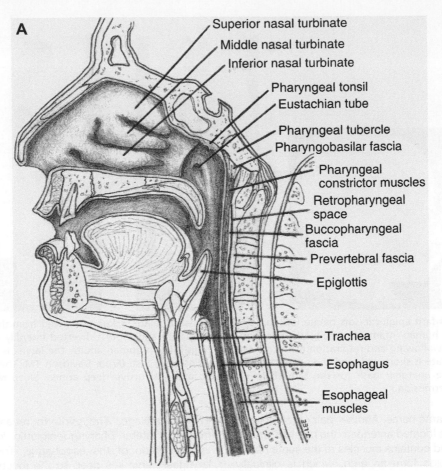

Fig. 8. (*A*) Sagittal view of pharynx. (*B*) Opened posterior view of pharynx otolaryngology. (*From* Van De Water TR, Staecker H. Otolaryngology. New York: Thieme; 2006. p. 554 (A), 553 (B); with permission.)

3. Inferior constrictor
4. Stylopharyngeus
5. Salpingopharyngeus
6. Palatopharyngeus.

The superior constrictor muscle arises from the posterior border of the lower part of the medial pterygoid plate, the pterygoid hamulus, the pterygomandibular raphe, the posterior part of the mylohyoid line of the mandible, and by fibers from the side of the tongue (**Fig. 9**). The fibers of the superior constrictor pass backward in a broad sheet and are inserted into the median raphe. The interval between the superior border of the muscle and the base of the skull is closed by fascia.

The middle constrictor muscle arises from the whole length of the superior border of the greater horn of the hyoid bone, from the lesser horn, and from the inferior end of the stylohyoid ligament. The fibers branch exteriorly to be inserted into the median raphe. As they spread downward

from the greater horn of the hyoid bone, they form a fan-shaped sheath to their insertion.

The inferior constrictor, the thickest of the constrictor muscles, is composed of 2 parts: thyropharyngeus and cricopharyngeus. The thyropharyngeus part of the inferior constrictor arises from the oblique line of the thyroid cartilage, from the tendinous band across the cricothyroid muscle, from the lateral surface of the cricoid cartilage at the upper edge of the tendinous band, and from the inferior horn of the thyroid cartilage. The cricopharyngeus portion of the inferior constrictor rises from the side of the cricoid cartilage. The fibers run horizontally and posteriorly, encircling the junction between the pharynx and esophagus to insert on the opposite side of the cricoid cartilage. The cricopharyngeus fibers are continuous with the circular fibers of the esophagus and are believed to act as a sphincter, regulating material entering the esophagus.

Human pharyngeal constrictor muscles appear to be organized into functional fiber layers, as

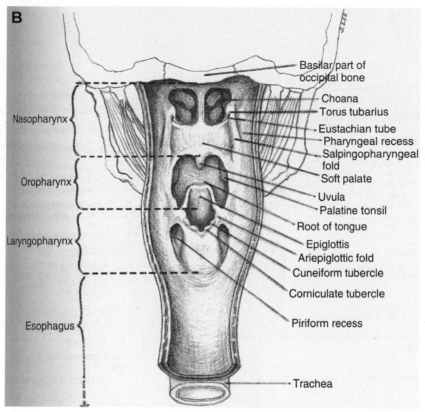

B

Basilar part of occipital bone

Choana

Torus tubarius

Nasopharynx

Eustachian tube

Pharyngeal recess

Salpingopharyngeal fold

Soft palate

Oropharynx

Uvula

Palatine tonsil

Root of tongue

Epiglottis

Laryngopharynx

Ariepiglottic fold

Cuneiform tubercle

Corniculate tubercle

Piriform recess

Esophagus

Trachea

Fig. 8. (*continued*)

indicated by distinct motor innervation and specialized muscle fibers. The slow inner layer appears to be a specialized layer that is unique to normal humans. The presence of the highly specialized, slow-tonic, and alpha-cardiac myosin heavy chain isoforms, together with their absence in human newborns and nonhuman primates, suggest that the specialization of the slow inner layer fibers maybe related to speech and respiration. This specialization may reflect the sustained contraction needed in humans to maintain stiffness in pharyngeal walls during respiration and to shape the wall for speech articulation. In contrast, the fast outer layer fiber is adapted for rapid movement as seen during swallowing.[15]

ANATOMY OF THE LARYNX

The larynx connects the pharynx with the trachea. It functions as a valve that separates the trachea from the narrow digestive tract and maintains a patent airway. It also provides an instrument for vocalization. The larynx is made up of cartilages, ligaments, and membranes that connect the cartilages and muscles to cause movement

of various parts. It is lined with a mucous membrane of columnar ciliated cells and contains many mucous glands.

There are 3 unpaired cartilages (thyroid, cricoid, and epiglottic) and 3 paired cartilages (arytenoid, corniculate, and cuneiform).

The thyroid cartilage has a peculiar shape, with 2 large plates anteriorly and laterally placed and fused in the midline anteriorly but open posteriorly. Projections extending superiorly and inferiorly from the posterior edges are called superior and inferior horns. The superior edge of the lamina presents a notch in the midline referred to as the thyroid notch. A structure called the oblique line is formed on the lateral surface of the thyroid cartilage. This line is important for the understanding of muscle attachments.

The cricoid cartilage is the only complete ring found in the respiratory system. It is larger posteriorly and anteriorly. The posterior portion is formed by 2 laminae, whereas the anterior portion presents an arch. Near the base of each lamina is found a facet for articulation with the inferior horn of the thyroid cartilage. On the superior surface of the lamina are facets for the articulation of the

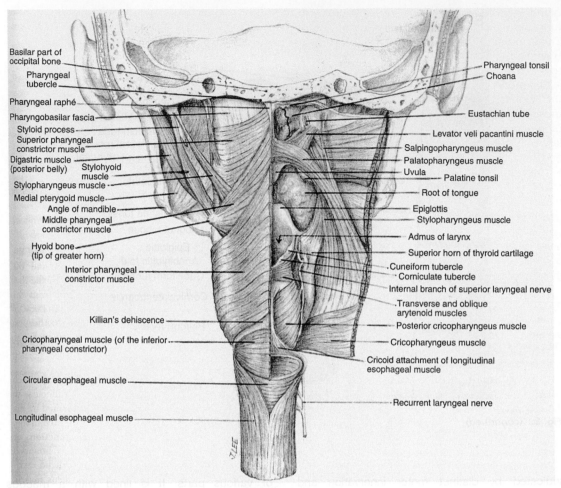

Fig. 9. Section through pharynx viewed from posterior otolaryngology. (*From* Van De Water TR, Staecker H. Otolaryngology. New York: Thieme; 2006. p. 555; with permission.)

arytenoid cartilages. The posterior surface of the lamina shows 2 hollow areas on either side of the midline for the posterior cricoarytenoideus muscles.

The epiglottic cartilage is a leaf-shaped structure. The base of the epiglottic cartilage is attached to the inside of the thyroid cartilage at the midline by the thyroepiglottic ligament.

The 3 paired cartilages—arytenoid, corniculate, and cuneiform—are small cartilages. The laryngeal folds consist of (1) paired aryepiglottic folds extended from the epiglottis posteriorly to the superior surface of the arytenoids, (2) paired vestibular folds (false vocal cords) extended from the thyroid cartilage posterior to the superior surface of the arytenoids, and (3) paired vocal folds (true vocal cords) extended from the posterior surface of the thyroid plate to the anterior part of the arytenoids. The interarytenoid fold bridges the arytenoid cartilages. The thyrohyoid

fold extends from the hyoid bone to the thyroid cartilage. The sensory innervation is the recurrent laryngeal nerve to the supraglottic larynx and the internal branch of the superior laryngeal nerve to the infraglottic larynx.

The larynx is the guardian of the airway. Functioning in this role, the larynx can initiate a wide range of reflexes with significant physiologic effects. Laryngeal chemoreflexes that are initiated when chemical substances contact the laryngeal mucosa include apnea, swallowing, hypertension, and changes in peripheral resistance. All of these reflexes can have fatal consequences. The larynx also contains various mechanoreceptors in its muscles and joints, which respond to and influence laryngeal function. These mechanoreceptors can be further divided into 2 groups. The first group consists of touch receptors, which may act to identify foreign bodies in the airway and modulate phonation. The second group consists of mechanoreceptors responsive to airflow, transmural pressure change, and pharyngeal receptors. These probably have a role in reflex control of breathing. Last but not least, there are proprioceptors that act as muscle spindle receptors.[16]

The motor innervation is the external branch of the superior laryngeal nerve to the cricothyroid muscle and the recurrent laryngeal nerve to all other laryngeal muscles. The blood supply to the larynx is provided by branches of the superior and inferior thyroid arteries.

There are 2 joints within the larynx, the cricothyroid joint and the cricoarytenoid joint, that provide the necessary articulation for laryngeal movement. The ligaments and membranes connecting the cartilages of the larynx to one another and to the hyoid bone are important because they fill the gaps between the cartilages, thereby completing the walls of the hollow organ.

The ligaments and membranes are: (1) thyrohyoid membrane, (2) hyoepiglottic ligament, (3) cricothyroid ligament, (4) vocal ligament, (5) conus elasticus, (6) vestibular ligament, and (7) cricotracheal ligament.

The thyrohyoid membrane is attached superiorly to the body and horns of the hyoid bone and inferiorly to the superior horn and superior edges of the thyroid cartilage. Thyrohyoid membrane is pierced by the internal branch of the superior laryngeal branch of the vagus nerve and by the superior laryngeal blood vessels.

The hyoepiglottic ligament extends from the hyoid bone to the anterior surface of the epiglottis. This is an important ligament participating in the movement of the epiglottis during swallowing.

The vocal ligament is attached anteriorly to the inside of the thyroid cartilage near the midline and posteriorly to the vocal process of the arytenoid cartilage. The vocal ligament is covered with mucous membrane. The conus elasticus extends superiorly from the superior border of the cricoid cartilage to attach to the vocal ligament. The weak vestibular ligament is situated posterior to the vocal ligament and extends from the thyroid cartilage anteriorly to the lateral surface of the arytenoid cartilage posteriorly. These are called the false vocal cords or vestibular cords.

MUSCLES OF THE LARYNX

The muscles of the larynx can be divided into 2 broad groups: extrinsic muscles and intrinsic muscles. The extrinsic muscles of the larynx can be subdivided into 2 groups: suprahyoid and infrahyoid muscles. The suprahyoid group of muscles is composed of (1) the anterior belly of the digastric muscle, which draws the hyoid forward; (2) the

posterior belly of the digastric muscle, which stabilizes and draws the hyoid back; (3) the genioglossus muscle, which elevates and advances the hyoid bone and lowers the mandible; (4) the stylohyoid muscle, which raises the hyoid and larynx and also serves to fix the hyoid bone during swallowing; and (5) the mylohyoid muscle, which raises the floor of the mouth and hyoid and lowers the mandible. The unique feature of the suprahyoid musculature is that these muscles have the capability of reversing origin and insertion, depending on demand.

The other group of extrinsic muscles of the larynx is referred to as the infrahyoid muscles. This group is composed of the (1) omohyoid muscle, which lowers the hyoid and opposes upward movement of the larynx; (2) the sternohyoid muscle, which lowers the hyoid and opposes upward movement of the larynx; (3) the sternothyroid muscle, which lowers the hyoid and opposes upward movement of the larynx; and (4) the thyrohyoid muscle, which lowers the hyoid and raises the larynx if the hyoid is fixed.

The intrinsic muscles of the larynx connect the various cartilages and membranes between the cartilages and allow for movement of the cartilaginous skeleton. The intrinsic muscles of the larynx are: (1) cricothyroid, (2) posterior cricoarytenoid, (3) lateral cricoarytenoid, (4) transverse arytenoid, (5) oblique arytenoid, (6) thyroarytenoid, (7) thyroepiglottic, and (8) aryepiglottic. All of these names reveal the muscle attachments. The cricothyroid muscle pulls the thyroid cartilage anteriorly and inferiorly in a rocking motion, thereby increasing the tension on the vocal cords. The posterior cricoarytenoid muscle contracts to widen the space between the 2 vocal cords (the rima glottidis). The lateral cricoarytenoid rotates or pulls the vocal process medially, thereby decreasing the width between the 2 vocal cords. The transverse arytenoid muscle pulls the arytenoid cartilages closer together by a gliding motion and is used in closing the rima glottidis. The oblique arytenoid muscle is used to bring the arytenoid cartilages closer together and to tighten the aryepiglottic fold. This muscle is used in the process of swallowing. The thyroarytenoid muscle can be used in contracting a portion of the vocal cord in production of high tones. When these muscles contract, they bring the arytenoid cartilage closer to the thyroid cartilage, thereby decreasing the tension on the vocal cords. A portion of this muscle, which is located on the lateral side of the vocal ligament, is called the vocalis muscle. It is thought that this muscle can be used in contracting a portion of the vocal cord in production of very high tones. The thyroepiglottic muscle aids the ar-yepiglottic muscle in tightening the aryepiglottic fold and in bringing the epiglottic cartilage into closer contact with the arytenoid cartilages during the process of closing the opening into the larynx during swallowing.[14]

DISCUSSION

The oral apparatus is the "gateway to the gut."[13] The oropharyngeal system is in unbroken conti-nuity with the pharynx and funnels food directly into the esophagus. The structure of the food channel is complicated by the peculiar crossing of the airway at the larynx. The oral apparatus not only prepares food but also initiates swallow-ing. It is designed to function in close coordina-tion with the pharynx. The oropharyngeal system is meticulously integrated with the production of speech. One of the major reasons the upper respiratory tract of man developed as it did is partly to facilitate speech. As man assumed an upright posture compared with quadripeds, the eyes, face, and mouth rotated downward and forward so that the interpupillary line of the eyes would be maintained parallel with the horizon. For the eyes and face to assume this anatomic position, the maxilla and mandible and also the ethmoid and palatine bones had to migrate poste-riorly. This led to a shortening of the face and the dental arches anterior-posteriorly. The resulting movement of the maxilla and mandible posteriorly forced the tongue to shift from its position residing solely in the oral cavity to a position where the distal portion of the tongue protruded into the pharynx. As the larynx descended and the soft palate shortened, the epiglottic–soft palate lockup, which is seen in other primates, was lost. The soft palate and uvula became more flaccid to facilitate speech.

With the descent of the larynx and the develop-ment of the oropharynx and the support of speech, certain disadvantages of morphology developed. There are 3 distinct roles of the pharynx, which require different muscular activities. The roles are respiration, deglutition, and phonation. For deglu-tition, the pharynx assumes the role of a flexible tube, the muscles of which force food from the oral cavity into the esophagus. For phonation, the pharynx is a muscular tube that can change length and shape to alter sounds passing through it. For air passage, the pharynx must remain as a rigid tube without collapse, especially during sleep. No muscle or group of muscles assumes this function as a primary role, leaving the pharynx subject to collapse and obstruction during certain conditions of respiration.

One reason the upper respiratory tract of man developed or evolved as it did is partly to facili-tate speech. The pharynx was narrowed to form a narrow, descendible tube for better sound modulation by rotation of the foramen magnum inferiorly, migration of the palate posteriorly, and shifting of the tongue into the oral pharynx. Orobuccal speech was generated as the larynx descended and the soft palate shortened, causing loss of the epiglottic–soft palate lockup. Cranial-based angulations further improved vocal quality.

The obstructing anatomy is clearly a soft tissue phenomenon, as it is absent during the day and present at night. The soft tissue is suspended and supported by the underlying skeleton. Soft tissue obstruction sites during sleep include the nose, upper and lower pharynx, and occasionally the larynx. Perhaps there are other contributing soft tissue changes, such as floppy epiglottis or lax pharyngeal musculature. The descended larynx, the oral pharyngeal tongue, and the acute cranial-based angulations are primary contribu-tors to sleep disorder breathing.[9]

REFERENCES

1. Davidson TM. The great leap forward: the anatomic basis for the acquisition of speech and obstructive sleep apnea. Sleep Med 2003;4:185–94.
2. Sadler TW. Langman's medical embryology. 8th edition. Baltimore (MD): Lippincott Williams & Wil-kins; 2000. p. 345–81.
3. Schoenwolf GC. Larson's embryology. 4th edition. Philadelphia: Elsevier; 2009. p. 543–582.
4. Humphrey T. The development of mouth opening and related reflexes involving the oral area of human features. Ala J Med Sci 1968;5(2):126–57.
5. Humphrey T. The relation between human fetal mouth opening reflexes and closure of the palate. Ala J Med Sci 1969;125(3):317–44.
6. Auvenshine RC. The relationship between structure and function in the development of the squamoman-dibular joint in rats. Dissertation for PhD, Department of Anatomy, LSU Medical School of Graduate Studies. 1976. New Orleans, LA.
7. Pitsillides AA. Early effects of embryonic move-ments. J Anat 2006;208(4):417–31.
8. Enlow DH, Hans MG. Essentials of facial growth. 2nd edition. Ann Arbor (MI): Needham Press; 2008. p. 1–19.
9. Barsh LI. The origin of pharyngeal obstruction during sleep. Sleep Breath 1999;3:17–21.
10. Newman LA. Anatomy and physiology of infant swallow, swallowing, and swallowing disorders. March 2001:3–4.

11. Crelin ES. The human vocal tract: anatomy, function, development and evolution. New York: Vantage; 1987. p. 97, 220, 223, 224.
12. Negus VE. The comparative anatomy of physiology of the larynx. New York: Grune and Stratton; 1949. p. 21, 187.
13. DuBrul EL. Sicher and DuBrul's oral anatomy. 8th edition. St Louis (MI): Ishiyaku EuroAmerica, Inc; 1988.
14. Crafts RC. Textbook of human anatomy. New York: Ronald Press Company; 1966. p. 553–69.
15. Mu L, Sanders I. Neuromuscular specializations within human pharyngeal constrictor muscles. Ann Otol Rhinol Laryngol 2007;116(8):604–17.
16. Van De Water TR, Staecker H. Otolaryngology. New York: Thieme; 2006. p. 552–65.

Cone Beam Computed Tomography: Craniofacial and Airway Analysis

David C. Hatcher, DDS, MSc[a,b,c,*]

KEYWORDS

- Cone beam CT (CBCT) • Volumetric imaging
- Degenerative joint disease • TMJ • Airway
- Retroglossal • Retropalatal • Facial growth

Imaging plays a role in the anatomic assessment of the airway and adjacent structures. Obstructive sleep-disordered breathing (OSDB) is not diagnosed with imaging, but imaging can identify patients with airways who are at risk for obstruction and other anatomic characteristics that may contribute to OSDB. The airway extending from the tip of the nose to the superior end of the trachea can be visualized on conventional computed tomography (CT) and cone beam CT (CBCT) scans. Because these scans also include the jaws, teeth, cranial base, spine, and facial soft tissues, there is an opportunity to evaluate the functional and developmental relationships between these structures. The skeletal support for airway is provided by the cranial base (superiorly), spine (posteriorly), nasal septum (anterosuperiorly), jaws, and hyoid bone (anteriorly). The airway valves include the soft palate, tongue, and epiglottis (**Fig. 1**). Airway obstructions or encroachments are of interest because they increase airway resistance that may contribute to OSDB; therefore, visualization and calculation of the airway dimensions are important. Common airway encroachments include turbinates, adenoids, long soft palate, large tongue, and pharyngeal and lingual tonsils. Less common airway encroachments include polyps and tumors.

This article discusses the use of 3-dimensional (3D) imaging (CBCT) to evaluate the airway and

selected regional anatomic variables that may contribute to OSDB. Optimal treatment outcomes begin with a complete and accurate diagnosis. Imaging may assist in delineating attributes that contribute to OSDB in patients who do not have a phenotype (such as high body mass index) that is routinely associated with OSDB.

CBCT AND IMAGE ANALYSIS

Technological advances in computing power, sensor technology, and reconstruction algorithms have merged and resulted in the introduction of a CBCT (also known as volumetric imaging). Volumetric imaging is synonymous with 3D imaging because the information has depth in addition to length and width. The 3D imaging domain includes radiograph (CT and CBCT) and magnetic resonance imaging technologies. The 2 principal differences that distinguish CBCT from traditional CT are the type of imaging source-detector complex and the method of data acquisition. The radiograph source for CT is a high-photon, output rotating anode generator, whereas for CBCT it can be a low-energy fixed anode tube similar to that used in dental panoramic machines. CT uses a fan-shaped x-ray beam from its source to acquire images and records data on solid-state image detectors that are arranged in a 360° array

[a] University of Southern Nevada, 11 Sunset Way, Henderson, NV 89014, USA
[b] Arthur A. Dugoni School of Dentistry, 2155 Webster Street, San Francisco, CA 94115, USA
[c] Private Practice, Diagnostic Digital Imaging, 99 Scripps Drive, #101, Sacramento, CA 95825, USA
* University of Southern Nevada, 11 Sunset Way, Henderson, NV 89014.
E-mail address: David@ddicenters.com

Sleep Med Clin 5 (2010) 59–70
doi:10.1016/j.jsmc.2009.11.001

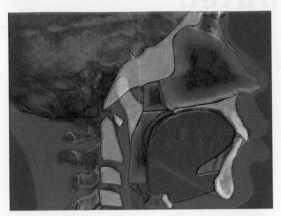

Fig. 1. Airway zones that are visible using CBCT (*blue and green*). These zones extend from the nasal tip to the epiglottis and are divided in the nasal, nasopharyngeal, and oral airways. The airway is supported posteriorly by the spine; superiorly by the cranial base; and anteriorly by the maxilla, mandible, and hyoid (*white*). The mobile elements associated with the airway include the tongue, soft palate, and epiglottis (*red*).

around the patient. CBCT technology uses a cone-shaped x-ray beam with a special image intensifier and a solid-state sensor or an amorphous silicon plate for capturing the image.

Conventional medical CT devices image patients in a series of axial plane slices that are captured either as individual stacked slices or using a continuous spiral motion over the axial plane. Conversely, CBCT presently uses one rotation sweep of the patient similar to that used for panoramic radiography. Image data can be collected for either a complete dental/maxillofacial volume or a limited regional area of interest. Scan times for these vary from 8 to 40 seconds for the complete volume. CBCT has a significantly lower radiation burden than a comparable scan using a conventional CT. CBCT has a favorable risk/benefit ratio for many craniofacial applications, including imaging of the airway and associated craniofacial structures.

ANATOMIC ACCURACY

An ideal imaging goal is to accurately represent the anatomy as it exists in nature, that is, the anatomic truth. The projection geometry associated with 2D techniques does not produce accurate anatomic images. 3D digital techniques using back projection algorithms create the opportunity to produce anatomically accurate images.

Current 3D imaging techniques allow an anatomically accurate capture of the surface and subsurface structures.[1–4] One measure of image

quality is the ability to detect small anatomic features. The variables that have significant influence on the quality of a CBCT include voxel size (smallest element in a 3D digital image), dynamic range (number of gray levels), signal, and noise. In general, the best quality image is composed of small voxels, large number of gray levels, high signal, and low noise. CBCT voxels are isotropic (equal size in all dimensions x, y, and z) and range in size from 0.1 to 0.4 mm. The captured field of view (FOV) can be scaled to match the regions of interest (ROIs). The ROI can include the entire craniofacial region or a selected subsection of the craniofacial anatomy. The display of the captured FOV or subset of image data can be viewed from any angle using various display techniques (**Fig. 2**). For example, the entire craniofacial skeleton may be captured using a CBCT scan, but using software tools, an ROI (such as the airway) may be selected, displayed, and analyzed. Several software companies have developed application-specific display and analysis software that result in the measurement (linear, area, volume, angular) of segmented and integrated anatomic structures. Of particular interest is the metric analysis of the airway and the adjacent structures. Specialized software for metric analysis of the airway has been calibrated using orthogonal and oblique airway phantoms, and has been validated for accuracy and precision.[2,3] The convergence of CBCT with the application software is very beneficial in understanding and diagnosing OSDB and its relationship to craniofacial anatomy.

FACIAL GROWTH AND THE AIRWAY

Alterations from the normal pattern of nasal respiration occurring during active growth can affect the development of the craniofacial skeleton in humans and experimental animals.[5–8] Severely reduced nasal airflow may induce compensations that include an inferior mandibular rest position, parting of the lips, increased interocclusal space, lower or more forward tongue position, lower positioning of the hyoid bone, a modal shift from nasal breathing to mouth breathing, anterior extension of the head and neck, increased anterior face height, increase in the mandibular and occlusal plane angles, narrow alar base, narrow maxillary arch, high palatal vault, posterior crossbite, class II occlusion, and clockwise facial growth pattern. These compilations of craniofacial and occlusal traits produce a facial phenotype that has been cited in the orthodontic literature as "adenoidal facies," thus ascribing an etiology and expressing a bias that hypertrophic adenoidal tissues are the cause of an obtunded nasal airflow that results in

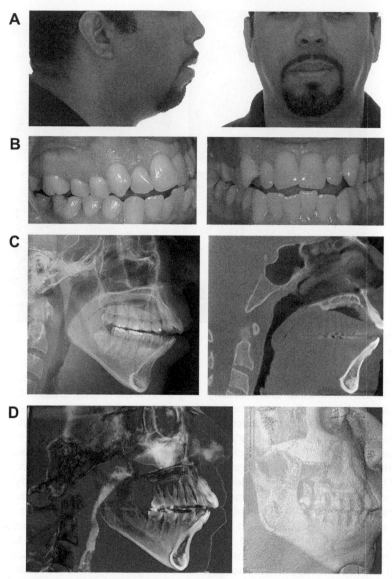

Fig. 2. Craniofacial and airway visualization. Various CBCT and patient visualization options. (*A, B*) Convex facial profile, narrow maxilla, anterior open bite, and forward head and neck posture. (*C*) Midsagittal airway (*right image*) and a standard cephalometric image generated from the CBCT volume using specialized software. (*D*) Volume-rendered and shaded surface display image of the head and neck skeleton along with the airway-skin boundaries. (*E*) Analysis of the airway. The midsagittal airway view is mapped (*left image*), and a series of cross-sectional areas (CSAs) of the mapped regions are generated (*right image*). The CSA and distance measurements are calculated and displayed for each of the cross-sectional intervals. The smallest cross-sectional area was identified to be 38.94 mm^2. (*F*) A reconstructed panoramic projection. The data volume can be reconstructed in any user-defined orthogonal, oblique, or curved plane to match the clinical investigation objective. Note the small condyles and forward posture of the mandible.

a specific pattern of craniofacial deformation. However, this facial phenotype may also occur secondary to aberrant mandibular growth. The end result in several craniofacial growth scenarios may be associated with alterations in airway dimensions, airway resistance, and functional airway patency, but the cause-and-effect

relationships need to be considered. For example, does an anatomic reduction in airway function cause the craniofacial compensations or does abnormal craniofacial growth result in compromised airway function? The anteroposterior dimensions of the airway have been shown to have a proportional relationship to jaw growth

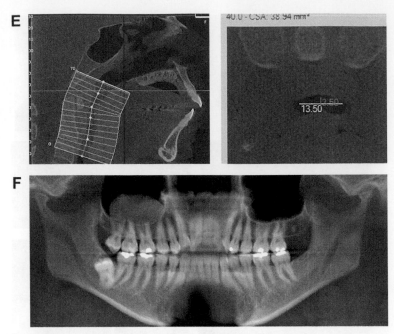

Fig. 2. (*continued*)

and facial growth pattern.[9] The airway is largest when there is normal mandibular and maxillary growth and when facial growth pattern occurs with a counter-clockwise rotation. Conversely, the airway is smaller with deficient maxillary and mandibular growth and when there is a clockwise facial growth pattern. Because mandibular growth has been linked to condylar growth and degenerative joint disease (DJD, also known as osteoarthritis) affects condylar growth, it is reasonable to postulate that a developmental onset of DJD may limit airway dimensions (**Figs. 3** and **4**).

Current 3D imaging techniques available for routine imaging provide the opportunity to use a "systems approach" to visualize and evaluate the functional and developmental relationships between proximal craniofacial regions. It has been reported that a developmental insult to the temporomandibular joints (TMJs) may have a regional effect on the growth of the ipsilateral side of the face, including the mandible, maxilla, and base of the skull.[10–18] Similarly, there is a direct relationship between jaw growth and airway development.[9] The notion that there are functional and growth relationships between adjacent anatomic regions creates the desire for a robust method to visualize and analyze them.

MANDIBULAR GROWTH

The mandible forms by using a combination of endochondral and intramembranous processes of bone formation. The condyles do not control growth of the entire mandible, but condylar growth contributes to the process of mandibular growth, primarily the condylar processes and rami, and secondarily the body and alveolar ridges. Mesenchymal cell differentiation into articular cartilage followed by endochondral ossification contributes to the condylar growth. There are several mandibular growth sites (growth fields), including the condyles, alveolar process, rami, body, and coronoid process. These growth sites have genetic potential for growth through mesenchymal cell differentiation and cell division, but the growth can be modulated through external or environmental (epigenetic) factors. These external factors include neighboring growth sites, hormones, tissue stress and strain, and tissue damage. The craniofacial complex generally grows in harmony. Changes occurring in one area of the craniofacial complex induce a response in the adjacent areas. A model proposed by Petrovic and coworkers[12,13] suggests that distant craniofacial changes (such as maxillary growth) are transformed into local (mandibular) growth signals by a complex interplay of muscle adaptation, neural input, connective tissue response, blood supply, biochemical growth activation, and suppression. Condylar fibrocartilage, during growth, is responsive to growth stimuli from various systemic and local influences. Ideally, condylar growth is modulated to keep pace with facial growth. Fibrocartilage in the adult condyle

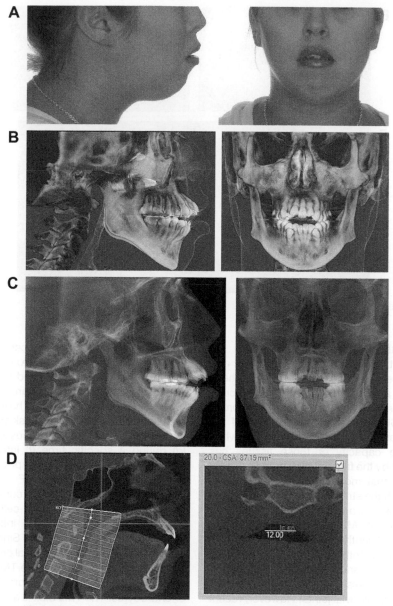

Fig. 3. Temporomandibular joint (TMJ), facial growth, and airway. A craniofacial phenotype that occurs after a developmental onset of TMJ DJD. The DJD limited or arrested the development of the condyles, and this resulted in reduced mandibular growth along with other craniofacial compensations (*F*). The condyles were located in the anteroinferior regions of their fossa when in habitual occlusion (*F*). Note the convex facial profile (*A–C*), the anterior open bite (*B–D, E, F*), and the forward head and neck posture. The mediolateral development of the maxilla and mandible was reduced (*B, C, E*), and the tongue was postured down and away from the depth of the palate. There was diffuse narrowing of the airway with the smallest cross-sectional area measuring 87.19 mm². The forward posture of the mandible may be a compensation to improve airway patency. Selective muscle recruitment is required to resist the clockwise rotation of the mandible and maintain airway patency.

has an adaptive function to maintain the mandible in its functional role. Reduced adaptive capacity of the fibrocartilage (such as DJD) during growth and development has been shown to limit growth of the ipsilateral half of the mandible. DJD in adulthood that results in significant hard tissue loss may be associated with a change in mandibular

posture, occlusion, and condyle/fossa spatial relationships.

DEGENERATIVE JOINT DISEASE

DJD (also known as degenerative arthritis, degenerative arthrosis, osteoarthritis, and osteoarthrosis)

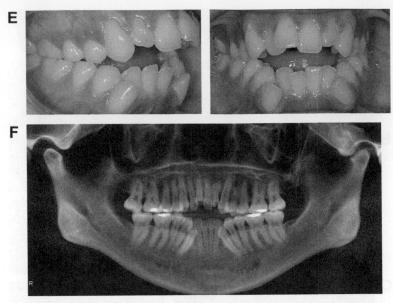

Fig. 3. (*continued*)

affects all joints, including the TMJ. There are several factors that can initiate the pathologic and imaging features associated with DJD. These factors create a situation whereby the articular structures can no longer resist the applied forces to the joint. DJD involves the destruction of the hard and soft articular tissues, and occurs when the remodeling capacity of those tissues has been exceeded by the functional demands. Therefore, scenarios that modulate and increase joint loads or diminish the strength or adaptive capacity of the articular tissues are of interest in discovering the pathogenesis of TMJ DJD. The understanding of DJD has significantly evolved during the past 30 years. Until recently, DJD of the TMJ was considered a wear and tear phenomenon that occurred in individuals older than 40 years, as observed in other synovial joints. However, recent investigations and clinical observations have discovered significant differences in the occurrence and behavior of TMJ DJD in comparison with other joints. TMJ DJD has been recognized to have a predilection for women and can be identified at all ages after puberty, and is not limited to individuals older than 40 years. It has been suggested that sex hormones and hormone receptors may play a role in the early age onset and sex predilection of this phenomenon. DJD onset and the associated complaints in women occur from puberty through menopause. The TMJ is a diarthrodial joint like other synovial joints; however, the expression of DJD differs from other joints. Key distinctions between the TMJ anatomy and other synovial joints include the predominance of

fibrocartilage in lieu of hyaline cartilage and motion mechanics that include rotation and translation. The TMJ is a loaded joint, and the joint loads or stress concentrations (force/area) may be equal to other load-bearing joints.[18] The functional movement of the condyle over the disk creates a contact force (F) applied in a direction (cos θ) over a distance (d) during a specific time (t) interval. The disk/condyle interactions can be expressed in terms of work (W) or power (P); $W = F \times d \times \cos \theta$ and $P = W/t$.[19–22] Investigators are currently examining the mechanobiology or single-cell biomechanics, that is, how physical forces influence biologic processes in the TMJ.[23–26] Single-cell biomechanics depend on their material properties relative to the surrounding matrix. The TMJ disk cells are a heterogeneous mixture of fibroblasts and fibrochondrocytes. The TMJ disk is a fibrocartilaginous tissue, but it is not a homogeneous tissue. The disk is composed mostly of collagen (type I), proteoglycans (glycosaminoglycan chains that are primarily chondroitin sulfate and dermatan sulfate), and water. The distribution and arrangement of the disk components are not uniform. This disk has been divided into 3 areas or zones: the anterior band, the intermediate zone, and the posterior band. These zones, like anatomic regions, create material property differences, and therefore the single-cell biomechanics between these zones may vary. The anatomic variations between the zones ideally reflect a structural relationship to the functional demands in terms of work and power. The work imparted on the tissues (cells) initiates a mechanotransduction pathway (mechanism by

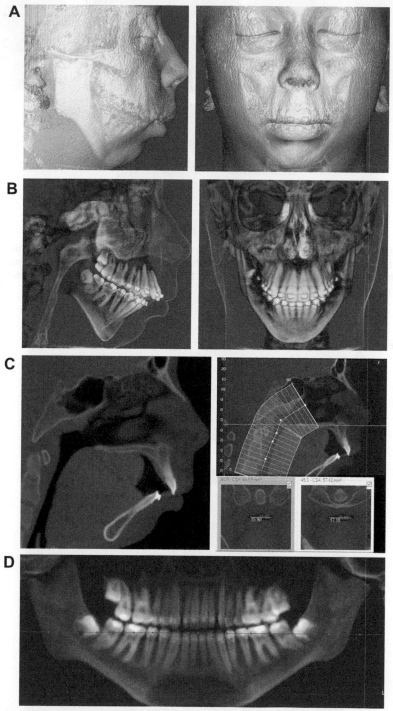

Fig. 4. (*A–D*) TMJ, facial growth, and airway. A craniofacial phenotype that occurs after a developmental onset of TMJ juvenile rheumatoid arthritis (JRA). The regional compensations to the JRA were similar to those observed in **Fig. 3** for DJD. There was a convex facial profile, clockwise facial growth pattern, steep mandibular and occlusal planes, obtuse gonial angles, small mediolateral jaw dimensions, inferior positioning of hyoid bone, anterior open bite, and small airway. The airway dimensions were diffusely narrowed with the smallest cross-sectional area measuring 49.59 mm².

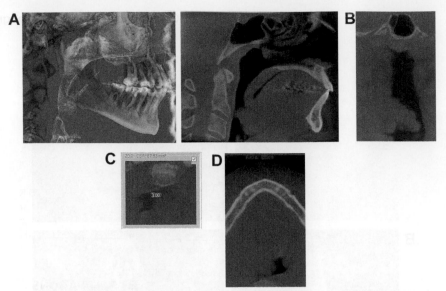

Fig. 5. Tumor; airway encroachment. (*A*) A soft tissue density extending from the tongue base region and encroaching on the airway space. (*B–D*) Soft tissue density extending from the right lateral wall of the oral pharynx. This soft tissue encroachment was determined to be a squamous cell carcinoma that had reduced the cross-sectional area to 87.93 mm².

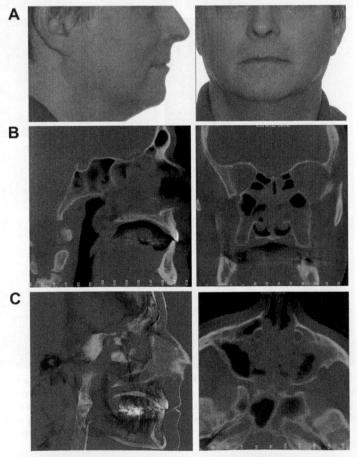

Fig. 6. Inflammatory disease; upper airway encroachment. A patient with severe rhinosinusitis (*A*). The ostiomeatal units and the nasal fosse were not patent. A polyp was extending into the nasopharynx (*B, left image*). A discontinuity of the airway spaces of the nose and the oral pharynx (*C, left image*) (air shown as white).

which cells convert a mechanical stimulus into a chemical activity) that results in gene expression. Gene expression initiates several pathways to produce (1) extracellular matrix proteins, (2) matrix metalloproteinases, (3) proinflammatory cytokines, or (4) apoptosis regulators. The extracellular matrix protein synthesis creates extracellular matrix and tissue regeneration. The production of matrix metalloproteinases and proinflammatory cytokines results in extracellular matrix degradation. Extracellular matrix degradation and apoptosis are pathways that can result in DJD. The variations in mechanotransduction pathways may be related to the tissue anatomy, tissue quality, and power (work/time). Several variables affect work, including peak forces, force vectors, velocity, and work cycles. The tissues' anatomy and quality will relate to the adaptive capacity of those tissues. Both mechanotransduction and signal transduction by hormones (β-estradiol, relaxin, progesterone) are currently being explored.[27,28] In vivo testing on rabbits using disk explants has demonstrated that increased serum levels of relaxin, β-estradiol and relaxin, and β-estradiol result in the loss of glycosaminoglycans and collagen from fibrocartilaginous sites (ie, TMJ and pubic symphysis) but not from hyaline cartilaginous sites. Relaxin and β-estradiol induced the matrix metalloproteinase expression of collagenase-1 and stromelysin-1. It was also shown that progesterone prevented the loss of matrix molecules. This hormone-induced, targeted matrix degradation may be the key to the understanding of why TMJ DJD is most commonly seen in women during their reproductive years. There is likely interplay between mechanotransduction and hormonal transduction of matrix degradation proteinases during the onset and progression of DJD.

DJD: IMAGING OBSERVATIONS

Current imaging modalities have revealed several stages associated with DJD that progress along a continuum from normal, failure, repair, and stability.[18] It has been observed that soft tissue changes occur first, and this progresses to the involvement of hard tissues in a small percentage of individuals. It has been proposed that DJD progresses until the functional forces (work and

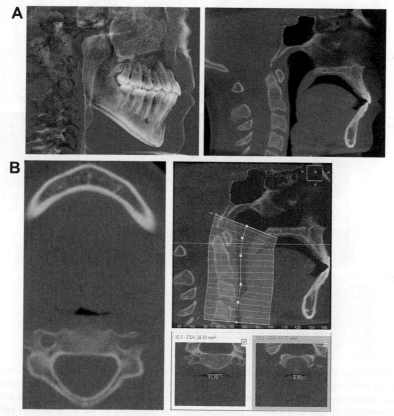

Fig. 7. Lingual tonsils; base of tongue encroachment. (*A, B*) The airway of a patient with large lingual tonsils. The airway at base of the tongue was calculated to be 13.77 mm².

power) are modulated by tissue changes to be within the adaptive capacity of targeted tissues.

AIRWAY

3D imaging is a very efficient method to inspect and identify diffuse narrowing (narrowing disturbed over a large distance) or focal narrowing (encroachments) of the airway. A reduction in airway radius increases the airway resistance as described by Poiseuille's law ($R = 8 nl/pr^4$) where R is resistance, n is viscosity, l is length, and r is radius. Airflow maintenance requires increased inspiration effort as the resistance to airflow increases as described by Ohm's law ($V = P_{mouth} - P_{alveoli}/R$) where V is flow, P is pressure, and R is resistance. The increased inspiration effort results in a greater differential pressure

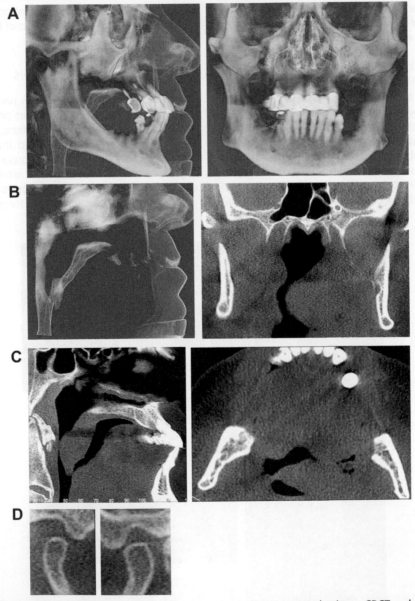

Fig. 8. (A–D) Tumor; upper airway encroachment. This individual was scanned using a CBCT and displayed using multiplanar sections and volume rendering. The condyles were in an acquired anteroinferior position within their fossa. A soft tissue mass was identified, extending from the left lateropharyngeal wall and extending into and enlarging the dimensions of the soft palate. This mass was determined to be a squamous cell carcinoma. The mass had reduced the airway dimensions, and the patient found it necessary to hold the jaw forward to maintain airway patency.

between the mouth and the alveoli. The airway, an elastic tube, is collapsible and is susceptible to the generation of a large pressure gradient between the lung alveoli and mouth. Mobility of the selected airway valves, such as the tongue, nares, soft palate, and epiglottis, may increase under the influence of increased respiratory pressure. Increased resistance in the airway requires a greater inspiratory pressure to maintain airflow predisposing to airway collapse.

Multivariate analysis shows both retroglossal ($P = .027$) and retropalatal spaces ($P = .0036$) to be predictive of respiratory disturbance index. Li and colleagues[29] have also demonstrated a relationship between the airway area and the likelihood of obstructive sleep apnea (OSA). There is a high probability of severe OSA if the airway area is less than 52 mm^2, an intermediate probability if the airway is between 52 to 110 mm^2, and a low probability if the airway is greater than 110 mm^2.[30–32] Lowe and colleagues[30] demonstrated that most constrictions occur in the oropharynx with a mean airway volume of 13.89 $\pm$ 5.33 cm^3. Barkdull and colleagues[33,34] demonstrated a correlation between the retro-lingual cross-sectional airway and OSA when this area was less than 4% of the cross-sectional area of the cervicomandibular ring. Encroachments that increase resistance can occur anywhere along the length of the airway and include rhinitis, deviate septum, polyps, tonsils, adenoids, and tumors (see **Fig. 4**; **Figs. 5–8**).

SUMMARY

Incorporation of 3D imaging into daily practice will allow practitioners to readily evaluate and screen patients for phenotypes associated with OSDB. This is particularly important in the adolescent population where many already seek orthodontic treatment for dentofacial deformities associated with OSDB.

The introduction and availability of CBCT has created the opportunity to serially examine individuals and acquire accurate 3D anatomic information. The "systems approach" of observing and testing the interactions and influence that adjacent regions have on each other will be a key to the understanding of the biomechanical influences on craniofacial form and the role they play in OSDB.

REFERENCES

1. Stratemann S, Huang J, Makik K, et al. Comparison of cone beam computed tomography imaging with physical measures. Dentomaxillofac Radiol 2008; 37(2):80–93.
2. Schendel SA, Hatcher D. CBCT semiautomated 3D airway analysis. J Oral Maxillofac Surg 2010. [Epub ahead of print].
3. Aboudara C, Nielsen I, Huang JC, et al. Comparison of airway space with conventional lateral head films and 3-dimensional reconstruction from cone-beam computed tomography. Am J Orthod Dentofacial Orthop 2009;135(4):468–79.
4. Aboudara CA, Hatcher D, Neilsen IL, et al. A three-dimensional evaluation of the upper airway in adolescents. Orthod Craniofac Res 2003;6(Suppl 1):173–5.
5. Woodside D, Linder-Aronson S, Ludstrom A, et al. Mandibular and maxillary growth after changed mode of breathing. Am J Orthod Dentofacial Orthop 1991;100:1–18.
6. Yamada T, Tanne K, Miyamoto K, et al. Influences of nasal respiratory obstruction on craniofacial growth in young *Macaca fuscata* monkey. Am J Orthod Dentofacial Orthop 1997;11:38–43.
7. Solow B, Siersback-Nielsen S, Greve E. Airway adequacy, head posture, and craniofacial morphology. Am J Orthod 1984;86:214–23.
8. Vargervik K, Miller A, Chierici G, et al. Morphologic response to changes in neuromuscular patterns experimentally induced by altered modes of respiration. Am J Orthod 1984;85:115–24.
9. Stratemann S. 3D craniofacial imaging: airway and craniofacial morphology [Unpublished MSc thesis], Department of Growth and Development. University of California San Francisco; 2005.
10. Legrell PE, Isberg A. Mandibular length and midline asymmetry after experimentally induced temporomandibular joint disk displacement in rabbits. Am J Orthod Dentofacial Orthop 1999; 115(3):247–53.
11. Legrell PE, Isberg A. Mandibular height asymmetry following experimentally induced temporomandibular joint disk displacement in rabbits. Oral Surg Oral Med Oral Pathol Oral Radiol Endod 1998; 86(3):280–3.
12. Stutzmann JJ, Patrovic AG. Role of the lateral pterygoid muscle and menisco temporomandibular frenum in spontaneous growth of the mandible and in growth stimulated by the postural hyperpropulsor. Am J Orthod Dentofac Orthop 1990;97:381–92.
13. Petrovic AG. Heritage paper. Auxologic categorization and chronobiologic specific for the choice of appropriate orthodontic treatment. Am J Orthod Dentofac Orthop 1994;105(2):192–205.
14. Nebbe B, Major PW. Prevalence of TMJ disc displacement in a pre-orthodontic adolescent sample. Angle Orthod 2000;70(6):454–63.
15. Flores-Mir C, Akbarimaned L, Nebbe B, et al. Longitudinal study on TMJ disk status and its effect on mandibular growth. J Orthod 2007;34(3):194–9.

16. Flores-Mir C, Nebbe B, Heo G, et al. Longitudinal study of temporomandibular joint disc status and craniofacial growth. Am J Orthod Dentofacial Orthop 2007;131(5):575–6.

17. Nebbe B, Major PW, Prassad N. Female adolescent facial pattern associated with TMJ disk displacement and reduction in disk length: part I. Am J Orthod Dentofacial Orthop 1999;116(2):168–76.

18. Hatcher DC, McEvoy SP, Mah RT, et al. Distribution of local and general stresses in the stomatognathic system. In: McNeill C, editor. Science and practice of occlusion. Chicago: Quintessence Publishing Co; 1997. p. 259–72.

19. Mah RT, McEvoy SP, Hatcher DC, et al. Engineering principles and modeling strategies. In: McNeill C, editor. Science and practice of occlusion. Chicago: Quintessence Publishing Co; 1997. p. 153–64.

20. Gallo LM, Chiaravolloti G, Iwaskai LR, et al. Mechanical work during stress field translation in the human TMJ. J Dent Res 2006;85(11):1006–10.

21. Nickel JC, Iwasaki LR, Beatty MW, et al. Static and dynamic loading effects on temporomandibular joint disc tractional forces. J Dent Res 2006;85(9):809–13.

22. Nickel JC, Iwaskai LR, Beatty MW, et al. Laboratory stresses and tractional forces on the TMJ disc surface. J Dent Res 2004;83(8):650–4.

23. Lammi M. Current perspective on cartilage and chondrocyte mechanobiology. Biorheology 2004; 41:593–6.

24. Turner CH. Biomechanical aspects of bone formation. In: Bronner F, Farach-Carson MC, editors. Bone formation. London: Springer Press; 2004. p. 79–105.

25. Carter DR, Beaupré GS, Wong M, et al. The mechanobiology of articular cartilage development and degeneration. Clin Orthop Relat Res 2004;(Suppl 427):S69–77.

26. Huang H, Kamm RD, Lee RT, et al. Cell mechanics and mechanotransduction: pathways, probes, and physiology. Am J Physiol Cell Physiol 2004;287: C1–C11.

27. Hashem G, Zhang Q, Hayami T, et al. Relaxin and beta-estradiol modulate targeted matrix degradation in specific synovial joint fibrocartilages: progesterone prevents matrix loss. Arthritis Res Ther 2006;8(4):R98.

28. Naqvi T, Duong T, Hashem G, et al. Relaxin's induction of metalloproteinases is associated with loss of collagen and glycosaminoglycans in synovial joint fibrocartilaginous explants. Arthritis Res Ther 2005; 7(1):R1–R11.

29. Li HY, Chen NH, Wang CR, et al. Use of 3-dimensional computed tomography scan to evaluate upper airway patency for patients undergoing sleep-disordered breathing surgery. Otolaryngol Head Neck Surg 2003;1294:336–42.

30. Lowe AA, Gionhaku N, Takeuchi K, et al. Three-dimensional CT reconstructions of tongue and airway in adult subjects with obstructive sleep apnea. Am J Orthod Dentofacial Orthop 1986; 90(5):364–74.

31. Avrahami E, Englender M. Relation between CT axial cross-sectional area of the oropharynx and obstructive sleep apnea syndrome in adults. AJNR Am J Neuroradiol 1995;16(1):135–40.

32. Ogawa T, Enciso R, Shintaku WH, et al. Evaluation of cross-section airway configuration of obstructive sleep apnea. Oral Surg Oral Med Oral Pathol Oral Radiol Endod 2007;103(1):102–8.

33. Chen NH, Li KK, Li SY, et al. Airway assessment by volumetric computed tomography in snorers and subjects with obstructive sleep apnea in a Far-East Asian population (Chinese). Laryngoscope 2002; 112(4):721–6.

34. Barkdull GC, Kohl CA, Patel M, et al. Computed tomography imaging of patients with obstructive sleep apnea. Laryngoscope 2008;118:1486–92.

Orthodontic Considerations Related to Sleep-Disordered Breathing

R. Scott Conley, DMD

KEYWORDS

- Orthodontics • Growth and development • Class I
- Class II • Class III • Obstructive sleep apnea

When the diagnosis of chronic obstructive sleep apnea (OSA) is made, the patient feels relief that he or she may finally be able to have a restful night of sleep. The diagnosis may have taken weeks, months, or years.[1] Following the overnight polysomnography (PSG) examination the seriousness of the condition is explained and a plan of treatment is initiated.[2,3] With so many disciplines involved in treatment, each area has its preferred method of treatment. Because the gold standard for OSA care is generally considered continuous positive air pressure (CPAP), the patient may be given a prescription for a machine and instructions on its use.[4] However, many other forms of treatment including orthodontics are possible.[5–9]

The orthodontist is rarely on the patient's mind when the diagnosis of chronic OSA is delivered. Some patients and physicians may remember orthodontics from when they had treatment to align their teeth as an adolescent. Others may reflect back on the time when their children needed treatment. However, the scope of orthodontic care is broader than the mere alignment of teeth. When orthodontists work with their medical colleagues several additional and successful forms of treatment are available to the patient with OSA. New evidence demonstrates that specific forms of orthodontic therapy at younger ages are successful in treating pediatric OSA. More research is needed, but even so the orthodontist can provide some treatment that may reduce the chances of the patient's developing OSA at a later age.

Several considerations must be explored in the patient with OSA based on each patient's age and stage of development. To explore the role played by each of these considerations, a brief review of cephalometrics and normal facial growth and development is essential. Because many adult patients with OSA display a similar skeletal pattern, aberrations in growth must also be discussed. An understanding of lateral cephalometric analysis provides objective measures to help distinguish normal from abnormal growth. These cephalometric surveys may encompass 1 or 2 specifically targeted measures or encompass full facial analysis in the sagittal dimension. Because patients are three-dimensional, posterior-anterior cephalometrics and now cone beam computed tomography (CBCT) play an increasingly important role. Because orthodontic treatment traditionally focuses on the teeth and their position, careful model analysis must also be considered. Most orthodontists are accustomed to working with an oral and maxillofacial surgeon to prepare patients for orthognathic surgery. Modifications of this surgical treatment have been demonstrated to be

Department of Orthodontics and Pediatric Dentistry, University of Michigan School of Dentistry, 1011 North University Avenue, Ann Arbor, MI 48109-1078, USA
E-mail address: rsconley@umich.edu

Sleep Med Clin 5 (2010) 71–89
doi:10.1016/j.jsmc.2009.10.005

1 of the most successful forms of OSA treatment. Indications for jaw surgery, the range of surgical options, and specific types of jaw surgery to avoid are discussed later. Pediatric patients are still growing so additional treatment options aimed at modifying the remaining growth can be considered. At least 1 form of treatment that is routinely performed with adolescent patients has been shown to be particularly beneficial in the treatment of OSA.

CLINICAL EXAMINATION AND STUDY MODEL EVALUATION

Before performing any clinical examination the medical history should be reviewed. Although most patients reporting to the orthodontic office are typically healthy and free of significant medical complications, pediatric and adult patients with sleep apnea have complex medical histories. For the pediatric population the orthodontist should follow up on attention deficit disorder/attention deficit and hyperactivity disorder, cor pulmonale, failure to thrive, and mouth breathing.[10] The medical history evaluation should also ask questions regarding snoring, nocturnal gasping, and bed-wetting. Each is a common sign of OSA in the pediatric population. In adults the orthodontist can insert the Epworth Sleepiness Scale form into the medical history survey.[11] Additional health questions should include past motor vehicle accidents and workplace accidents, as these can be related to sleep-disordered breathing.[12,13]

In the pediatric patient the orthodontist should examine the oropharynx because the primary cause of OSA is tonsilar and adenoid hypertrophy. The lingual and pharyngeal tonsils are visible intraorally although the adenoids are not. Tonsilar size ranges from type I, in which the tonsils are barely visible in the pharyngeal pillars, to type IV, in which the right and left tonsilar tissues almost approximate each other in the midline (referred to as "kissing tonsils").[14] When hypertrophic tonsils are observed clinically, radiographic evaluation should also be conducted. The pharyngeal tonsils and lingual tonsils will be seen in the lateral cephalometric radiograph in the region of the mandibular angle near the dorsum of the tongue. The hypertrophic adenoids, which were not visible intraorally, appear as a moderately radiopaque mass above the soft palate. Tonsilar and adenoid tissue normally shrinks in volume after the age of 6 years.[15] This shrinkage may result in spontaneous improvement of mild OSA. However, the hypertrophic tonsilar and adenoid tissue may be so large that the normal tissue reduction either does not occur or is not sufficient to improve the patient's obstruction. If this finding is noticed early by the orthodontist a referral should be made to the otolaryngologist for possible removal as early removal can reduce the tendency for patients to develop the adverse effects of mouth breathing. The classic long-term effects of mouth breathing ("adenoid facies") are patients with long faces, open bites, and narrow maxillary and mandibular dental arches.[16]

When the orthodontist evaluates late adolescent and adult dentition, the patient should ideally have a class I (normal) dental relationship, in which the mesiobuccal cusp of the upper first molar rests in the buccal groove of the lower first molar. In addition, the upper canine should be centered between the lower canine and the first premolar. In a class II relationship the upper first molar is forward of the buccal groove and the upper canine is forward of the lower canine. For a class III the upper first molar is behind the lower buccal groove and the upper canine is behind the lower canine (**Fig. 1**A–C).

The pediatric patient may present in the primary dentition (all baby teeth present) or the mixed dentition (a combination of baby teeth and adult teeth). In both the normal bite relationship is termed a "flush terminal plane." When viewed from the side the most posterior surface of the upper molar is in line with the most posterior surface of the lower molar. When the last primary teeth are lost and the child develops to adult dentition, ideally the lower molar shifts forward into a class I relationship. Not every patient with a flush terminal plane experiences this shift. Approximately 65% of flush terminal plane patients develop into a normal class I relationship, whereas the other 35% develop into a mild class II relationship.[17] Typically this amount of class II is mild and does not result from an underlying jaw discrepancy. Full cusp class II and the full cusp class III relationships are more significant concerns. Neither is ideal, and both often result from a malpositioned maxilla, mandible, or both.

Early recognition of adverse bite relationships should cause the orthodontist to examine closely the facial attributes of the child. Significant skeletal jaw imbalances, when present, should be recognized early as it is advantageous to attempt growth modification while growth is still present. If left untreated, skeletal imbalances will at best remain the same, but can become worse. If left untreated until the patient is skeletally mature, the only remaining way to correct the jaw discrepancy is jaw surgery. Orthodontic camouflage, in which teeth are extracted to mask the skeletal discrepancy, may provide the patient with a functional bite, but may not produce an ideal skeletal

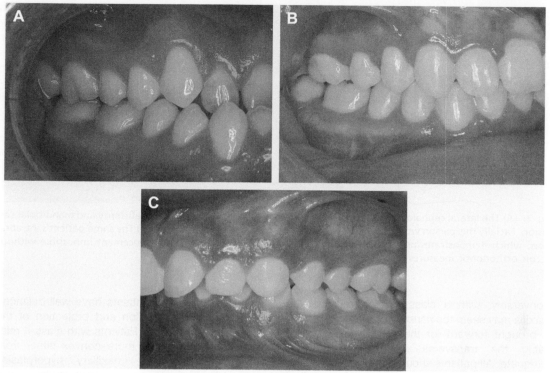

Fig. 1. Lateral intraoral occlusal views. (*A*) A class III relationship, in which the lower first molar is mesial or forward of the ideal position. (*B*) The "normal" or ideal occlusion, in which the mesiobuccal cusp of the upper first molar sits in the buccal groove of the lower first molar. (*C*) A class II relationship, in which the lower first molar is distal or behind the ideal position.

relationship. This combined dental and skeletal assessment is important because some patients will have a normal bite relationship (dental occlusion) yet have unfavorable skeletal classification (**Fig. 2**). These imbalances present a unique challenge when discussing treatment options for these patients. Assessment of the skeletal relationship begins during the clinical examination but for quantification, lateral cephalometric analysis must be performed.

When the dentition is being evaluated attention should also be directed toward the transverse or crossarch dimension. Many patients with OSA, particularly pediatric patients, demonstrate a maxillary transverse deficiency (crossbite) in which the upper teeth are too narrow to occlude properly with the mandibular teeth.[18] This deficiency can present as a single tooth crossbite, a unilateral crossbite in which the right or left side is too narrow, or a bilateral crossbite in which both sides are too narrow. With the unilateral crossbite, one must determine whether this is a true unilateral crossbite (no shift) or whether the patient has a bilateral crossbite with a lateral shift of the occlusal relationship. In pediatric

patients, what seems to be a unilateral crossbite is commonly a bilateral crossbite with a shift. In adults, the shift has often been present so long the patient no longer shifts perceptibly. To distinguish the difference one must observe the patient opening and closing. In a bilateral crossbite with a shift the patient starts in complete crossbite on 1 side with the lower dental midline deviated to that side. During opening the lower dental midline shifts back into alignment with the maxillary midline. During closing one often observes the patient hit prematurely on 1 side that deflects the jaw. A true unilateral crossbite is rare and when present the patient bites in crossbite with the midlines off and opens without any noticeable shift. At the fully open position the midlines are off the same amount as when biting down.

The presence of a crossbite can be positively or negatively affected by the sagittal bite relationship. Class II patients (maxillary molar and canine positioned more forward than the mandibular molar and canine) may seem to have appropriate transverse dimension. However, when the mandible is positioned more anteriorly to simulate growth or surgical correction a crossbite can be observed.

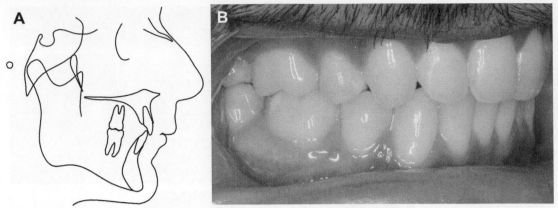

Fig. 2. (*A*) The lateral cephalometric tracing depicts an individual with mandibular deficiency and mandibular retrusion. Facially this person would benefit from mandibular advancement surgery. (*B*) The same patient's intraoral view, which demonstrates near ideal occlusion, making surgical mandibular advancement impossible without heroic orthodontic measures.

Conversely, with a class III malocclusion, the maxilla may seem too narrow but when the maxilla is brought forward (or the mandible is brought back) the transverse relationship may be adequate. All patients should be examined in their initial bite position and in the anticipated final sagittal bite position.

CEPHALOMETRIC EVALUATION

Cephalometric radiographic analysis enables skeletal and dental assessment by comparing the patient to a set of normative values. Lateral cephalometric analysis provides information only on 2 dimensions: vertical and sagittal. The third dimension (transverse) is unanalyzed unless the practitioner uses a posterior anterior cephalometric radiograph (PA film). The primary cephalometric analysis used in this article is the cephalometrics for orthognathic surgery (COGS).[19] A sample lateral cephalometric tracing that includes the common lateral cephalometric landmarks is shown as **Fig. 3**. **Table 1** lists the lateral cephalometric landmark with its anatomic definition. **Table 2** lists the male and female adult normative values used in the COGS analysis. The COGS analysis is broken down into 5 main categories.

1) Cranial base measures
2) Horizontal maxillary and mandibular skeletal measures
3) Vertical maxillary and mandibular skeletal and dental measures
4) Intramaxillary and intramandibular measures
5) Dental measures.

When a patient's measures are compared with the COGS standards, the patient is assigned the appropriate skeletal diagnosis. Class I (normal)

skeletal relationship patients have well-balanced faces with good position and projection of the maxilla and mandible. Patients with class II relationships are typically more convex either from maxillary overgrowth (maxillary hyperplasia), a mandibular undergrowth (mandibular hypoplasia), or a combination of the two. The class III skeletal patient demonstrates the exact opposite problem; maxillary hypoplasia, mandibular hyperplasia, or a combination of the two (**Fig. 4**A–C)

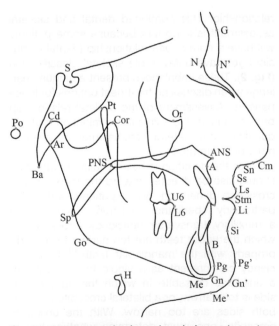

Fig. 3. A representative lateral cephalometric tracing. The individual landmarks are marked with red dots. For a complete anatomic description of the landmarks, see **Table 1**.

demonstrates the lateral cephalometric tracings representative of the 3 different skeletal classifications.

Mild skeletal deviations from ideal generally do not constitute an increased risk of OSA. However, significant jaw abnormalities, particularly mandibular micrognathia, have been linked to OSA, especially within the pediatric population.[20] When performing the cephalometric analysis, class II patients beyond 1 standard deviation (SD) smaller than the ideal measurement may be considered mandibular deficient (also referred to as retrognathic or hypoplastic). At 2 SDs or beyond they are classified as severely mandibular deficient or micrognathic. To put this into proper context, the normal adult mandibular position (N–B) is −5.3 mm. A measure of −12.0 mm results in a patient who displays significant mandibular hypoplasia. A measure of −18 mm would be an extreme situation. One can imagine from examining the cephalometric tracing in **Fig. 5** how this mandibular deficiency can result in a functional airway deficit. In some cases this marked mandibular deficiency may be caused by a craniofacial anomaly such as Pierre Robin syndrome or Marfan syndrome.[21] Pierre Robin syndrome is characterized by a cleft palate, glossoptosis, and severe mandibular deficiency. Patients with Marfan syndrome present with long faces, downward and backward rotated mandibles, and narrow dental arches.

Many investigators have reported several cephalometric indicators that can be used to indicate the potential for OSA. Although cephalometric analysis alone is insufficient to diagnose OSA, it can suggest the need for additional testing. One cephalometric measure is the linear distance from the mandibular plane to the hyoid bone (MP–H). A distance greater than 15.4 mm indicates a person at risk for OSA.[22,23] Increased values indicate a collection of soft tissue, frequently adipose tissue, in the submental area (submental lipomatosis). Generally the adipose tissue is not confined to the submental area but may also be present around the airway. This collection of tissue creates pressure, making airway collapse more likely.

Another reported cephalometric measure that indicates a greater risk of OSA is an increased mandibular plane angle. This measure is frequently associated with a steep occlusal plane, overerupted posterior dentition, a large gonial angle, and anterior open bite. This collection of features is historically referred to as "adenoid facies" and more recently as vertical maxillary excess.[24] In addition to the skeletal markers that potentially indicate a greater risk of OSA, some soft tissue measures, especially those associated with soft palate dimensions, are reported. A longer soft palate[22,23] and a wider soft palate can combine to reduce the posterior air space (PAS).[25–27] The combination of these factors is represented in a figure by Cistulli that uses side-by-side figures to demonstrate a patient with a normal airway and a second patient with a reduced airway (**Fig. 6**).[27]

As clinicians have become more aware of OSA, attempts have been made to assess the facial and skeletal characteristics comprehensively. Many articles report that maxillary deficiency alone, mandibular deficiency alone, or combined maxillomandibular deficiency can predispose a patient to OSA.[28] No clear, accurate, and comprehensive examinations have been performed. Although maxillary and mandibular deficiency can contribute to the disease process, investigators focus on mandibular deficiency. A series of cephalometric evaluations of patients with OSA concluded that mandibular deficiency was present in 16% to 60% of their study group populations.[22,28–31] This conclusion means that 40% to 84% of the study population consisted of patients without mandibular deficiency, confirming that the facial profile or cephalometrics cannot be relied on solely to diagnose OSA.

Another risk factor for OSA is obesity.[32] In several cephalometric studies obese patients with OSA have been shown to exhibit only minimal skeletal differences from patients who do not have OSA.[25,33,34] As a result, the predisposing factor in the development of OSA is considered to be the increased parapharyngeal adipose tissue stemming from obesity rather than an underlying skeletal discrepancy. The most severely affected patients, however, tend to demonstrate obesity and an underlying skeletal discrepancy. In these individuals it seems as if the obesity and the resulting adipose tissue around the airway work synergistically with the mandibular or maxillary deficiency to create a more severe presentation of the disease. These trends of mandibular deficiency and obesity seem to be maintained across different cultures, as shown in reports from China, Japan, and other countries.[33,34]

GROWTH AND DEVELOPMENT

Much of what is known about facial growth and development has come from cephalometric analysis of annual radiographs. Brush and Bolton (1926)[35] developed the first longitudinal growth study at Case Western Reserve with several other well-known studies following theirs. Longitudinal

Table 1
COGS landmarks

Skeletal (bony) landmarks	
S	Sella; the geometric center of the sella turcica
N	Nasion; the intersection of the nasal bones and the frontal bone in the midsagittal plane
ANS	Anterior nasal spine; the most anterior point of the bony maxilla
PNS	Posterior nasal spine; the most posterior point of the bony maxilla
A	"A" point; the deepest point on the anterior surface of the bony maxilla between ANS and the upper incisor
U1	Upper incisor; the most inferior point on the upper central incisor
U6	Upper first molar; the most mesial portion of the upper first molar
L1	Lower incisor; the most superior point of the lower central incisor
L6	Lower first molar; the most mesial portion of the lower first molar
B	"B" point; the deepest portion on the anterior contour of the mandible between the lower incisor and pogonion
Pg	Pogonion; the most prominent point on the anterior surface of the mandible
Gn	Gnathion; a constructed point midway between pogonion and menton
Me	Menton; the most inferior point on the bony chin
Go	Gonion; the most posterior-inferior point on the gonial angle of the mandible
Ar	Articulare; the radiographic superimposition of the ascending ramus and the cranial base
Cd	Condylion; the most posterior-superior point on the mandibular condyle
Cor	Coronoid process; the most superior point on the coronoid process
Ptm	Most posterior-superior point of the pterygomaxillary fissure
Po	Porion; the midpoint of the superior aspect of the external auditory meatus
HP	Horizontal plane
MP	Mandibular plane
NF	Nasal floor
OP	Occlusal plane

Soft tissue landmarks	
G	Glabella; the most anterior point of the forehead above the nose
N'	Soft tissue nasion
Cm	Columella
Sn	Subnasale; the junction of the inferior aspect of the nose and superior component of the upper lip
Ss	Superior sulcus; the deepest point on the curvature of the upper lip
Ls	Labrale superius; the most prominent point of the upper lip
Stm	Stomion; the intersection of the upper and lower lips (when the lips do not contact, stomion is the midpoint between the upper and lower lip)
Li	Labrale inferius; the most prominent point of the lower lip
Si	Sulcus inferius; the deepest point on the curvature of the lower lip. Also known as soft tissue "B" point or the mentolabial fold
Pg'	Soft tissue pogonion; the most prominent point on the anterior contour of the soft tissue chin
Gn'	Soft tissue gnathion; a constructed point midway between soft tissue pogonion and soft tissue menton
Me'	Soft tissue menton; the most inferior point of the soft tissue chin

growth analysis reveals that children are not "little adults." The shape of an infant face is generally round. As one reaches skeletal maturity the face is generally much longer and narrower than an infant's face. Growth changes the size and shape. Several theories of growth and development have been espoused, each identifying and focusing on 1 aspect of facial growth. The most complete picture, however, likely involves components from each theory of growth.[36–39]

Growth takes place in all 3 dimensions simultaneously. However, growth peaks, slows, and ultimately ceases at different times in ,the different planes of space and the different regions of the skull (**Fig. 7**). For example, 1 of the most remarkable and rapid changes in size and shape of the head occurs in the cranial vault between birth and the age of 2 years. During this time, the cranial vault has established nearly 90% of is growth.[40] Following the age of 2 years significantly less growth occurs in the vault and most growth occurs in the cranial base and the face. Within the face maxillary growth generally occurs earlier, proceeds faster, and stops sooner than mandibular growth. This earlier maxillary growth results in the normal convex appearance of the face during prepubertal years. As the child approaches the pubertal years, maxillary growth slows and mandibular growth begins to accelerate, enabling the transition from a convex face to the straighter, more adult face. Another generally accepted growth trend is that transverse facial growth (facial width) ceases first, followed by anteroposterior (sagittal) growth, with vertical growth ceasing last. The sequential cessation of growth is 1 reason different treatment strategies are used at different times during sleep apnea treatment in pediatrics.

Every individual demonstrates a unique growth pattern, making his or her facial characteristics unique. Variations in growth patterns lead to convex, concave, and straight facial appearances. As stated earlier, patients with OSA tend to have greater facial convexity, resulting from an underlying mandibular deficiency. Other patients with OSA may present with concave facial and skeletal characteristics from midface deficiency, which can also lead to airway insufficiency. When an adverse growth pattern is recognized while growth is still occurring, treatment should attempt to correct the unfavorable growth pattern. Of particular importance is minimizing the effects of mouth breathing. Left untreated many mouth breathers develop a long face, a narrow maxilla and mandible, anterior open bite, and mandibular deficiency. If mouth breathing is caught early and treated

Table 2
COGS normativx2e values (see Table 1 for abbreviations)

			Date		
			COGS Standards		
Patient	Male	Standard Deviation	Female	Standard Deviation	Patient
Cranial base					
Ar-Ptm (//HP)	37.1	2.8	32.8	1.9	
Ptm-N (//HP)	52.8	4.1	50.9	3.0	
Horizontal (skeletal)					
N-A-Pg angle	3.9	6.4	2.6	5.1	
N-A (//HP)	0.0	3.7	−2.0	3.7	
N-B (//HP)	−5.3	6.7	−6.9	4.3	
N-Pg (//HP)	−4.3	8.5	−6.5	5.1	
Vertical (skeletal, dental)					
N-ANS (I HP)	54.7	3.2	50.0	2.4	
ANS-Gn (I HP)	68.6	3.8	61.3	3.3	
PNS-N (I HP)	53.9	1.7	50.6	2.2	
MP-HP (angle)	23.0	5.9	24.2	5.0	
1-NF (I NF)	30.5	2.1	27.5	1.7	
1-MP (I MP)	45.0	2.1	40.8	1.8	
6-NF (I NF)	26.2	2.0	23.0	1.3	
6-MP (I MP)	35.8	2.6	32.1	1.9	
Maxilla, Mandible					
PNS-ANS (//HP)	57.7	2.0	52.6	3.5	
Ar-Go (linear)	52.0	4.2	46.8	2.5	

	Mean	Standard Deviation	Patient	
Go-Pg (linear)	83.7	4.6	74.2	5.8
B-Pg (//MP)	8.9	1.7	7.2	1.9
Ar-Go-Gn (angle)	119.1	6.5	122.0	6.9
Dental				
OP upper-HP (angle)	6.2	5.1	7.1	2.5
1-NF (angle)	111.0	4.7	112.5	5.3
1-MP (angle)	95.0	5.2	95.9	5.7
A-B (//OP)	−1.1	2.0	−0.4	2.5

Soft tissue analysis: adult standards

Facial form	Mean	Standard Deviation	Patient
Facial convexity angle G-Sn-Pg'	12	4	
Maxillary projection G-Sn	6	3	
Mandibular projection G-Pg'	0	4	
Vertical height ratio G-Sn/Sn-Me	1		
Lower face throat angle (Sn-Gn'-C)	100	7	
Lower vertical height/depth ratio (Sn-Gn'/C-Gn')	1.2		
Lip position and form			
Nasolabial angle Cm-Sn-Ls	102	8	
Upper lip protrusion Ls to (Sn-Pg')	3	1	
Lower lip protrusion Li to (Sn-Pg')	2	1	
Mentolabial sulcus Si to (Li-Pg')	4	2	
Vertical lip/chin ratio Sn-Stm/Stm-Me' (HP)	0.5		
Maxillary incisor exposure Stm-1	2	2	
Interlabial gap Stms-Stmi	2	2	

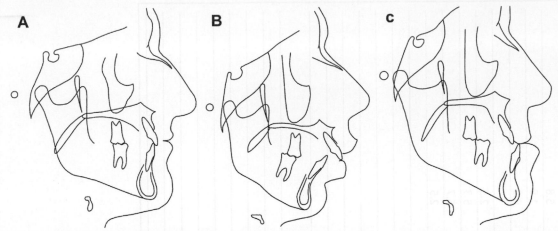

Fig. 4. Lateral cephalometric views of 3 distinct skeletal malocclusion. (*A*) A patient with nearly ideal skeletal and dental balance. (*B*) A patient with a class II skeletal malocclusion. Note the significant mandibular deficiency, the everted lower lip, and the significant horizontal distance between the upper and lower incisors. (*C*) The opposite, a skeletal class III patient with mandibular hyperplasia and maxillary hypoplasia. Note the reverse overlap of the incisors; the upper incisor is behind the lower incisor.

appropriately, it might be possible to prevent or minimize these adverse growth effects. In adults in whom growth has ceased, surgery is the only way to alter these craniofacial characteristics permanently.

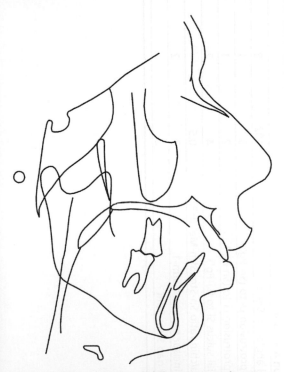

Fig. 5. In this mandibular-deficient patient, the airway is also drawn. Note the significant narrowing of the airway extending from the tip of the soft palate inferiorly toward the epiglottis. This airway can become narrower in the supine position during sleep.

TREATMENT MODALITIES

Proper treatment of the patient with OSA must use a team-based approach. Although the team composition differs based on the situation or the institution, the patient's best interests should be of the highest priority. By combining different medical and dental specialists into a team each practitioner is free to focus on his or her area of expertise. Following patient examination by each discipline the seemingly disparate pieces of information are reviewed and the best treatment strategy is developed. When every team member participates on an equal footing each patient receives the best possible care because the best care often results from combining several forms of treatment.

No matter what treatment or combinations of treatment are selected it is essential to assess the patient's progress. Failure to evaluate care with a follow-up PSG can lead to incomplete correction of the disease and keep the patient at an increased risk of myocardial infarction, stroke, cardiac arrhythmia, and even death. If 1 treatment method fails, the patient must be reassessed and new treatment or treatment combinations employed.

PEDIATRIC ORTHODONTIC TREATMENT APPROACHES

CPAP is 1 of the most successful forms of treatment. However, in the pediatric and adolescent population anecdotal discussion has emerged about growth disturbances as a result of long-term use of CPAP. From a biomechanical

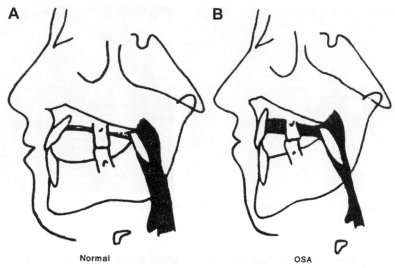

Fig. 6. (*A*) A "normal" airway with normal skeletal positioning of both jaws. (*B*) A patient with a longer face height, mildly deficient jaw position, and narrower airway. (*From* Cistulli PA. Craniofacial abnormalities in OSA: implications for treatment. Respirology 1996;3:167; with permission.)

standpoint there is some validity to these concerns. The elastic straps that hold the CPAP mask in place apply an inhibitory force on normal maxillary and mandibular forward growth. This

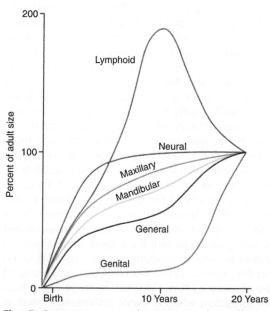

Fig. 7. Scammon curves demonstrate the different rates of growth of the different tissues in the body. Note the excessive lymphoid tissue overgrowth that shrinks as continued development occurs. The maxilla grows more along the neural growth curve and the mandible follows the general growth curve. (*From* Proffit WR. Later stages of development. In: Proffit WR, Fields HW Jr, Sarver DM. Contemporary orthodontics. 4th edition. St Louis (MO): Elsevier; 2007. p. 108; with permission.)

force is similar to the restrictive effect that orthodontic headgear has on maxillary growth in class II children. However, when orthodontic headgear is employed it is selected to restrain exuberant maxillary growth. The goal of CPAP, however, is to maintain airway patency; growth restraint is not desired. A potential worst-case scenario occurs when a maxillary-deficient (class III) adolescent patient with OSA is prescribed CPAP, which could adversely affect the already deficient maxillary skeletal development. In an attempt to minimize potential growth disturbances from CPAP, some clinicians are providing maxillary protraction headgear during waking hours to combat the pressure placed on the maxilla from the mask with nightly CPAP.

It is unclear whether the anecdotal reports of midface deficiency result from CPAP use or whether an underlying skeletal anomaly was present before prescribing CPAP. To answer this question, a prospective randomized clinical cephalometric study needs to be performed to determine whether CPAP has an adverse effect on the developing face. If a negative effect is observed the next question will be to determine which is more harmful: creating a facial growth disturbance or the adverse effects of not treating the OSA.

A recent publication reports on the positive effects of rapid maxillary expansion in children diagnosed with OSA (**Fig. 8**).[41] The paper has a small sample size and the respiratory disturbance index (RDI) is low but some clinical implications can be inferred. If basal bone can be expanded in the maxilla, additional space may be made in the oropharyngeal airway. If the

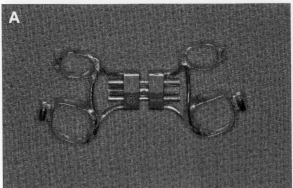
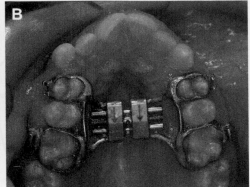

Fig. 8. (*A*) A rapid maxillary expansion appliance. (*B*) The same appliance after cementation to the maxillary first molars and first premolars bilaterally.

oropharyngeal airway is increased, airflow should increase and airway resistance should decrease. If airflow is improved, fewer obstructive episodes should occur, potentially resolving the OSA, increasing daytime alertness, and decreasing long-term morbidity. These results are supported by previous orthodontic research in which rapid maxillary expansion was reported to result in correcting bed-wetting.[42] At that time, OSA was largely unknown and undiagnosed and the connection to bed-wetting and rapid maxillary expansion was unclear. However, because bed-wetting is 1 of the clinical manifestations of OSA clinicians can now infer that the improvement in bed-wetting resulted from correcting the OSA.

The precise mechanisms for decreasing obstructive events via rapid maxillary expansion are not fully understood. The improvement may stem from treating multiple causes and multiple sites. As the maxilla expands the palate and floor of the nasal cavity also expand, which theoretically increases the volume of the nasal cavity. This increase has now been supported by clinical research that performed a three-dimensional CBCT radiographic assessment.[43] However, PSG was not performed. Another possible cause is a change in tongue position resulting from the direct expansion of the maxillary dentition. This larger upper arch may allow the tongue greater space and allow for more forward positioning of the tongue. The effect of widening the maxillary basal bone on the velum of the palate, superior pharyngeal constrictors, and the surrounding orofacial musculature cannot be overemphasized. Increased muscle tone is impossible to assess radiographically or clinically but could be performed with EMG. To date, these studies have not been conducted. Although each component (increased nasal floor, increased upper arch size, and increased muscle tone) may contribute only

a small amount to the correction, the combination seems to be clinically significant and beneficial to the patients in studies reported to date.

In patients without a crossbite rapid palatal expansion may not be indicated. However, the importance of upper and lower arch development should not be underestimated. Although OSA should not automatically place a patient into a nonextraction arch development form of treatment, extraction therapy should not be construed as always having a negative effect on sleep architecture. Sound clinical judgment that draws on biomechanics, diagnosis, and treatment planning along with biology of tooth movement must be combined with the patient's desires, esthetics, and sleep health to make the decision to extract or not to extract. Careful and complete analysis of tooth mass/arch length (crowding) must also be performed to determine how much (if any) arch development is necessary. The treatment goal must include a stable functional occlusion with the teeth positioned within the alveolus. When a stable nonextraction result can be achieved in adolescent patients for whom the decision to extract or not to extract is borderline, arch development treatment may be preferred. Such a development would give the patient the largest arch dimension possible. Arch development methods that focus on the skeleton rather than the teeth alone should be considered first. However, teeth can and must be extracted when a stable orthodontic result is not determined to be possible.

For patients with an underlying skeletal discrepancy the final jaw position must be determined. An individual's growth pattern used to be considered immutable, but reevaluation of growth mechanisms and the resulting successful growth modification therapies (orthodontic headgear, functional appliances) have changed orthodontic beliefs and treatment plans.

A direct cause-and-effect relationship cannot be drawn between patients' orthodontic treatment and subsequent development of OSA as adults. However, it is well documented that mandibular anterior repositioning appliances can be effective in the adult population for patients with mild to moderate OSA. Although no studies have been made one should consider treating the growing adolescent patient with class II OSA with a mandibular anterior repositioning appliance. This type of treatment is an effective adult OSA therapy and is already commonly prescribed for adolescent class II treatment to address mild mandibular deficiency. Such therapy may also positively treat the OSA. It is impossible to state definitively whether this functional appliance treatment during the adolescent time period prevents future development of OSA as an adult even if it successfully resolves the OSA during adolescence, because OSA is multifactorial. Several other contributing factors, especially weight gain, can affect the chances of developing OSA. One advantage of mandibular anterior repositioning treatment performed during adolescence is that it preserves arch dimensions rather than reducing them with extraction.

Initially the class III malocclusion was considered a result of mandibular overgrowth, but it is now believed that a class III malocclusion results more from deficient maxillary growth. There may be a component of mandibular overgrowth in some cases.[44] Each patient must be diagnosed individually. If airway concerns are present, it is advisable to encourage maxillary growth rather than move the mandible back.

In adult patients studies have been conducted in class III patients examining the short-term airway changes following mandibular setback surgery.[45,46] Each of these has demonstrated a decrease in airway. Most patients accommodated these changes well, but they were typically not patients at high risk of developing OSA. One study reported a sample size of only 10 patients, all of whom were young women of normal weight.

In severe skeletal class II or class III adolescent patients jaw surgery must be considered. Before initiating the surgical orthodontic care a diagnostic sleep study should be performed. Although this might add a cost to the patient's treatment, if OSA is diagnosed, significant changes to the surgical treatment plan may result and the cost and surgical morbidity are less than those of a second stage of jaw surgery later. When severe skeletal discrepancies are observed surgical orthodontic treatment can be performed in preadolescent or adolescent patients. In preadolescent patients, a technique termed distraction osteogenesis using a rigid external distractor can be considered for class III patients. For class II patients distraction osteogenesis can be performed with either an internal or an external distractor to enhance the mandibular size and position.

ADULT ORTHODONTIC TREATMENT APPROACHES
Oral Appliances

For the adult patient with mild to moderate OSA several oral appliances are available. The orthodontist is not the only dental practitioner able to provide this type of care; general dentists, prosthodontists, and orthodontists may provide similar appliances. Before selecting a particular oral appliance, however; the patient must undergo PSG to determine the type, severity, and location of the obstruction. If the site is the upper airway (nasal cavity or retropalatal area) efficacy of mandibular protrusion appliances and tongue-retaining devices may be limited. In patients with hypertrophic tonsils and adenoids and a tongue obstruction the efficacy of the oral appliance may be improved by tonsillectomy and adenoidectomy. Before fabricating the appliance it is essential to obtain pretreatment records, including a panoramic radiograph, lateral cephalometric radiograph, photographs (extraoral and intraoral), and study models. These records will serve as baseline records and for future patient assessment.

Tongue-positioning Appliances

In the supine position all gravity-dependent tissues, including the tongue, tend to collapse posteriorly. The tongue base normally is held anteriorly by the genial tubercles (the site of attachment of the genioglossus and geniohyoid muscles). If this support is insufficient, a tongue-retaining device may be considered.

Mandibular Anterior Repositioning Appliances

A second class of removable appliances is available to protrude the mandible and assist in maintaining this forward position during sleep (see article on Oral Appliances). Because all anterior repositioning appliances function in a like manner the patient and clinician can choose the most appropriate and comfortable appliance based on cost, convenience, durability, adjustability, and patient comfort. Including the patient in this decision can enhance compliance.

Potential complicating factors include changes in the bite with long-term use.[47,48] Some research reports minimal dental movement whereas other research demonstrates dental and unexpected skeletal changes in the mandible. In patients with a class II malocclusion before treatment the dental and skeletal changes are positive, and some patients even obtain a class I dental relationship. Class I patients may become mildly class III. Because the primary function of the appliance is to resolve the sleep apnea, occlusal changes may be left untreated. It is unclear whether these occlusal changes persist if appliance use is discontinued.

To measure the effect of the appliance objectively and screen for bite changes, follow-up lateral cephalometric radiography and PSG should be performed. These examinations may evolve into using three-dimensional imaging with CBCT, which can demonstrate airway changes with greater detail and accuracy. A recent report demonstrates an increase in the transverse dimension of the airway.[49] Although these images clearly demonstrate measurable airway changes the radiographic airway dimensional change may not reflect a positive PSG change. If incomplete resolution is observed the appliance must be retitrated. If complete resolution is still not observed alternative forms of treatment may need to be considered. In other cases the PSG may demonstrate complete resolution, requiring continued observation but no additional treatment.

SURGICAL ORTHODONTIC APPROACH

For the newly diagnosed adult with moderate to severe OSA, the noncompliant patient receiving CPAP, the patient who has received incomplete treatment with an oral appliance, and the patient with refractory OSA several surgical orthodontic treatment options are available. The surgical treatment plan must be based on a comprehensive assessment of the patient's dental occlusion or malocclusion and the underlying skeletal and facial characteristics.

ISOLATED GENIOPLASTY

A first-tier surgical therapy for OSA is an advancement genioplasty.[50] The best candidates have a functional occlusion, good maxillomandibular skeletal positioning, and deficient chin projection (called retrogenia or microgenia). Retrogenia must be differentiated from retrognathia. In retrognathia the mandible is small and in a poor sagittal position, but the bony chin button may be adequate. The term retrogenia describes a small bony chin button.

The small chin button can be found in a normal-size, deficient, or excessive mandible.

In some patients a standard inferior border genioplasty osteotomy is performed. Other osteotomy designs include advancing a full-thickness core of the mandibular symphysis that contains the genial tubercles. Once the lingual cortex of the block of bone is advanced beyond the buccal cortex of the mandibular body the block is rotated 90° to maintain the advanced position.

Whatever the osteotomy design, the genial tubercles must be present in the advanced segment to increase the resting muscle length of the genioglossus and geniohyoid muscles. This increased length induces increased muscle activity and increased tension, resulting in decreased tongue obstruction. Even with well-designed and appropriate genioplasties most patients experience only partial resolution of the symptoms. Therefore, a second surgical phase of treatment (or a more aggressive first stage of treatment) that advances the mandible alone or the maxilla and the mandible must be performed.

MANDIBULAR ADVANCEMENT

In 1980 Bear and Priest[51] first reported on surgical mandibular advancement, which had limited success for 2 reasons. Without presurgical orthodontics the width of the maxilla is typically too narrow to accommodate the advanced mandible, forcing the surgeon to advance the mandible into a posterior crossbite. The new crossbite can result in lateral shifts (either to the right or the left), leading to instability of the surgical result and adversely affecting temporomandibular joint health. The second problem is the mandible may not be able to be advanced far enough to resolve the OSA.

MAXILLOMANDIBULAR ADVANCEMENT

Jaw surgery to advance the maxilla and the mandible has become the gold standard in surgical orthodontic care for OSA.[52] This gives the surgeon the ability to maintain a functional occlusion in class I patients or enhance the functional occlusion in class II and class III patients while simultaneously improving the profile. Because most patients with OSA wish to pursue maxillomandibular advancement (MMA) quickly for resolution of their symptoms they may not wish to pursue the necessary presurgical orthodontic treatment. As a result 1 of the published risks associated with MMA is postoperative malocclusion. To prevent this a preferred approach uses CPAP short term during the presurgical orthodontic phase. Orthodontics produces complementary dental arches for the surgeon who performs MMA to resolve OSA. Following surgery CPAP is often no longer required.

PRESURGICAL ORTHODONTIC PREPARATION

Presurgical orthodontic therapy for MMA must focus on all 3 planes of space just as with any other surgical orthodontic patient. The orthodontist must plan the ideal transverse, sagittal, and vertical position of the teeth within the respective jaws. This enables the surgeon to position each jaw ideally relative to the cranial base and relative to the airway. Special consideration by the orthodontist must be given to arch width, arch form, leveling, and arch length deficiency. Each individual aspect will be addressed separately for ease of discussion but should be considered in a combined and coordinated manner.

TRANSVERSE DIMENSION AND ARCH FORM

The interarch transverse relationship is especially important; without adequate attention to this dimension the final mandibular position is adversely affected. To maximize improvement the orthodontist and oral surgeon must assess the transverse dimension in the current bite position and the planned postsurgical bite position. Maxillary transverse excess rarely occurs, but when it is present it can be managed by fabricating a stainless steel lingual arch that is activated to narrow the maxillary arch. Because a smaller arch leaves less room for the tongue (which may exacerbate the sleep apnea), consideration should be directed instead toward increasing the dimension of the mandibular basal bone via transverse mandibular symphyseal distraction osteogenesis.[53–55]

If maxillary transverse deficiency is observed several treatment remedies are possible. Mild maxillary transverse deficiencies (1–3 mm) can be addressed with orthodontic therapy using mildly expanded arch wires. A more efficient orthodontic technique uses a mildly expanded transpalatal arch (TPA) (**Fig. 9**A, B). In moderate transverse deficiency (3–6 mm), transverse expansion occurs surgically, with interdental osteotomies performed between the lateral incisor and canine bilaterally (**Fig. 10**). The maxillary dentition is aligned in 3 segments: second molar to canine bilaterally and a separate lateral incisor to lateral incisor segment. Segmental maxillary surgery has several potentially negative consequences. First, interdental cuts risk damaging 1 or both teeth adjacent to the osteotomy site. Secondly, a kink in the vascular pedicle may occur, which can result in the loss of 1 or more maxillary segments. Finally, the amount of expansion is limited, with more expansion observed in the molar region, and the stability of segmental maxillary procedures is poor.

In severe maxillary transverse deficiency (>6 mm) transverse maxillary distraction osteogenesis (previously referred to as surgically assisted rapid maxillary expansion) is the preferred approach (**Fig. 11**A, B). Canine and molar expansion are routinely achieved in a proportion of nearly 1:1. By widening the palate the floor of the nose is also widened. Improved breathing from surgical expansion alone can be observed just as nonsurgical rapid maxillary expansion has been shown to improve OSA in children.

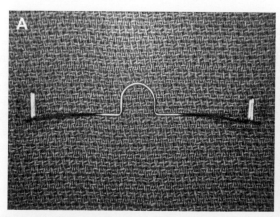
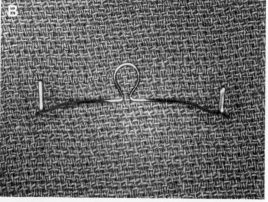

Fig. 9. (*A*) The expanded TPA. The adjustment loop has been opened to produce the desired amount of maxillary expansion. Unless used in a skeletally immature patient, this will expand only the teeth, not the palate. (*B*) The passive, unexpanded TPA.

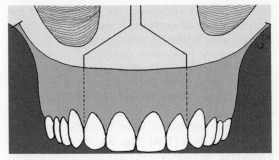

Fig. 10. A segmented Le Fort I osteotomy. The osteotomy is performed between the maxillary lateral incisors and the maxillary canines to obtain canine and molar expansion. Care must be taken to prevent kinking the gingival pedicle to preserve tissue and tooth health.

VERTICAL DIMENSION AND LEVELING

Patients with OSA may have deep overbite, moderate overbite, or an open bite; they may have a long face or short face; they may present with 1 occlusal plane or multiple occlusal planes. When multiple maxillary occlusal planes are present (typically in a patient with a long face), the patient who does not have sleep apnea is best treated with a segmented Le Fort I osteotomy to level the maxillary arch. The osteotomy site is determined primarily by the location of the "step" in the occlusal planes. If the occlusal plane "step" occurs in the canine area the maxilla is segmented distal to the canine. If the "step" is in the incisor area only, the arch is segmented between the maxillary canine and lateral incisor. The same risks mentioned for segmental maxillary surgery for transverse expansion apply to the vertical considerations described here. Though leveling with segmented surgery is more stable in the vertical plane of space the surgeon may prefer orthodontic leveling of the dental arches so a less risky single piece Le Fort I osteotomy can be performed.

Because surgical segmentation may not be possible orthodontic segmentation of the maxillary arch can be performed for more efficient arch leveling. Following segmental tooth alignment, specially fabricated intrusion or extrusion arches are placed. The intrusion arch results in superior (upward) movement of the maxillary incisors and inferior positioning of the maxillary posterior teeth.[56] The opposite occurs when an extrusion arch is used. The efficiency of both specially activated arch wires can be enhanced with interarch vertical elastics; however, care must be taken not to deliver too much eruptive force. Once level arches are obtained a continuous, rigid stainless steel arch wire is placed to maintain the level occlusal plane for the surgeon.

For the patient with a short face and deep bite it is often more efficient to open the bite during surgery rather than level the mandibular arch with presurgical orthodontics. This approach also allows earlier surgical mandibular advancement for OSA. With this technique the surgical splint is thicker, particularly in the midarch region. During immediate postsurgical fixation the splint remains wired to the maxillary arch. Once the wires are removed vertical intermaxillary elastics are used from the rigid maxillary arch wire to a more flexible mandibular arch wire. Leveling is efficient because the lower teeth erupt into the newly created space rather than into the opposing arch. All of the bands or brackets must be firmly in place; if not, the tooth or group of teeth without brackets does not erupt and is left behind.

If the surgeon prefers presurgical leveling, an alternative orthodontic approach must be considered. Once the maxillary arch is aligned a maxillary impression is taken to fabricate an anterior bite

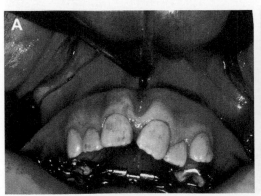

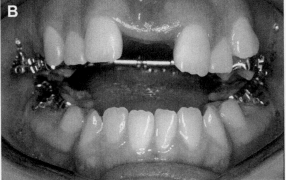

Fig. 11. (*A*) The intraoperative view of surgically assisted rapid palatal expansion. A circumferential cut is made above the level of the maxillary tooth roots. Finally, the osteotome is placed in the midsagittal region to split the suture. (*B*) The significant amount of expansion that can be obtained following activation of the appliance.

plate. The mandibular incisors strike the acrylic, creating interocclusal space posteriorly. With a rigid maxillary arch, bite splint, and light mandibular arch wire the mandibular dentition is erupted as described earlier. This approach has the advantage of creating level arches that fit well for the surgeon. The disadvantages are the additional presurgical orthodontics and the additional patient compliance needed with the splint and elastics. Patients with sleep apnea need to proceed to surgery quickly and if compliance with the bite splint and elastics is poor, the surgical correction will be unnecessarily delayed.

SAGITTAL DIMENSION: MOLAR CLASSIFICATION, CROWDING, AND SPACING

The pretreatment sagittal relationship (class I, II, or III) assists in determining the amount of jaw movement required for the patient receiving MMA. Skeletally balanced patients (class I) are typically planned for approximately 10 mm advancement in both arches.[8] Patients with nearly ideal occlusion may undergo jaw surgery with arch bars and not require orthodontic treatment. However, most patients do not present with this type of occlusion.

More commonly patients present with class II molar, canine, and skeletal relationships, which means the mandible needs to be advanced further than the maxilla. To determine how much further, the current molar relationship, skeletal relationship, and dental crowding must be considered. When examining dental crowding one should strive to maintain (or preferably augment) the dental arch dimensions in patients with OSA. Smaller arches provide less room for the tongue. As a result nonextraction orthodontic treatment in borderline situations is preferred but the teeth must be positioned within basal bone and sound periodontal health must be maintained. If the crowding is so significant that either of these goals is unattainable extractions must be performed.

If extractions are deemed appropriate the management of the extraction space is important. The goal of MMA is to produce significant jaw advancement; therefore, the direction of space closure is different. In class II mandibular-deficient patients with OSA with 7 mm or more dental crowding the orthodontist should retract the lower front teeth at least to maintain and preferably to increase the class II relationship, enabling the largest possible mandibular advancement to be performed for the greatest potential airway improvement.

POSTSURGICAL FINISHING

Accomplishing the presurgical orthodontic objectives enables the surgeon to accomplish the surgical objectives. When the surgeon achieves a class I molar and canine relationship, final arch form coordination, interdigitation of the posterior occlusion, and detailing of the bite is faster. With the surgical splint removed final finishing is accomplished with complementarily shaped orthodontic arch wires. Elastics are used to obtain final leveling and adjusting of the dental arches. Once the occlusion is acceptable the orthodontic appliances are removed and orthodontic retainers are placed.

MAXILLARY AND MANDIBULAR TRANSVERSE DISTRACTION OSTEOGENESIS

Given the reports in the pediatric or adolescent literature demonstrating improvement in OSA resulting from expansion, one must theorize that surgical expansion of the adult dental arches will produce similar improvement. A recent case report[53] illustrates the successful incorporation of bimaxillary transverse distraction osteogenesis in combination with MMA in an adult male with severe OSA. The pretreatment RDI of 60 was reduced to a posttreatment RDI of 4. No interim sleep study was performed, so it is not clear how much correction resulted from the transverse distraction osteogenesis and how much resulted from the maxillomandibular advancement.

A clinically useful guideline when considering bimaxillary transverse distraction osteogenesis is that the mandible can be expanded a maximum of 10 mm. If the patient presents with narrow arches but no crossbite, expansion of both arches must be planned. If a crossbite exists the maxilla must be expanded more than the mandible. Custom-made rapid maxillary and rapid mandibular expansion appliances must be constructed. The standard design should be used in the maxilla. In the mandible, the expansion screw body should be placed lingual to the mandibular incisors and oriented approximately 45° to the occlusal plane to facilitate activation of the appliance. If adequate interdental space is present between the maxillary and mandibular central incisors, limited predistraction movement is required to diverge the roots. As progress is made with transverse distraction osteogenesis, additional information will be developed. A new testing protocol using a preexpansion/postexpansion and postmaxillomandibular advancement sleep study must be initiated, which improves understanding of the amount of correction from the transverse expansion and the amount from the MMA.

SUMMARY

OSA has developed from an unknown condition to one that affects multiple medical and dental disciplines including orthodontics. Orthodontists must screen for OSA in their examinations of new pediatric and adult patients. When signs or symptoms of OSA are observed the orthodontist must implement appropriate referrals for definitive diagnosis. Early recognition of mouth breathing and airway obstruction by the orthodontist can facilitate early treatment and potential correction of OSA in the pediatric population. Once the diagnosis has been made, treatment protocols that have been consistently applied for orthodontic malocclusion may be applied for resolution of OSA. When treating an adult orthodontic patient (particularly an adult orthognathic surgery patient) who has signs and symptoms of OSA orthodontists must consult diligently with their medical colleagues. Presurgical sleep studies aid sound surgical orthodontic treatment decisions; as Benjiman Franklin said, "an ounce of prevention is worth a pound of cure."

REFERENCES

1. Smith R, Ronald J, Delaive K, et al. What are obstructive sleep apnea patients being treated for prior to this diagnosis? Chest 2002;121(1):164–72.
2. Strollo PJ Jr, Rogers RM. Obstructive sleep apnea. N Engl J Med 1996;334(2):99–104.
3. Young T, Palta M, Dempsey J, et al. The occurrence of sleep-disordered breathing among middle-aged adults. N Engl J Med 1993;328(17):1230–5.
4. Sanders MH, Kern NB, Stiller RA, et al. CPAP therapy via oronasal mask for obstructive sleep apnea. Chest 1994;106(3):774–9.
5. Smith PL, Gold AR, Meyers DA, et al. Weight loss in mildly to moderately obese patients with obstructive sleep apnea. Ann Intern Med 1985;103(6 (Pt 1)):850–5.
6. Cohen R. Obstructive sleep apnea: oral appliance therapy and severity of condition. Oral Surg Oral Med Oral Pathol Oral Radiol Endod 1998;85(4): 388–92.
7. Coleman JA Jr. Laser-assisted uvulopalatoplasty: long-term results with a treatment for snoring. Ear Nose Throat J 1998;77(1):22–4, 26–9, 32–4.
8. Prinsell JR. Maxillomandibular advancement surgery for obstructive sleep apnea syndrome. (1939). J Am Dent Assoc 2002;133(11):1489–97.
9. Scrima L, Broudy M, Nay KN, et al. Increased severity of obstructive sleep apnea after bedtime alcohol ingestion: diagnostic potential and proposed mechanism of action. Sleep 1982;5(4):318–28.
10. Marcus CL. Sleep-disordered breathing in children. Am J Respir Crit Care Med 2001;164(1):16–30.
11. Johns MW. Reliability and factor analysis of the Epworth Sleepiness Scale. Sleep 1992;15(4):376–81.
12. George CF. Reduction in motor vehicle collisions following treatment of sleep apnoea with nasal CPAP. Thorax 2001;56(7):508–12.
13. Powell NB, Riley RW, Schechtman KB, et al. A comparative model: reaction time performance in sleep-disordered breathing versus alcohol-impaired controls. Laryngoscope 1999;109(10):1648–54.
14. Friedman M, Tanyeri H, La Rosa M, et al. Clinical predictors of obstructive sleep apnea. Laryngoscope 1999;109(12):1901–7.
15. Proffit WR. Later stages of development. In: Proffit WR, Fields HW Jr, Sarver DM, editors. Contemporary orthodontics. 4th edition. St Louis (MO): Elsevier; 2007. p. 108.
16. Harvold EP, Tomer BS, Vargervik K, et al. Primate experiments on oral respiration. Am J Orthod 1981; 79(4):359–72.
17. Moyers R. Handbook of orthodontics. 3rd edition. Chicago: Mosby - Year Book; 1973.
18. Cistulli PA, Palmisano RG, Poole MD. Treatment of obstructive sleep apnea syndrome by rapid maxillary expansion. Sleep 1998;21(8):831–5.
19. Burstone CJ, James RB, Legan H, et al. Cephalometrics for orthognathic surgery. J Oral Surg 1978; 36(4):269–77.
20. Wittenborn W, Panchal J, Marsh JL, et al. Neonatal distraction surgery for micrognathia reduces obstructive apnea and the need for tracheotomy. J Craniofac Surg 2004;15(4):623–30.
21. Cistulli PA, Sullivan CE. Sleep apnea in Marfan's syndrome. Increased upper airway collapsibility during sleep. Chest 1995;108(3):631–5.
22. Riley R, Guilleminault C, Herran J, et al. Cephalometric analyses and flow-volume loops in obstructive sleep apnea patients. Sleep 1983;6(4):303–11.
23. Fleisher KE, Krieger AC. Current trends in the treatment of obstructive sleep apnea. J Oral Maxillofac Surg 2007;65(10):2056–68.
24. Lowe AA, Santamaria JD, Fleetham JA, et al. Facial morphology and obstructive sleep apnea. Am J Orthod Dentofacial Orthop 1986;90(6):484–91.
25. Tsuchiya M, Lowe AA, Pae EK, et al. Obstructive sleep apnea subtypes by cluster analysis. Am J Orthod Dentofacial Orthop 1992;101(6):533–42.
26. Tangugsorn V, Skatvedt O, Krogstad O, et al. Obstructive sleep apnoea: a cephalometric study. Part II. Uvulo-glossopharyngeal morphology. Eur J Orthod 1995;17(1):57–67.
27. Cistulli PA. Craniofacial abnormalities in obstructive sleep apnoea: implications for treatment. Carlton, Vic. Respirology 1996;1(3):167–74.
28. Tangugsorn V, Skatvedt O, Krogstad O, et al. Obstructive sleep apnoea: a cephalometric study. Part I. Cervico-craniofacial skeletal morphology. Eur J Orthod 1995;17(1):45–56.

29. Halperin E, Lavie P, Alroy G, et al. The hypersomnia-sleep apnoea syndrome (HSAS): ENT findings. Sleep Res 1979;8:188.

30. deBerry-Borowiecki B, Kukwa A, Blanks RH. Cephalometric analysis for diagnosis and treatment of obstructive sleep apnea. Laryngoscope 1988;98(2):226–34.

31. Lyberg T, Krogstad O, Djupesland G. Cephalometric analysis in patients with obstructive sleep apnoea syndrome. I. Skeletal morphology. J Laryngol Otol 1989;103(3):287–92.

32. Ferguson KA, Ono T, Lowe AA, et al. The relationship between obesity and craniofacial structure in obstructive sleep apnea. Chest 1995;108(2):375–81.

33. Sakakibara H, Tong M, Matsushita K, et al. Cephalometric abnormalities in non-obese and obese patients with obstructive sleep apnoea. Eur Respir J 1999;13(2):403–10.

34. Yu X, Fujimoto K, Urushibata K, et al. Cephalometric analysis in obese and nonobese patients with obstructive sleep apnea syndrome. Chest 2003;124(1):212–8.

35. Behrents RG, Broadbent Jr BH. A chronological account of the Bolton-Brush growth studies – in search of truth for the greater good of man 1984. Available at: http://dental.case.edu/bolton-brush/chronological.pdf.

36. Lavergne J, Petrovic A. Discontinuities in occlusal relationship and the regulation of facial growth. A cybernetic view. Eur J Orthod 1983;5(4):269–78.

37. Moss ML. The primacy of functional matrices on orofacial growth. Dent Pract 1968;19:65.

38. Scott JH. Growth at facial sutures. Am J Orthod 1956;42:381.

39. Sicher H. Oral anatomy. St Louis (MO): CV Mosby; 1952.

40. Ranly DM. A synopsis of craniofacial growth. 2nd edition. Norwalk (CT): Appleton & Lange; 1988.

41. Villa MP, Malagola C, Pagani J, et al. Rapid maxillary expansion in children with obstructive sleep apnea syndrome: 12-month follow-up. Sleep Med 2007;8(2):128–34.

42. Timms DJ. Rapid maxillary expansion in the treatment of nocturnal enuresis. Angle Orthod 1990;60(3):229–33 [discussion: 234].

43. Oliveira De Felippe NL, Da Silveira AC, Viana G, et al. Relationship between rapid maxillary expansion and nasal cavity size and airway resistance: short- and long-term effects. Am J Orthod Dentofacial Orthop 2008;134(3):370–82.

44. Bailey LT, Proffit WR, White RP Jr. Trends in surgical treatment of Class III skeletal relationships. Int J Adult Orthodon Orthognath Surg 1995;10(2):108–18.

45. Kawamata A, Fujishita M, Ariji Y, et al. Three-dimensional computed tomographic evaluation of morphologic airway changes after mandibular setback osteotomy for prognathism. Oral Surg Oral Med Oral Pathol Oral Radiol Endod 2000;89(3):278–87.

46. Saitoh K. Long-term changes in pharyngeal airway morphology after mandibular setback surgery. Am J Orthod Dentofacial Orthop 2004;125(5):556–61.

47. Almeida FR, Lowe AA, Otsuka R, et al. Long-term sequelae of oral appliance therapy in obstructive sleep apnea patients: Part 2. Study-model analysis. Am J Orthod Dentofacial Orthop 2006;129(2):205–13.

48. Almeida FR, Lowe AA, Sung JO, et al. Long-term sequelae of oral appliance therapy in obstructive sleep apnea patients: Part 1. Cephalometric analysis. Am J Orthod Dentofacial Orthop 2006;129(2):195–204.

49. Haskell JA, McCrillis J, Haskell BS, et al. Effects of mandibular advancement device (MAD) on airway dimensions assessed with cone-beam computed tomography. Semin Orthod 2009;15(2):132–58.

50. Riley RW, Powell NB, Guilleminault C. Obstructive sleep apnea syndrome: a review of 306 consecutively treated surgical patients. Otolaryngol Head Neck Surg 1993;108(2):117–25.

51. Bear S, Priest J. Sleep apnoea syndrome: correction with surgical advancement of the mandible. J Oral Surg 1980;38:543–9.

52. Waite PD, Shettar SM. Maxillomandibular advancement: a cure for obstructive sleep apnea. Oral Maxillofac Surg Clin North Am 1995;7:327.

53. Conley RS, Legan HL. Correction of severe obstructive sleep apnea with bimaxillary transverse distraction osteogenesis and maxillomandibular advancement. Am J Orthod Dentofacial Orthop 2006;129(2):283–92.

54. Conley RS, Krug AY. Mandibular distraction osteogenesis with a new ratchet screw. J Clin Orthod 2006;40(4):219–23 [quiz 231].

55. Conley R, Legan H. Mandibular symphyseal distraction osteogenesis: diagnosis and treatment planning considerations. Angle Orthod 2003;73(1):3–11.

56. Burstone CR. Deep overbite correction by intrusion. Am J Orthod 1977;72(1):1–22.

Oral Appliance Therapy in Sleep Medicine

Dennis R. Bailey, DDS[a,b,*], Aarnoud Hoekema, DMD, PhD[c]

KEYWORDS

- Oral appliances • Sleep-related breathing disorders
- Mandibular repositioning appliances
- Mandibular advancement device
- Mandibular repositioning devices • Standards of practice

Oral appliance therapy provided by the dentist has become a well recognized means by which patients who have a sleep-related breathing disorders (SRBD) may have an alternative to continuous positive airway pressure (CPAP) or surgery for their management.[1] Oral appliances aim at relieving upper airway obstruction and snoring by modifying the position of the mandible, tongue, and other oropharyngeal structures. Oral appliance treatment of SRBD has gained considerable popularity because of its simplicity and supposed reversibility. In 1902, the French physician Pierre Robin laid the foundation for oral appliance therapy. With a monobloc appliance, Robin[2] treated children who suffered from breathing difficulties and glossoptosis caused by hypoplasia of the mandible. The first case of an oral appliance that repositioned the mandible in an adult patient with obstructive sleep apnea (OSA) was not reported until 1980.[3] The first patient series of oral appliance therapy for OSA was reported in 1982 and described the effects of an appliance that repositioned the tongue.[4] Currently, well over 90 different oral appliances are marketed for the treatment of snoring and OSA.[5]

Oral appliances have become an optional consideration for patients with mild-to-moderate sleep apnea and for those who simply snore. The role of the dentist actually starts with the ability to recognize patients who may be at risk for any type of sleep disorder and especially sleep apnea.[6] It is incumbent on anyone in health care to be attuned to symptoms that may indicate a sleep disorder, and dentistry is no exception. Over the last decade, the number of dentists who have sought advanced training in the use of oral appliances and have become educated in sleep medicine has grown significantly. Additionally, sleep medicine specialists and primary care physicians now seek out dentists with specialized training and experience in the field of dental sleep medicine along with expertise in the use of these appliances and who possess the training needed to comanage sleep apnea patients.

MECHANISM OF ACTION

The effect of oral appliances and how they specifically work is not totally understood. At this time, oral appliances are believed to be effective in improving the airway by repositioning the mandible in such a way that they move the tongue forward and prevent the mandible and correspondingly the tongue from collapsing back into the airway during sleep. Regardless of which appliance is used, the overall process is intended to prevent the collapse of the tongue base back into the oropharynx, while at the same time there

[a] Orofacial Pain and Dental Sleep Medicine, Dental Sleep Medicine Mini–Residency, UCLA School of Dentistry, Los Angeles, CA, USA
[b] 7901 East Belleview Avenue, Suite 200, Englewood, CO 80111, USA
[c] Department of Oral and Maxillofacial Surgery, University Medical Center Groningen, Hanzeplein 1, Post Office Box 30.001, 9700 RB, Groningen, The Netherlands
* Corresponding author. 7901 East Belleview Avenue, Suite 200, Englewood, CO 80111.
E-mail address: RMC4E@aol.com (D.R. Bailey).

Sleep Med Clin 5 (2010) 91–98
doi:10.1016/j.jsmc.2009.10.007
1556-407X/10/$ – see front matter © 2010 Published by Elsevier Inc.

is associated tension placed on the pharyngeal musculature and stabilization of this musculature to help support the airway and thereby further prevent collapse (**Figs. 1** and **2**).

In addition to improving the oropharyngeal and retroglossal airway, nasal patency may be improved. The repositioning of the mandible the tongue moves the tongue base down and forward. This in effect moves the superior surface of the tongue away from the inferior surface of the soft palate. Hence there is improvement at this airway space (retropalatal area), and there is often associated improvement in nasal airway patency overall.

TYPES OF ORAL APPLIANCES

There are many different oral appliances on the market today. In **Table 1**, there is a listing of many of the better known oral appliances typically used by dentists. The early design of oral appliances was what is termed a monobloc design. These appliances were one piece that had the upper and lower components joined solidly together. This prevented the mandible from being able to freely move, and the appliance was very difficult to adjust or modify. Today for the most part all of the available oral appliances work in a similar manner as has been described and are separate components for the mandible and the maxilla. The difference that sets one apart from another is the manner by which they are joined together. Some have a more rigid method by which they are fixed together, whereas others use more of an elastic effect. In addition, there are some that are adjusted by the patient on an as-needed basis, and some

Obstructed Airway in Sleep Apnea

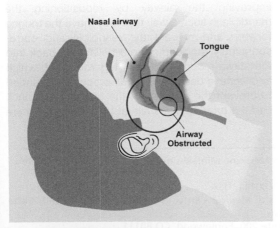

Fig. 1. Demonstrates an airway that is closed or obstructed. Circled area shows the collapse of the soft palate and the tongue base into the airway.

Airway Improved Using Oral Appliance

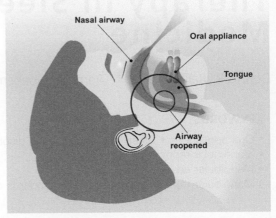

Fig. 2. With an oral appliance (MRA) in place, the airway is now open; tongue base is forward and held out of the airway.

require adjustment by the dentist. Another characteristic is the size or bulk of the appliance. They are not all the same when it comes to how large the appliance may be and how much room is consumed in the mouth as a consequence.

In general and for the sake of clarity, oral appliances may be divided into two broad types: tongue retainers and MRAs that are also known as MADs or in other cases mandibular repositioning devices (MRDs). In reality, the term mandibular repositioning is more applicable, because the action of advancing the mandible also requires some degree of vertical opening of the mouth and allows for separation of the teeth. Regardless, the use of the term dental appliance is not applicable to these appliances, because they are considered medical devices and are used for the management of a medical condition and not treating a dental or dentally related condition.

The tongue retainers often times do not fit tightly to the teeth even though they also create some degree of mandibular repositioning. Their main function is to pull and hold the tongue forward and thus prevent the tongue base from collapsing into the oropharyngeal airway space during sleep. The amount of mandibular movement with these devices is very restricted.

The MRA type appliances are designed such that they fit securely on the teeth and should be very retentive so that with any type of mandibular movement the appliance is held securely in place. Some of the appliances allow for a small degree of mandibular movement that is side to side, and others are very restrictive. In addition, some of the appliances allow for some degree of

Table 1
Commonly used oral appliances[a]

Tongue-Retaining Appliances	Phone Contact	Web Site
Tongue stabilizer device (TSD)	800-828-7626	http://www.aveotsd.co.nz
Tongue retaining device	262-638-8353	None
Mandibular repositioners (mandibular repositioning device [MRD]/mandibular advancement device [MAD])		
Thornton anterior positioner (TAP)	866-AMI-SNOR	http://www.TAPINTOSLEEP.com
Myerson elastic mandibular advancement (EMA)	800-423-2683	http://www.openairway.com
Therasnore	800-477-6673	http://www.distar.com
SUAD herbst	888-447-6673	http://www.strongdental.com
Nocturnal airway patency appliance (NAPA)		http://www.johnsdental.com http://www.greatlakesortho.com
Elastomeric	800-828-7626	http://www.greatlakesortho.com
Good air oral airway dilator	877-770-7623	http://www.goodair.com
PM positioner (2 types)	800-253-1196	http://www.adjustablepmpositioner.com
Somnodent	888-447-6673	http://www.somnomed.com
Oral/nasal airway system (OASYS)	888-866-2727	http://www.oasyssleep.com
SilentNite	800-854-7256	http://www.glidewelldental.com
Silencer	604-576-0952	http://www.the_silencer.com
Klearway	800-828-7626	http://www.klearway.com

[a] This is not a complete listing of oral appliances. Those that are listed are the ones that are well known to most of the dentists involved with dental sleep medicine in North America. For a more complete listing see the US Food and Drug Administration (FDA) Web site listed in the text.

vertical or mouth opening while worn, and others do not. Another characteristic that is variable with different appliances that needs to be considered is the amount of tongue space and the ability to achieve a comfortable lip seal. This is variable based on the size of the device and in some cases by the manner by which they are joined together.

MEDICAL DEVICES

Oral appliances are now viewed by the FDA as class 2 medical devices and as such must adhere to more detailed standards along with special controls.[7] This classification clearly views them as devices that are indicated for the treatment of a medical condition, and they have received what is termed a 510K. Oral appliances before the changed ruling in 2002 were categorized separately for snoring and sleep apnea. At this time they are all combined into the same group that is designated by the user code LRK. By going to the FDA's Webs site and putting in the user code, the appliances that have been cleared by the FDA can be found: http://www.accessdata.fda.gov/scripts/cdrh/cfdocs/cfPMN/pmn.cfm.

APPLIANCE SELECTION

The selection of an oral appliance often is based on user preference and may be associated with the specific training the dentist has received. It is, however, necessary to consider several factors that may impact the use of an oral appliance for not only effectiveness but also for patient comfort. Several factors that may be considered in selecting an oral appliance can be found in **Table 2**. Most appliances available today are a two-piece design as has been described previously in an attempt to address many of these selection criteria.

EFFECTIVENESS

The effectiveness of oral appliance is based on both patient satisfaction with symptom improvement and the outcome of follow-up testing with polysomnography. This allows for an assessment of the improvement and normalization of the apnea–hypopnea index (AHI) or respiratory disturbance index (RDI) along with improvement in the blood oxygen levels of the patient. Many patients may experience an improvement symptomatically but may not have

Table 2
Factors to consider in oral appliance selection

Factor	Importance
Adjustable	Allows for modification if restorative dental work is needed such as a crown or other restoration
Titratable	The ability to modify the vertical opening or the position of the mandible on a horizontal plane (advancement) for optimum airway opening and effect
Full tooth coverage	Making certain the upper and lower teeth are fully engaged in the appliance to prevent undesirable tooth movement
Posterior support	The upper and lower components of the appliance should have contact in the posterior aspect for stabilization of the temporomandibular joints (TMJs) (similar to a stabilization splint) and may be beneficial for patients with sleep bruxism
Mandibular (jaw) mobility	Allows for free movement of the mandible during sleep and also may be beneficial for patients with sleep bruxism
Open nasal airway	Improves breathing—improves oxygen levels during sleep
Adequate lip seal	Improves nasal breathing, reduces tendency to mouth breathe and may prevent drying of the mouth
Adequate tongue space	Assists in preventing the collapse of the tongue into the oropharyngeal airway

substantial improvement on the polysomnography or with their blood oxygen levels.

A review article published in 2007 evaluated many studies on oral appliance therapy and its associated effectiveness.[8] The average effectiveness for patients with mild-to-severe sleep apnea was found to be 52%. This level of effectiveness was based on the oral appliance adequately controlling the sleep apnea. In this review, pretreatment Epworth Sleepiness Scale (ESS) scores were compared with the post-treatment scores. It was found that the general improvement in the ESS was from 11.2 down to 7.8.

Another study published in 2007 found that oral appliances, when used to treat mild sleep apnea, are effective in 75% of the cases. Additionally, they are 65% effective in patients with moderate sleep apnea and 52% effective on those patients with severe sleep apnea.[9] In this study, the mean AHI before treatment was 26 plus or minus 17.7 and with the oral appliance, the mean AHI was 4.8 plus or minus 5.3. Out of the 83 patients in the study, 53 (62%) were treated successfully with an oral appliance. In this study, two different appliances were used, and these focused primarily on mandibular advancement. In a more recent study that compared oral appliances with CPAP therapy, it was demonstrated that oral appliance therapy was not inferior to CPAP in effectively treating OSA.[10] This study, however, indicated that CPAP was more effective in the treatment of patients with severe sleep apnea. In

patients with mild-to-moderate sleep apnea, oral appliance therapy was effective in 84% of patients, whereas in patients with severe disease, oral appliance therapy was effective in 69% of the patients. Studies on the long-term effects of oral appliances in the treatment of OSA suggest high success rates after follow-up periods ranging from 2 to 5 years.[11–14] Approximately 80% of patients who were successfully treated initially also experienced a satisfactory effect on snoring with long-term oral appliance therapy. In the long-term, a gradual decline in treatment effect therefore should be anticipated. These numbers may reflect bias, because not all patients originally treated were included in these analyses. Long-term effectiveness of oral appliance therapy in unselected OSA patients therefore may be lower. The main reasons for an attenuation of the treatment effect following an initially successful treatment relate to a failure of maintaining advancement of the mandible in the prescribed position and an increase in body weight during the follow-up period.[10,15]

To establish when an oral appliance may be effective is a difficult task given all of the possible variables affecting the outcome. Long-term studies would be needed to establish this. Such studies would evaluate many of the possible characteristics of patients with sleep apnea. It has been advocated that oral appliance therapy may have the most favorable outcome in patients with milder sleep apnea, who have less obesity and possess certain craniofacial findings, particularly mandibular retrognathism.[16] Based on these criteria in approximately 80% of patients, it could be established whether an oral appliance would be effective.

Effectiveness also may need to be considered in terms of improvement in the patient's medical status. As it relates to cardiovascular disease and specifically blood pressure, there are three studies that found an improvement.[17-19] In one such study in 161 patients, there was an improvement after 60 days of use of the oral appliance. The mean blood pressure went from 132 over 82 down to 128 over 79. In addition, it has been reported that the improvement in the blood pressure with the use of an oral appliance was nearly the same as that found with CPAP. In another study, oral appliance therapy was found to improve endothelial function along with improvement in the AHI and a reduction in the ESS score.[20] This indicates that oral appliance therapy may have some impact on oxidative stress.

Oral appliance outcomes also may be based on their effectiveness in relation to surgery and CPAP therapy. In relation to surgery, a review article found that oral appliances are superior to upper airway surgery in treating OSA effectively.[8] This review made up of primarily case studies found that after 1 year those that had UPPP surgery had an AHI of less than 10, 51% of the time whereas with oral appliance use 78% had an AHI of less than 10. The data was worse after four years of treatment. At that point only 3% of the surgery group had an AHI less than 10 as compared with 63% in the oral appliance group. With CPAP, the effectiveness was better as compared with oral appliance therapy. With the use of an oral appliance, however, the compliance was more favorable as well as being the preferred method for the management of the OSA by the patient.[21]

An additional concern, as it relates to outcomes, is the use of a custom fabricate oral appliance as compared with the use of one that is noncustom fabricated. The latter device often is termed a semicustom appliance, a thermoplastic appliance, or by dentists it is referred to as a boil and bite device. The semicustom oral appliance often is purchased over the Internet and in some cases may be purchased by the dentist and fabricated in one visit without the need to have it custom-made by a dental laboratory. It has been found that these so-called thermoplastic devices are not as effective when compared with the custom-fabricated oral appliances.[22]

ADVERSE EFFECTS

One of the major concerns with the use of oral appliances is the potential for adverse effects. The main concern is with tooth movement, occlusal (bite) changes, jaw pain, and the presentation of temporomandibular dysfunction (temporomandibular joint [TMJ] or temporomandibular disorder). These conditions need to be evaluated on an ongoing basis by the dentist who is involved with the oral appliance therapy as is indicated in the practice parameters paper on oral appliances.[23]

The most likely complaint from patients using an oral appliance is that their bite feels off after using the device for an entire night. In most instances, this feeling resolves over a brief period of time, usually 30 to 60 minutes. Rarely does it last for a long time or through an entire day. When this is more of a long-term finding, it needs to be addressed promptly. This may involve tongue, neck, and jaw exercises or the use of muscle relaxation-type medications such as Flexeril or Skelaxin, two of the more commonly used medications. In some cases, a course of physical therapy for the head, neck, and jaw may be indicated. If the bite changes do not resolve, then the patient should be advised to discontinue use of the oral appliance. This may create a dilemma when the patient is responding favorably to the oral appliance and cannot use the CPAP. Therefore, the patient should be consulted with regarding other options, including continued use of the oral appliance despite ongoing adverse effects, and should be evaluated more frequently. Some patients they may express the feeling that they have had tooth movement. Although this may occur, it is not a very common complaint. Dentists should retain a record of the patient's teeth, termed diagnostic study models, so that this can be evaluated on an ongoing basis or when the patient feels this may be occurring. In rare situations, orthodontics may be needed to correct the bite. Because oral appliance therapy has been shown to be a good predictor for the outcome of maxillomandibular advancement surgery in OSA patients,[24] one may choose to proceed with this type of surgery in case of progressive bite changes.

Dysfunction involving the TMJs has not been found to be a common outcome with the use of an oral appliance. It has been found that after 1 year of use of an oral appliance, there were no anatomic changes of the joints and no evidence of TMJ pathology.[25] Often the patient will feel that he or she is having pain in the region of the TMJs. This is often muscle pain that is referring to the face or head. At this time, this should be investigated more completely and may be managed similar to how bite changes are addressed.

Another common outcome is an increased amount of saliva production or drooling. Often this occurs at the onset of treatment and will

Table 3
Indications for oral appliance treatment based on the practice parameters on oral appliances published February 2006

Treatment	Indicated	Contraindicated
Snoring only	Yes	No
Mild-to-moderate sleep apnea	Yes	No
Sleep apnea—patient prefers oral appliance	Yes	No
Severe sleep apnea (not as primary treatment)	No	Yes
Central sleep apnea	No	Yes

decrease once the oral appliance is used on a regular basis. If this continues, it may be indicative of excessive mouth breathing or an inadequate lip seal.

INDICATIONS FOR ORAL APPLIANCE THERAPY

The indication for oral appliances that are used to manage sleep-related breathing disorders is derived mainly from the standards of practice or practice parameters that were published by the American Academy of Sleep Medicine (AASM) in February of 2006. The practice parameters paper addresses the indications for oral appliance therapy and, the companion paper reviews the most current literature on this topic.[23,26] The findings in the review paper organized the data that were used for creating the indications for oral appliance therapy for managing sleep apnea and snoring.

The practice parameter paper indicates that based on the evidence that was available, the use of oral appliances is

- For patients with primary snoring where the presence of sleep apnea has been eliminated
- For patients with mild-to-moderate sleep apnea who wish to use an oral appliance as an alternative to CPAP or surgery and
- In patients with severe sleep apnea who have a documented intolerance to CPAP or where surgery has not been successful (**Table 3**).

In the instance of mild-to-moderate sleep apnea, many of these patients have attempted to use CPAP or have had a trial of it at the time of the sleep study and are unable to tolerate it or do not feel that CPAP is compatible with their lifestyle.

In the practice parameters for the use of oral appliances, it is indicated that

Table 4
Dental considerations for oral appliance therapy

Condition	Considerations
Poor dental status	Resolve dental disease Remove loose or compromised teeth Restore decayed or broken teeth
Periodontal (gum) disease	Reduce inflammation Improve oral hygiene Scale (clean) teeth Refer patient to a periodontist
Inadequate number of teeth to support oral appliance	No definite number required Consensus: 6 to 10 teeth per arch If inadequate number, consider dental implants
TMJ disorder	If limited (restricted) opening, manage temporomandibular disorder first Differentiate between muscle pain and joint-related pathology/dysfunction

"Oral appliances should be fitted by qualified dental personnel who are trained and experienced in the overall care of oral health, the temporomandibular joint, dental occlusion and associated structures."

It is further stated that the dental management aspect should be delivered by dentists with "serious training" in sleep medicine that focuses on diagnosis, treatment, and follow-up care. Therefore, before treatment several dental and oral health considerations need to be taken into consideration whenever an oral appliance is being considered (**Table 4**). To accomplish this, the dentist with an interest in managing sleep apnea with the use of an oral appliance needs to have advanced training beyond that which is presented in the 4 years of dental school, particularly as it relates to the management of TMJ disorders and orthodontic considerations.

SUMMARY

Since their introduction in the 1980s, oral appliances are being used increasingly for the treatment of SRBD. Mandibular repositioning appliances are the primary form of management in oral appliance treatment. Effectiveness of these appliances appears to be related primarily to the degree of mandibular advancement imposed by the appliance but some evidence suggests that the degree of vertical opening also may play a role.[27,28] It must be recognized that continuing to advance the mandible does not always result in a more optimum result. There may be a point of diminishing returns. Oral appliances are generally effective for treating snoring and in many cases for the treating OSA. However, a placebo effect related to symptom relief as opposed to normalization of the AHI or RDI and the improvement in oxygen saturation always should be considered. In addition, a gradual decline in treatment effect may be anticipated in the long-term. In the OSA patient, effectiveness of therapy always should be confirmed by polysomnography, both in the initial phase of treatment and when relapse is suspected during long-term follow-up examinations. Although usually not serious, oral appliance therapy may result in transient adverse effects on the craniomandibular and craniofacial complex when therapy is initiated. When continued, long-term adverse effects may involve changes in the dental occlusion that need to be monitored for as long as the oral appliance is being used. Although there is convincing evidence that oral appliance therapy is effective for the treatment of OSA, it is generally less effective than CPAP, particularly in more severe OSA. Nevertheless, many patients prefer an oral appliance to CPAP. Unfortunately, the ability to predict treatment outcome and preselect suitable patients for oral appliance therapy remains limited in clinical practice. Based on the current level of evidence, oral appliance therapy is recommended as primary treatment for snoring and as an option in patients with mild-to-moderate OSA. In severe disease, CPAP therapy should be considered first. Treatment of patients with oral appliances should be performed by a dentist with specialized training and supervised by a physician, both of whom have training and experience in the field of SRBD. To guarantee long-term efficacy and safety, as well as the management of any adverse effects, follow-up examinations should be conducted on a regular basis.

REFERENCES

1. Cistulli PA, Gotsopoulos H, Marklund M, et al. Treatment of snoring and obstructive sleep apnea with mandibular repositioning appliances. Sleep Med Rev 2004;8(6):443–57.
2. Robin P. Glossoptosis due to atresia and hypotrophy of the mandible. Am J Dis Child 1994;48:541–7.
3. Bear SE, Priest JH. Sleep apnea syndrome: correction with surgical advancement of the mandible. J Oral Surg 1980;38(7):543–9.
4. Cartwright RD, Samelson CF. The effects of a nonsurgical treatment for obstructive sleep apnea. The tongue-retaining device. JAMA 1982;248(6):705–9.
5. Hoekema A, Stegenga B, de Bont LG. Efficacy and comorbidity of oral appliances in the treatment of obstructive sleep apnea–hypopnea: a systematic review. Crit Rev Oral Biol Med 2004;15(3):137–55.
6. Schwarting S, Netzer NC. Abstract from Sleep Utah 2006 (0556), Annual meeting of APSS. Sleep apnea for the dentist—political means and practical performance. Salt Lake City, Utah, June 17–22, 2006.
7. Center for Devices and Radiologic Health, US Food and Drug Administration. Class II special controls guidance document: intraoral devices for snoring and/or obstructive sleep apnea: guidance for industry and FDA. Bulletin, November 12, 2002.
8. Hoffstein V. Review of oral appliances for treatment of sleep-disordered breathing. Sleep Breath 2007; 11(1):1–22.
9. Machado MA, Juliano L, Taga M, et al. Titratable mandibular repositioner appliances for obstructive sleep apnea syndrome: are they an option? Sleep Breath 2007;11:225–31.
10. Hoekema A, Stegenga B, Wijkstra PJ, et al. Obstructive sleep apnea therapy. J Dent Res 2008;87: 882–7.
11. Walker-Engström ML, Tegelberg A, Wilhelmsson B, et al. 4-year follow-up of treatment with dental

appliance or uvulopalatopharyngoplasty in patients with obstructive sleep apnea: a randomized study. Chest 2002;121(3):739–46.

12. Rose EC, Barthlen GM, Staats R, et al. Therapeutic efficacy of an oral appliance in the treatment of obstructive sleep apnea: a 2-year follow-up. Am J Orthod Dentofacial Orthop 2002;121(3):273–9.

13. Marklund M, Sahlin C, Stenlund H, et al. Mandibular advancement devices in patients with obstructive sleep apnea: long-term effects on apnea and sleep. Chest 2001;120(1):162–9.

14. Fransson AM, Tegelberg A, Leissner L, et al. Effects of a mandibular protruding device on the sleep of, patients with obstructive sleep apnea and snoring problems: a 2-year follow-up. Sleep Breath 2003; 7(3):131–41.

15. Marklund M, Stenlund H, Franklin KA. Mandibular advancement devices in 630 man and women with obstructive sleep apnea and snoring: tolerability and predictors of treatment success. Chest 2004; 125(4):1270–8.

16. Hoekema A, Doff MHJ, de Bont LG, et al. Predictors of obstructive sleep apnea–hypopnea treatment outcome. J Dent Res 2007;86(12):1181–6.

17. Barnes M, McEvoy RD, Banks S, et al. Efficacy of positive airway pressure and oral appliance in mild to moderate obstructive sleep apnea. Am J Respir Crit Care Med 2004;170:656–64.

18. Gotsopoulos H, Kelly JJ, Cistulli PA. Oral appliance therapy reduces blood pressure in obstructive sleep apnea: a randomized, controlled trial. Sleep 2004; 27:934–41.

19. Yoshida K. Effect on blood pressure of oral appliance therapy for sleep apnea syndrome. Int J Prosthodont 2006;19:61–6.

20. Itzhaki S, Dorchin H, Clark G, et al. The effects of 1-year treatment with a Herbst mandibular advancement splint on obstructive sleep apnea, oxidative stress, and endothelial function. Chest 2007;131:740–9.

21. Ferguson K, Ono T, Lowe A, et al. A randomized crossover study of an oral appliance vs nasal continuous positive airway pressure in the treatment of mild–moderate obstructive sleep apnea. Chest 1996;109:1269–75.

22. Vanderveken OM, Devolder A, Marklund M, et al. Comparison of a custom-made and a thermoplastic oral appliance for the treatment of mild sleep apnea. Am J Respir Crit Care Med 2008;178(2):197–202.

23. Ferguson KA, Cartwright R, Rogers R, et al. Oral appliances for snoring and obstructive sleep apnea: a review. Sleep 2006;29(2):244–62.

24. Hoekema A, de Lange J, Stegenga B, et al. Oral appliances and maxillomandibular advancement surgery: an alternative treatment protocol for the obstructive sleep apnea–hypopnea syndrome. J Oral Maxillofac Surg 2006;64(6):886–91.

25. de Almeida FR, Bittencourt LR, de Almeida CIR, et al. Effects of mandibular posture on obstructive sleep apnea severity and TMJ in patients fitted with an oral appliance. Sleep 2002;25(5):507–13.

26. Kushida CA, Morgenthaler TI, Littner MR, et al. Practice parameters for the treatment of snoring and obstructive sleep apnea with oral appliances: an update for 2005. Sleep 2006;29(2):240–3.

27. Frantz D. The difference between success and failure. Sleep Rev 2001;2:20–3.

28. Hoekema A. Oral appliance therapy in obstructive sleep apnea-hypopnea syndrome: a clinical study on therapeutic outcomes. The American Academy of Dental Sleep Medicine 2008. p. 77.

Ambulatory Testing for Adult Obstructive Sleep Apnea for the Dentist

Michael R. Littner, MD

KEYWORDS

- Sleep apnea • Polysomnography
- Ambulatory sleep testing • Home sleep testing

CASE PRESENTATION

The patient is a 45-year-old man who presents to his primary care physician with a complaint of daytime sleepiness.

History of the Present Illness

The patient has been somewhat sleepy during the day for many years. When questioned, he states that he has snored for as long as he can remember. In the past, his sleepiness has not interfered with his functioning at home or work. Recently, he has gained weight and needs an alarm clock to wake up in time for work as an accountant. He sleeps in on weekends.

The patient admits to feeling tired at the wheel of his car on several occasions, needing to stop and refresh himself every hour. He has never fallen asleep while driving. Before his loud snoring drove his wife to another bedroom, she told him that he sometimes stops breathing for short periods while asleep.

The patient awakens with a dry mouth and frequently, a mild headache. His sleep/wake cycle is regular, with an 11 PM bedtime. He routinely sleeps 7 hours a night. He awakens only mildly refreshed and drinks large amounts of caffeinated beverages during the day, starting early in the morning. He does not nap during the week but does so occasionally on weekends despite sleeping 8 to 9 hours at night.

Physical examination reveals an obese man (body mass index [BMI] of 33) with a blood pressure of 135/85 mmHg. Examination of the oropharynx reveals a visualized soft palate and an edematous base of the uvula, with the tongue protruding and without phonation. This is consistent with a class 3 Mallampati.[1] The patient has tonsils that are not enlarged. His examination was otherwise unremarkable.

The patient's previous physician had prescribed a diet and a nonsedating antihypertensive (an angiotensin enzyme inhibitor) for systemic hypertension. He has also been advised to reduce his caffeine intake after work.

The patient lives in a community that has an American Academy of Sleep Medicine (AASM) accredited Sleep Disorders Center, but the next available appointment is in 3 months. The patient's physician contacted the Center, and the director recommends consideration of an unattended portable sleep study in the patient's home (a home sleep test [HST]). The patient keeps an appointment during which he is evaluated by a physician sleep specialist for the probability of obstructive sleep apnea (OSA). The physician concludes that the patient probably has OSA based on his symptoms, including an Epworth Sleepiness Scale (ESS) score of 11 (normal <10) consistent with mild daytime sleepiness, a physical examination, and his BMI. The decision is made to educate the patient on how to use the portable monitor, which includes a pulse oximeter and also provides heart rate, a measure of respiratory effort, a measure of nasal/oral airflow, and a measure of body position. The patient used the monitor overnight and returned it the next day.

David Geffen School of Medicine at UCLA, 16111 Plummer Street, Sepulveda, CA 91343, USA
E-mail address: mlittner@ucla.edu

Sleep Med Clin 5 (2010) 99–108
doi:10.1016/j.jsmc.2009.09.004
1556-407X/10/$ – see front matter. Published by Elsevier Inc.

The portable study shows a respiratory disturbance index (RDI) of 20/h, which for this portable monitor equals apneas and hypopneas divided by recording time in hours. The RDI was 30/h when the patient was supine. Together with the patient's clinical history and physical examination, the sleep specialist reviewing the study considers this result to be consistent with a moderately severe OSA/hypopnea syndrome. The patient is offered one of several options that include a full night-attended polysomnogram (PSG) for continuous positive airway pressure (CPAP) titration, referral for an oral appliance (OA), or referral for upper airway surgery. The patient is counseled not to drive while sleepy, to lose weight, and to adhere to proper sleep hygiene practices, such as not drinking caffeine after midday, using the bed only for sleep and sex, and so forth. The patient elects to be referred to a dentist who specializes in treating patients with OSA with an OA, also called a mandibular advancement device.

A follow-up appointment 1 month after the fitting reveals that the patient is substantially less tired during the day, has stopped snoring, does not sleep in, and has become more productive at work. His wife now sleeps in the same bedroom. A repeat portable HST documents that the RDI is 4, which is consistent with elimination of significant OSA.

INTRODUCTION

OSA in adults is recognized predominantly by daytime somnolence and nighttime snoring, often in obese individuals.[2,3] The diagnosis is confirmed by demonstrating a sufficient number of obstructive apneas (absence of airflow with continued respiratory effort), obstructive hypopneas (reduction in airflow despite sufficient respiratory effort to produce normal airflow), or respiratory-effort–related arousals (RERAs; partial upper airway obstruction without significant reduction in airflow or saturation that terminates in an arousal) during sleep.[2] OSA seems to affect about 4% of men and 2% of women aged between 30 and 60 years.[4] The general nonspecificity of daytime sleepiness and snoring requires an objective measurement of apneas, hypopneas, and RERAs during sleep for confirmation of OSA.[3,5]

In general, confirmation involves an overnight sleep study while monitoring several respiratory channels, sleep staging by electroencephalogram (EEG), electrooculogram (EOG), and chin electromyogram (EMG), and leg movements may also produce frequent arousals.[6] The study is attended by a technician who performs and observes the study, ensures quality and safety, and makes needed interventions including application of CPAP, the most frequently used therapy. This approach is called attended PSG.

To increase access to diagnosis and potentially reduce cost, there has been an effort to produce monitors that incorporate part or all of the PSG and make it portable and ideally usable in the patient's home, without an attendant technician. Recent recommendations from the AASM and coverage determinations for CPAP from the Centers for Medicare & Medicaid Services (CMS) provide guidance for the use of portable monitors in the diagnosis of OSA.[7–9]

SUPERVISION OF AMBULATORY SLEEP MONITORING

Ambulatory sleep testing for OSA should be performed under the supervision of a sleep specialist. A sleep specialist is an individual who is certified in sleep medicine by either the American Board of Sleep Medicine or (since 2007) or is eligible to be certified by the American Board of Medical Specialties through one of the following boards: internal medicine, pediatrics, family medicine, otolaryngology, or psychiatry and neurology.[8] The following sections provide the rationale, procedures, and recommendations for the identification of patients, and types of ambulatory monitors, interpretation strategies, measurement of outcomes, and strategies for follow-up.

CLASSIFICATION OF METHODS FOR DIAGNOSIS OF SLEEP-DISORDERED BREATHING

The AASM in 1994[10,11] classified diagnostic sleep examinations into 4 types (**Table 1**). The classification begins with attended PSG (Type I) and subsequent types require no attendant (Type II) and fewer channels (Types III and IV) than are typically part of the attended and unattended PSG (Types I and II). The AASM recommendations of 2007[8] limited acceptable portable examinations to those that measured a minimum of airflow, oximetry, and respiratory effort, making a 3-channel monitor acceptable. However, all pulse oximeters measure heart rate, making such 3-channel monitors effectively 4-channel (a Type III examination). The CMS now accepts all 4 Types but has limited Type IV monitors to a minimum of 3 channels. CMS also does not require a direct measure of airflow to be part of a portable monitor.

Portable monitors are generally designed to be used unattended, usually in the patient's home. However, the monitors can also be used attended or unattended in the sleep laboratory.

THE PROPER STUDY DESIGN TO VALIDATE A PORTABLE MONITOR FOR HST

As discussed in a previous article,[12] validation of a particular monitor involves comparison to attended PSG, with determination of the sensitivity and specificity of the portable monitor. This comparison should be made in a patient population representative of the population using the method. Patient selection should be consecutive without undue referral biases or, at least, with the referral bias clearly defined and uninfluenced by the investigator or a small group of providers.

There are 2 approaches that should be used to validate a portable monitor. First, the sensitivity and specificity under ideal conditions should be determined in a simultaneous comparison with attended PSG using blinded assessment. If using the portable monitor with a technician to attend the study, then intervention is appropriate, whereas for unattended use, there should be no intervention to repair or correct possible data loss from the portable monitor. This provides the sensitivity and specificity for the diagnosis in direct comparison during the same real-time period as the PSG. The report should include the apneas and hypopneas during various patient positions for the PSG and portable monitor and the details of the intervention, if used. Ideally, the portable monitor should have a position monitor. If the monitor does not perform well in this setting, it is of questionable use. This comparison is for validation of attended or unattended in-laboratory use only.

The second step in the validation process is to compare the in-laboratory attended PSG (Type I in **Table 1**) to the portable monitor used in the intended environment in the patient's home, usually unattended. The study should be blinded and randomized and the PSG and portable monitor should be applied in every patient. The interval between studies should be short, preferably a week or less. Variables that may affect the results are body position, total sleep time, rapid-eye-movement (REM) sleep time, and environmental conditions, such as room temperature and extraneous noise. These contribute to normal night-to-night variability,[13] which may differ between laboratory and portable monitoring environment.

Table 1
AASM classification of types of studies of sleep apnea evaluation (with CMS modification)

	Type I	Type II	Type III	Type IV[a,b]
	Attended PSG	Unattended PSG	Modified portable sleep Apnea testing	Continuous single or dual bioparameter recording
Measures	Minimum of 7, including EEG, EOG, chin EMG, ECG, airflow, respiratory effort, and oxygen saturation	Minimum of 7, including EEG, EOG, chin EMG, ECG, airflow, respiratory effort, and oxygen saturation	Minimum of 4, including ventilation (at least 1 channel of respiratory movement and airflow), heart rate or ECG, and oxygen saturation	Minimum of 1: oxygen saturation, flow, or chest movement
Body position	Documented or objectively measured	Possible	Possible	No
Leg movement	EMG or motion sensor desirable but optional	Optional	Optional	No
Personnel	Yes	No	No	No
Interventions	Possible	No	No	No

Patterned after practice parameters for the use of portable recording in the assessment of obstructive sleep.[11] Six hours overnight recording is the minimum.

Abbreviation: ECG, electrocardiography.

[a] Type IV may also include any monitor that does not meet criteria for a higher type.

[b] CMS requires a Type IV monitor to measure at least 3 channels.

WHAT CAN BE EXPECTED FROM A COMPARISON OF A PORTABLE MONITOR WITH PSG

The concept that portable monitoring can be as diagnostically effective as PSG rests on the assumption that not all of the PSG-monitored channels are necessary to make a diagnosis of OSA. For this assumption to be valid, the definition of what constitutes a confirmatory study for OSA is important. The definition of an apnea is the cessation or near-cessation of airflow for 10 seconds or more that cannot be attributed to another cause or artifact. The definition of a hypopnea is more difficult. The current AASM manual on scoring requires one of the following to be true[1]: a 30% or greater reduction in airflow and a 4% desaturation or an EEG arousal[2] or a 50% or greater reduction in airflow and a 3% desaturation or an EEG arousal.[14] In addition, the AASM manual includes a RERA as

a respiratory event consistent with OSA. As discussed previously, a RERA does not require any obvious reduction in airflow or arterial oxygen saturation and is associated with an arousal. **Figs. 1–3** display typical tracings using 10-minute, 2-minute, and 1-minute epochs (time frames) that document apneas and hypopneas in patients with OSA on an HST using a Type III portable monitor. The longer time frame provides an overview of the patient's respiratory events, which is useful for counting the number of events and determining if a Cheyne-Stokes respiratory pattern (not seen in these figures) is present. The shorter time frame allows for close examination of each event for artifact and evidence, such as cardiac pulsations on the airflow channel to distinguish central from obstructive events. Only apneas and hypopneas can be detected with this approach.

Scoring of hypopneas differs between the AASM and CMS. The AASM criteria are the same

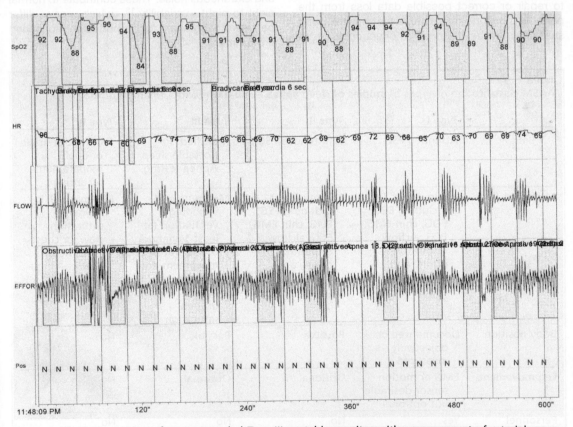

Fig. 1. A 10-minute tracing of an unattended Type III portable monitor with measurement of arterial oxygen hemoglobin saturation from a pulse oximeter (SpO2), heart rate (HR), nasal/oral airflow by nasal/oral pressure cannula (Flow), respiratory effort by chest wall movement (Effor), and supine (S) or nonsupine (N) position (Pos) by a position sensor. The tracing demonstrates a series of obstructive apneas (cessation or near cessation of airflow with continued respiratory effort) and hypopneas (30% or more reduced airflow with 4% arterial oxygen desaturations from preceding baseline), is typical of an entire night's tracing, and is consistent with severe OSA because the airflow is absent or reduced in the presence of continued respiratory effort.

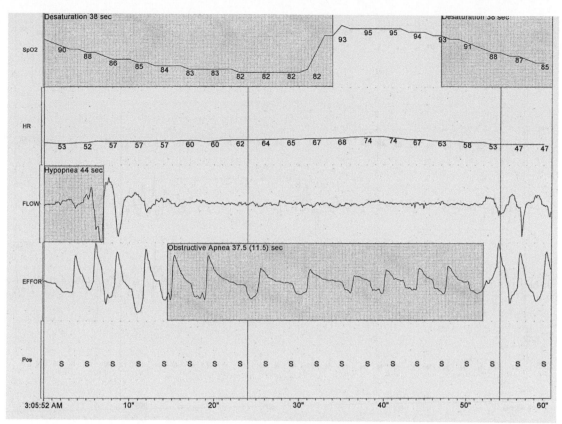

Fig. 2. A 1-minute tracing from a patient similar to that in **Fig. 1** to indicate the flexibility of the software of many portable monitors that permits review of the raw data and allows editing of the events, if necessary. In the example, a typical apneic episode is displayed. Abbreviations are the same as for **Fig. 1**.

for PSG and portable monitors. CMS criteria require that sleep be measured using traditional sensors in a facility-based sleep laboratory for PSG, they define hypopneas only as a 30% reduction in airflow or thoracoabdominal movement and a 4% desaturation, and they do not recognize RERAs. For portable monitors, CMS refers to an apnea/hypopnea index (AHI; apneas and hypopneas per hour of sleep or recording) and a respiratory disturbance index (RDI). The CMS scoring for the RDI may be identical to CMS scoring for AHI but may differ depending on the technology used, and it does not require a direct measure of airflow if the technology does not support it.[9]

If the goal is to define OSA by a combination of hypopneas associated with 4% desaturations and clear-cut apneas, a 2-channel monitor may be sufficient if the issues of sleep, central apneas (apneas without continued respiratory effort), and body position are not clinically relevant. On the other hand, if arousals are part of the definition of hypopneas, 2-channel and most Type III monitors would fall short in many patients, and if RERAs are also required, both monitors would most probably

be inadequate. The more types of events that are acceptable in making a diagnosis of OSA, the less likely it is that the portable monitor will detect most of them. Consequently, AASM requires at least airflow, respiratory effort, oximetry, and heart rate channels and CMS requires at least 3 channels for a portable monitor.

SLEEP STAGING

Portable monitors do not generally provide a measure of REM sleep and many do not provide body position. This makes it difficult to fully characterize the AHI or RDI result. For example, patients who snore and have severe daytime sleepiness may sleep mostly in the N2 and N3 non-REM stages, and they may have an AHI of 4 on one night but have normal stage R (REM) sleep on a second night with an AHI of 15. Most portable monitors do not have sleep staging and the interpretation of these 2 AHIs would be difficult. On the other hand, a PSG with sleep stages and with measurement of AHI, including arousals, and RERAs would

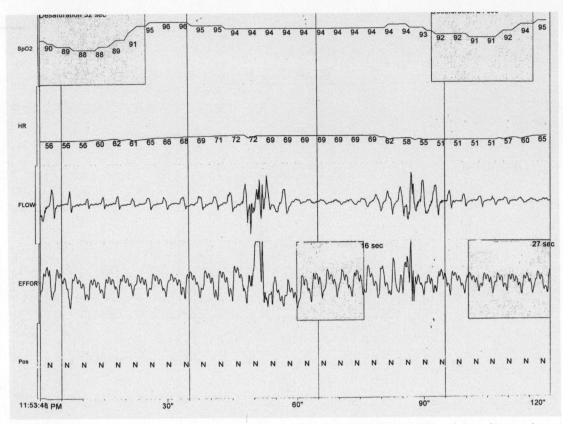

Fig. 3. A 2-minute tracing from a patient similar to that in **Fig. 1** to indicate the flexibility of the software of many portable monitors that permits review of the raw data and allows editing of the events, if necessary. In the example, a typical hypopneic episode is displayed at the 60-second mark with a resultant 4% arterial oxygen desaturation (from 95%–91%). The event preceding the hypopneic event does not qualify since the desaturation is only 2%. Abbreviations are the same as for **Fig. 1**.

provide important information in the interpretation of the study. In particular, an AHI of 4 in the first case would potentially prompt a second baseline study in a patient with a high probability of OSA, but in the case of the portable monitor an AHI or RDI of 4 might be interpreted as nonsignificant and the patient may not be properly evaluated. With a portable sleep study, because some patients may be awake for long periods during the night, a lack of sleep staging may lead to underestimation of the AHI or RDI during sleep.

THE APPROPRIATE AHI OR RDI DEFINITION OF OSA BY PORTABLE MONITORING

Historically, hypopneas (decreased airflow) and obstructive apneas have been used to characterize OSA, and studies have suggested that hypopneas may have the same clinical significance as apneas in many patients.[15] However, the standard method of measuring airflow with a thermistor may leave many hypopneas unrecognized.[16] Additionally, partial upper airway obstruction that leads to

increased amplitude of intrathoracic pressure can trigger an arousal (ie, a RERA), and such arousals may produce daytime sleepiness.[16,17]

Based on newer more sensitive technology, such as nasal pressure measurements instead of thermistors to measure airflow, definitions of hypopnea and respiratory events for research purposes were proposed, and they are now accepted by the AASM as set forth in the most recent scoring manual,[14] including syndrome definition using a composite AHI and RERAs greater than or equal to 5 for confirmation of OSA.[16]

As previously discussed, PSG is potentially capable of capturing all of the currently recommended respiratory events, whereas portable monitors, in general, capture only disturbances in airflow and saturation leading to an AHI or RDI, frequently underestimating the number of potential respiratory events during sleep (ie, apneas, hypopneas, desaturations, and RERAs). Depending on the technology and definitions used, AHI or RDI may vary considerably on the same night in the same patient.

CMS criteria require an AHI or RDI greater than or equal to 5 with symptoms of OSA, such as daytime sleepiness, or an AHI or RDI greater than or equal to 15, irrespective of symptoms. The recording must be for a minimum of 2 hours, and if sleep is recorded, the number must be the minimum that would be required for a 2-hour period of sleep.[9] A summary of the AASM and CMS diagnostic criteria for in-laboratory PSG and HST is provided in **Table 2**. Several situations are not currently defined.

The portable monitor user should be aware of its operating characteristics and must not rely on computer-generated scoring. The AASM requires that the data be displayed for manual scoring or editing of automated scoring. As mentioned previously, the portable monitor does not measure several events that may be recorded on the PSG, does not usually measure sleep, and may not measure position.[7]

Daytime sleepiness can occur in sleep disorders other than OSA.[3] The typical Type III portable monitor is of little use in these cases, and patients with daytime sleepiness and a negative portable monitor study should have the cause of the daytime sleepiness characterized. This will often require an attended PSG and possibly, a multiple sleep latency test (MSLT) that requires measurement of sleep staging.[3,18,19] MSLT testing consists of 4 or 5 attempted daytime naps, with measurement of the time taken to fall asleep on each nap being used as a measure of the patient's propensity to fall asleep during the day. Currently, the test is used mainly as a diagnostic test for narcolepsy, with a positive test result requiring REM periods to be recorded during at least 2 of the naps.[20]

TECHNICAL CONSIDERATIONS

As discussed earlier, the type of sensors may affect the results. For example, use of a thermistor is excellent for detection of apneas but fairly insensitive for detection of modest reductions in airflow.[14,16] Nasal pressure seems to be very

Table 2
Diagnostic criteria for treatments based on PSG or HST

Treatment	Procedure	CMS Asymptomatic and Without Associated Comorbid Conditions[a]	CMS Symptomatic or with Associated Comorbid Conditions	AASM Asymptomatic and Without Associated Comorbid Conditions	AASM Symptomatic or with Associated Comorbid Conditions
Positive airway pressure	Full-night diagnostic PSG	AHI ≥ 15	AHI ≥ 5	AHI ≥ 15	AHI ≥ 5
	Split-night diagnostic PSG	AHI ≥ 15	AHI ≥ 5	AHI ≥ 40	AHI ≥ 40[b]
	HST	AHI or RDI ≥ 15	AHI or RDI ≥ 5	Not indicated for diagnostic testing	AHI ≥ 15
Surgery	PSG or HST	Not specified	Not specified	AHI ≥ 15	AHI ≥ 5
Oral appliance	PSG or HST	Not specified	Not specified	Snoring or AHI ≥ 5	Snoring or AHI ≥ 5
Positional therapy	PSG or HST	Not specified	Not specified	Not specified	Snoring or AHI ≥ 5
Weight loss	PSG or HST	Not specified	Not specified	Not specified	Not Specified

[a] Asymptomatic means without daytime sleepiness or other symptoms typically associated with OSA. The patient may have snoring.
[b] AHI ≥ 20 based on clinical judgment (eg, if there are also repetitive long obstructions and major desaturations)— PSG; attended polysomnography in a facility-based sleep laboratory; HST: performed with an unattended Type II, III or IV monitor, for CMS, or an unattended home sleep test performed with a Type III monitor, for AASM; AHI: apnea/hypopnea/RERA index according to the criteria for AASM or apnea/hypopnea index according to the criteria for CMS; RDI: to be used when referring to apneas, hypopneas, and other technology-dependent events per recording or sleep hour, for CMS.

sensitive to reductions in airflow, but data loss may be a problem because of loss of signal or mouth breathing.[16] The AASM recommends that both be used in a portable monitor.[8]

Several studies have documented that the method of sampling the saturation signal with an oximeter is important in accurately measuring reductions in arterial oxygen saturation.[21,22] For example, an oximeter set at a 3-second recording rate produced almost twice as many 3% desaturations as a 12-second recording rate.[21] Furthermore, desaturations stored in oximeter memory may cause substantial underestimations of desaturations displayed in real time online at any recording rate.[22]

The method of scoring, manual versus automated, is also a consideration. Without the ability to manually review data, results will always be suspect because artifact may often mimic respiratory events. In general, automated scoring has been less accurate that manual scoring, which, however, takes considerably longer.[7] Additionally, the ability to independently calibrate and test the equipment is desirable for ensuring that equipment failure is not producing erroneous results.

THE EVIDENCE TO DATE

Based on the evidence from several reviews,[12,18] Type II and IV portable monitors, particularly unattended in the home, are not sufficiently accurate or validated for the AASM to recommend their use currently.[7] Type III monitors are useful when attended in the laboratory and of potential use when unattended in the laboratory or the home.

In October 2003, a joint task force of the AASM, the American College of Chest Physicians, and the American Thoracic Society published an evidence-based review (joint review) of portable monitors to determine if they can have an equivalent sensitivity and specificity to PSG.[12] Fifty-one publications with 54 studies were reviewed. Sensitivities and specificities were calculated in 49 of these studies. Since then, there have been several studies of Type III and IV monitors that have not substantially changed the evidence available for the use of portable monitors. Several of these studies up to 2006 have been summarized.[8,23] The studies do not support the use of Type III portable monitors in HST as a standalone approach to the diagnosis of OSA. However, the evidence does support the use of Type III portable monitors as part of a management approach, along with expert clinical evaluation and access to a sleep center, as necessary, to provide treatment for OSA and to further evaluate cases that are nondiagnostic on HST. This approach (as discussed in a previous publication and similar to that recommended by the AASM) is outlined in the following sections.

WHAT CAN BE SUPPORTED BY THE EVIDENCE

As discussed previously, based on the current evidence, attended and unattended Type III monitors with a minimum of airflow, oximetry, respiratory movement, and heart rate can be recommended under certain conditions. An additional sensor to measure body position and one to measure snoring is strongly recommended.

From evidence and strategic analyses, the use of a Type III portable monitor would seem to be more appropriate for diagnosing rather than excluding OSA for the following reasons:

1. A positive portable study (see **Figs. 1–3**), if properly performed in a patient with clinical features of OSA, has a high degree of specificity and positive predictive value.
2. A negative or nondiagnostic portable study should be followed usually with an attended PSG, because the portable monitor study
   (a) is less likely to detect other evidence of OSA, including RERAs and subtle hypopneas and does not allow the determination of REM AHI.
   (b) does not diagnose other disorders contributing to the patient's clinical presentation, such as periodic limb movement disorder.

Based on considerations similar to these , the AASM guidelines recommend that unattended Type III studies are acceptable for diagnosis if the AHI is greater than or equal to 15 based on manual scoring and if there is careful follow-up of negative studies including, in most cases, a PSG for confirmation.[7,8]

This article has concentrated on the diagnosis of OSA without considering that PSG is used to monitor CPAP titration during sleep. To date, there seems to be only one study that examined a Type III portable monitoring montage to titrate CPAP during an attended study.[24] The use of an attended portable monitor to make a diagnosis during the first half of the night followed by a CPAP titration during the second half of the night (split-night study) has also not been examined. For these reasons, use of a portable monitor to diagnose and titrate CPAP cannot be well-supported by evidence. To date, although there should not be any reason to doubt its utility, there is no data about the use of portable monitoring to diagnose OSA followed by treatment with an OA. However, AASM practice parameters and guidelines[8,18,25] recommend that treatment with an OA or surgery be followed with an attended PSG or portable monitor study, for evaluation of the efficacy of the treatment.

OTHER CRITERIA THAT SHOULD BE PRESENT TO CONSIDER THE USE OF AN HST

In the proper setting, with appropriate patient selection, and careful follow-up, including ready access to attended PSG, home portable studies are feasible and recommended by the AASM.[8] The following conditions are recommended:

1. A high pretest probability (ie, a high prevalence of OSA in the patient population). There are several equations that estimate pretest probability for OSA and use readily available data such as BMI, sex, history of snoring, neck circumference, and so forth or other data, such as radiographs of the upper airway with cephalometric measurements.[18,26–31]
2. The availability of attended PSG (Type I study) for patients with a strong clinical history and a negative or nondiagnostic portable monitoring study.
3. The availability of treatment and appropriate follow-up.
4. An experienced sleep practitioner, ideally a board-certified sleep specialist, who is capable of evaluating the clinical, portable monitoring and, if necessary, PSG information.

The approach to CPAP titration is beyond the scope of this article, but there has been a trend toward using autotitrating CPAP (APAP) machines unattended in the patient's home. Evidence-based guidelines published by the AASM[32] recommend such an approach as an option.

Cost-effectiveness should be considered but is beyond the scope of this article. However, it is not obvious that portable monitoring will inevitably reduce costs. One analysis of the use of a laboratory-attended Type III portable monitor suggests that this is may be more cost-effective than performing attended PSGs on all patients.[33]

The following points summarize the case that was presented at the beginning of this article. The patient had a history and physical examination that was consistent with OSA. There was a substantial delay in obtaining a laboratory-based PSG. It was reasonable to perform an unattended portable Type III study as an HST. The results were consistent with moderate OSA, and an OA is an option for treatment.[25] The overall approach was supervised by a sleep specialist and resources were available to ensure that the patient would be fully evaluated and treated. This study illustrates the use of portable monitoring as part of

an integrated clinical pathway in which the evaluation is pursued until a patient's diagnosis is obtained, therapy instituted, and appropriate follow-up organized.

REFERENCES

1. Mallampati S, Gatt S, Gugino L, et al. A clinical sign to predict difficult tracheal intubation: a prospective study. Can Anaesth Soc J 1985;32:429–34.
2. Bassiri AG, Guilleminault C. Clinical features and evaluation of obstructive sleep apnea-hypopnea syndrome. In: Kryger MH, Roth T, Dement WC, editors. Principles and practice of sleep medicine. 3rd edition. Philadelphia: W.B. Saunders Company; 2000. p. 869–78.
3. American Academy of Sleep Medicine. International classification of sleep disorders. In: Sateia MJ, editor. Diagnostic and coding manual. 2nd edition. Westchester (IL): American academy of sleep medicine; 2005. p. 51–5.
4. Young T, Palta M, Dempsey J, et al. The occurrence of sleep-disordered breathing among middle-aged adults. N Engl J Med 1993;328:1230–5.
5. Resta O, Foschino-Barbaro MP, Legari G, et al. Sleep-related breathing disorders, loud snoring and excessive daytime sleepiness in obese subjects. Int J Obes Relat Metab Disord 2001;25: 669–75.
6. Hening WA, Allen RP, Earley CJ, et al. Restless legs syndrome task force of the Standards of Practice Committee of the American Academy of Sleep Medicine. An update on the dopaminergic treatment of restless legs syndrome and periodic limb movement disorder. Sleep 2004;27:560–83.
7. Chesson AL Jr, Berry RB, Pack A. Practice parameters for the use of portable monitoring monitors in the investigation of suspected obstructive sleep apnea in adults. Sleep 2003;26:907–13.
8. Collop NA, Anderson WM, Boehlecke B, et al. Clinical guidelines for the use of unattended portable monitors in the diagnosis of obstructive sleep apnea in adult patients. J Clin Sleep Med 2007;3:737–47.
9. Continuous Positive Airway Pressure (CPAP). Therapy for Obstructive Sleep Apnea (OSA). Available at: http://www.cms.hhs.gov/transmittals/downloads/R96NCD.pdf. Accessed May 5, 2009.
10. Ferber R, Millman R, Coppola M, et al. Portable recording in the assessment of obstructive sleep apnea. Sleep 1994;17:378–92.
11. Practice parameters for the use of portable recording in the assessment of obstructive sleep apnea. Standards of Practice Committee of the American Sleep Disorders Association. Sleep 1994;17:372–7.

12. Flemons WW, Littner MR, Rowley JA, et al. Home diagnosis of sleep apnea: a systematic review of the literature: an evidence review cosponsored by the American Academy of Sleep Medicine, the American College of Chest Physicians, and the American Thoracic Society. Chest 2003;124: 1543–79.

13. Le Bon O, Hoffmann G, Tecco J, et al. Mild to moderate sleep respiratory events: one negative night may not be enough. Chest 2000;118:353–9.

14. Iber C, Ancoli-Israel S, Chesson A, et al. AASM manual for the scoring of sleep an associated events: rules, terminology and technical specifications. 1st edition. Westchester (IL): American Academy of Sleep Medicine; 2007. p. 45–50.

15. Gould GA, Whyte KF, Rhind GB, et al. The sleep hypopnea syndrome. Am Rev Respir Dis 1988;137: 895–8.

16. Anonymous. Sleep-related breathing disorders in adults: recommendations for syndrome definition and measurement techniques in clinical research. The Report of an American Academy of Sleep Medicine Task Force. Sleep 1999;22:667–89.

17. Guilleminault C, Stoohs R, Clerk A, et al. A cause of excessive daytime sleepiness. The upper airway resistance syndrome. Chest 1993;104: 781–7.

18. Kushida CA, Littner MR, Morgenthaler T, et al. Practice parameters for the indications for polysomnography and related procedures: an update for 2005. Sleep 2005;28:499–521.

19. Littner MR, Kushida C, Wise M, et al. Practice parameters for clinical use of the multiple sleep latency test and the maintenance of wakefulness test. Sleep 2005;28:113–21.

20. American Academy of Sleep Medicine. International classification of sleep disorders. In: Sateia MJ, editor. Diagnostic and coding manual. 2nd edition. Westchester (IL): American Academy of Sleep Medicine; 2005. p. 81–6.

21. Davila DG, Richards KC, Marshall BL, et al. Oximeter's acquisition parameter influences the profile of respiratory disturbances. Sleep 2003;26:91–5.

22. Davila DG, Richards KC, Marshall BL, et al. Oximeter performance: the influence of acquisition parameters. Chest 2002;122:1654–60.

23. Littner MR. Polysomnography and cardiorespiratory monitoring. In: Kushida CA, editor. Obstructive sleep apnea; diagnosis and treatment. New York: Informa Healthcare USA, Inc; 2007. p. 35–60.

24. Montserrat JM, Alarcón A, Lloberes P, et al. Adequacy of prescribing nasal continuous positive airway pressure therapy for the sleep apnoea/hypopnoea syndrome on the basis of night time respiratory recording variables. Thorax 1995;50: 969–71.

25. Kushida CA, Morgenthaler T, Littner MR, et al. Practice parameters for the treatment of snoring and obstructive sleep apnea with oral appliances: an update for 2005. Sleep 2006;29:240–3.

26. Gurubhagavatula I, Maislin G, Pack AI. An algorithm to stratify sleep apnea risk in a sleep disorders clinic population. Am J Respir Crit Care Med 2001;164: 1904–9.

27. Flemons WW, Whitelaw WA, Brant R, et al. Likelihood ratios for a sleep apnea clinical prediction rule. Am J Respir Crit Care Med 1994;150:1279–85.

28. Viner S, Szalai JP, Hoffstein V. Are history and physical examination a good screening test for sleep apnea? Ann Intern Med 1991;115:356–9.

29. Netzer NC, Stoohs RA, Netzer CM, et al. Using the Berlin Questionnaire to identify patients at risk for the sleep apnea syndrome. Ann Intern Med 1999; 131:485–536.

30. Kushida CA, Efron B, Guilleminault C. A predictive morphometric model for the obstructive sleep apnea syndrome. Ann Intern Med 1997;127:581–7.

31. Tsai WH, Remmers JE, Brant R, et al. A decision rule for diagnostic testing in obstructive sleep apnea. Am J Respir Crit Care Med 2003;167:1427–32.

32. Morgenthaler TI, Aurora RN, Brown T, et al. Practice parameters for the use of autotitrating continuous positive airway pressure devices for titrating pressures and treating adult patients with obstructive sleep apnea syndrome: an update for 2007. An American Academy of Sleep Medicine report. Sleep 2008;31(1):141–7.

33. Reuven H, Schweitzer E, Tarasiuk A. A cost-effectiveness analysis of alternative at-home or in-laboratory technologies for the diagnosis of obstructive sleep apnea syndrome. Med Decis Making 2001; 21:451–8.

Orofacial Myology and Myofunctional Therapy for Sleep Related Breathing Disorders

Abbey Cooper, MA, CCC-SLP

KEYWORDS
- Myofunctional therapy • Orofacial myology
- Mouth breather • Tongue thrust • Lip seal

In the management of sleep related breathing disorders, the role of the speech therapist or speech-language pathologist in orofacial myology or myofunctional therapy, is in the early stages of being recognized. The main goal of this treatment is to develop improved tongue posture and enhanced nasal breathing. This was demonstrated in a study where oropharyngeal exercises reduced the severity and primary symptoms of obstructive sleep apnea.[1] Because this form of treatment is little known and is not a standard of care, this article explores the role of orofacial myology in the management of patients with sleep breathing disorders.

OROFACIAL MYOLOGY AND MYOFUNCTIONAL THERAPY

Orofacial myology is the scientific study of the oral and facial muscles—how they work in harmony or demonstrate "abnormal variations of the function thereof".[2] The term "tongue thrust" is frequently associated with orofacial myofunctional disorders. Tongue thrust is the inappropriate or constant lingual pressure or contact on or between the teeth, at rest and during function. An orofacial myofunctional disorder is any pattern involving the oral/orofacial musculature that may lead to abnormal facial growth and function. Myofunctional therapy involves establishing, stabilizing, and reinforcing a healthy oral environment and facilitating the use of orofacial muscles to promote normal growth and development, and proper tongue posture and breathing patterns.

COMMON SIGNS OF MYOFUNCTIONAL DISORDER?

The International Journal of Orofacial Myology has published a list of the most common signs of myofunctional disorder in a patient.[3] Many of these signs are found in patients who are at risk for sleep apnea or have sleep-related breathing disorders. These signs are:

FACTORS IN HEAD AND NECK GROWTH AND DEVELOPMENT THAT INFLUENCE OROFACIAL STRUCTURES

The area of the head and neck is a key area for growth and development from infancy to adolescence.[4] Within this region, the tongue is a major muscle and a large component in head and neck development. Throughout adult life, the genioglossus (GG) muscle affects and modulates the head and neck system in relation to breathing. Poor positioning of the tongue affects breathing and allows a series of events to occur that can affect the orofacial complex.[4] During an evaluation, a patient generally presents with decreased tone and mobility in the cheek, tongue, lip, and soft

Front Range Speech-Language Pathology, Inc, 7901 East Belleview Avenue, Suite 200, Englewood, CO 80111, USA
E-mail address: rmc4e@aol.com

Sleep Med Clin 5 (2010) 109–113
doi:10.1016/j.jsmc.2009.10.002
1556-407X/10/$ – see front matter © 2010 Published by Elsevier Inc.

- Predominately vertical facial growth
- High narrow palate
- Narrow nostrils

- Maxillary hypodevelopment
- Class II, overjet, crossbite, openbite
- Incisal protrusion
- Hypofunction of the mandibular muscles
- Hypofunction of the lips and cheeks

- Hypertrophy of gums/tissue, frequent bleeding
- Dry, chapped lips, sores on lips

- Short, retracted upper lip with a large, outward lower lip or lip placed between teeth
- Articulation errors in speech, excessive saliva, anterior or lateral lisping

- Altered oral sensation
- Allergic shiners

- Poor head/neck posture, forward and tipped posture
- Shoulders rolled forward
- Mouth breathing
- Audible tongue thrust, forward protrusion of the tongue
- Excessive contraction of the mentalis muscle

- Ineffective chewing and swallowing pattern causing choking and excessive belching, gas, and "stuck" sensation
- Vocal quality changes

palate, and sensory alterations with poorly coordinated nasal breathing.[5]

In a baby, tongue position encompasses nearly the entire oral cavity or mouth, as the infant's main objective is to suck for nutrition and comfort. Babies are unable to breathe through their mouths unless they are screaming, when the seal between the soft palate and the epiglottis is broken, and in turn, pulls the larynx downward.[4] In the condition referred to as soft palatal epiglottal lock-up in infants, the epiglottis and the inferior tip of the soft palate are in contact.[6] This epiglottal lock-up is lost as a direct result of the acquisition of speech and the descent of the larynx. It has been suggested that the loss of the epiglottal lock-up contributes to airway compromise by causing the tongue base to collapse more readily into the oropharyngeal airway.

From 2- to 6 years, the child learns to balance, to use body muscles to be upright, and to use the tongue and facial muscles for speech. During this period the hyoid descends to a position approximately two-thirds of the way down the pharynx, causing the attachment of the base of the tongue to be repositioned. This repositioning allows the articulation of vowels and consonants. This is also the time when the mixed dentition is present. The shift of the larynx is completed between 5-and 6 years, and the tongue, hyoid, and larynx rest in the adult position between C5 and C6. At age 6 years, the tongue should be resting in a natural position with most of the weight following the anterior wall of the throat, and the body of the tongue connecting with the hard and soft palates.[4]

The upward and forward thrust of the tongue is the main feature of the well-positioned hyoid. When the hyoid is positioned too high, it disrupts the breathing and phonatory processes. The muscles important for speech, swallowing, nose breathing, and facial expression, are the temporalis, masseter, zygomaticus major, buccinator, and levator labii superioris. The movement of these muscles facilitates the widening of facial structures to allow air to pass through the nasal cavity and the opening of the pharynx, allowing air to be pulled into the lungs with the contraction of the diaphragm.[4] The act of chewing requires the tongue to be in the floor of the mouth and to move in a forward-downward pattern to allow the food to remain in-between the teeth. The muscles important for chewing include the temporalis and masseter muscles and the ptyerygoid muscles, that are aids to the masseter muscle. When the tongue is in a low-forward position for tasks such as breathing, swallowing, and speech, it must be adjusted to ensure stability for all these functions.

MYOFUNCTIONAL THERAPY

What are the goals of myofunctional therapy? The goals of therapy depend on the patient and should be customized accordingly. In general, the goals include control of the extrinsic tongue muscles to correct, stabilize, and maintain breathing, speech, swallowing, and chewing, and the enhancement of tone and mobility of the oral, orofacial, and cervical structures[5] to place the tongue in a "proper posture during function and at rest."[7]

Myofunctional therapy is primarily a series of exercises designed to improve tongue position and tongue function, improve the lip seal, and enhance nasal breathing. Oropharyngeal exercises target the tongue, soft palate, lateral pharyngeal wall, and lips and are derived from the principles of speech language pathology.[1,5] The first step in therapy is the elimination of noxious habits including thumb or digit sucking, mouth breathing, biting or chewing on objects, and improper head, neck and body posture.

Mouth breathing places the pharynx and upper esophageal sphincter in a negative relationship and thus promotes deficits. These include shallow clavicular breathing, tonguethrust swallowing, poorly coordinated tongue posture, non- precise speech, and phonation-breathy, low toned voice due to poor respiratory function and support.[8] Snoring and apnea patients present with a significant reduction in the tone and sensory awareness of the upper airway musculature due to the persistent negative pressure and weight of these structures during the night.[5] Upper airway dilator muscles are important in maintaining the pharyngeal airway opening.[1] At the same time, the styloglossus muscle raises the tongue to make a seal with the soft palate to allow for nasal breathing and prevent unnecessary mouth breathing.[4]

Swallowing exercises and therapy are important to allow for smooth deglutition. When the hyoid rests too high or the muscles are extremely tense, the swallow reflex is initiated too soon. In addition, the mastication phase is shortened and does not allow enough time for the food to be ground and mixed with saliva;and this, in turn, causes the oral stage of swallowing to be incomplete. As a result, dysphagia, aspiration, reflux, globus sensation, and other digestive problems can occur. Proper swallowing also allows for the aeration of the middle ear via the Eustachian tube and can decrease the occurrence of otitis media.[8]

Tongue thrust occurs along with the swallowing mechanism. When a person has tongue thrust, there is increased tone in the palate affecting the velopharyngeal area, the hyoid, the mentalis, the buccinator, and the neck and chest muscles. Due to increased tone in the chest cavity, a small expiration of air that follows the act of swallowing is missed. This release of air is necessary to allow the larynx to lower and return to a natural resting position.[8]

A study published by Guimaraes and colleagues in 2009[1] in the American Journal of Respiratory and Critical Care Medicine, stated that upper airway dilator muscles play a major role in the maintenance of the pharyngeal wall and are a factor in the origin of obstructive sleep apnea syndrome (OSAS). Participants in this study presented with moderate OSAS, were between the ages of 25 yearsand 65 years, and had completed a course of myofunctional therapy. The participants received oropharyngeal treatment including passive and active exercises involving the soft palate, tongue, and facial muscles, executed for 20 minutes each, 2 times a day. After 2 months, the control group experienced no change whereas patients in the treatment group had decreased neck circumference, snoring symptoms, perceived daytime sleepiness, and apnea hypopnea index (AHI) scores. Their scores on the Epworth Sleepiness Scale decreased by 6 points. There was evidence that oropharyngeal exercises reduced pharyngeal collapsibility during sleep and improved perceived daytime symptoms. This is presumably related to improved tongue position or posture, better nasal breathing with reduced mouth breathing and associated improvement in maintaining a comfortable and relaxed lip seal.

TONGUE MUSCLE PHYSIOLOGY

Much of the rationale for myofunctional therapy is based on the effects of negative pharyngeal pressure in the airway that is associated with sleep related breathing disorders and their adverse effect on tongue posture. Under normal conditions, in the supine position the GG muscle presents high amplitude background activity, and during inspiration promotes transient bursts of activity to facilitate the opening of the airway. This activity produces forward posturing or protrusion of the tongue. In quiet sleep the activity of the GG is similar to that seen while awake.[9] Horner[10] has reported that the GG is controlled by various neuromodulators responding via the hypoglossal motor nucleus. The neurochemicals histamine, norepinephrine, acetylcholine, orexin, and serotonin have a direct effect on GG activity through this motor nucleus. However, when the activity of these neurochemicals is decreased or the stimulus lost, there is a decreased level of muscle activity. This may be associated with neurogenic changes that are associated with changes in the output from the hypoglossal motor nucleus[11] and ultimately leads to the collapse of the GG into the pharyngeal airway during sleep. In OSAS patients, associated with these changes is an increase in GG activity during wakefulness.[12]

The muscles of importance in the area of the tongue are the GG, the muscles related to the hyoid, and the muscles that control the soft palate. The activity of these muscles is related to the activity of the diaphragm. If there is an increase in the activity of the diaphragm, then the muscles that act to dilate and stiffen the airway become more active. The pharyngeal muscles are affected by negative pressure that may develop within the airway with apnea. This is referred to as the negative pressure reflex (NPR).[13] As negative pressures develop, there is also an increase in the NPR that leads to an increase in muscle dilator activity. This increased activity is unable to sustain the airway against the increase in negative pressure.

The nasal airway is also important, as it affects the activity of the GG. With mouth breathing, the upper airway muscles exhibit a decreased level of electromyographic (EMG) activity.[14]

The upper airway muscles have an increase in EMG activity when the route of breathing is solely through the nose. The hypothesis is that receptors in the nasal mucosa may modulate this muscle activity. With nasal breathing there is an increase in GG activity and decrease in the tendency for the airway to collapse.[15] Mouth breathing leads to a decreased level of EMG activity in the upper airway that can lead to its collapse. This is further complicated by the fact that in the supine position, with mouth breathing, the mandible is displaced posteriorly and thus additionally compromises the airway.

The activity of the GG muscle is also affected by the various levels of PO_2 and PCO_2. As repetitive hypoxic episodes occur there is a decrease in GG activity. However with sustained hypoxia there is no decrease in GG activity. This may explain why some patients with sleep apnea present an improvement with the use of supplemental oxygen. In contrast, with an increase in CO_2 levels (hypercapnia), there is an increase in GG activity as well as an associated increase in activity of the diaphragm.[13]

The GG muscle has been shown to have an increase in type II fast twitch fibers in the sleep apnea patient.[16] These fibers are more susceptible to fatigue in patients with sleep apnea when compared with normal subjects,[16] since increased GG activity is potentially the equivalent of an increase in negative pressure in the airway.[17] In addition, as demonstrated by Douglas, during non-rapid eye movement (NREM) sleep when there is an increase in airway resistance, the GG does not show increase in activity.[18] In fact, GG activity via a negative-pressure reflex responded adequately and appeared to be maintained to some degree during NREM sleep, but decreased during rapid eye movement (REM) sleep.[19] It was found that an inhibitory reflex to GG activity appeared in NREM sleep and seemed to become more prevalent in REM sleep. In NREM sleep, suppression of GG activity was more profound than in REM sleep.[10] Increased levels of

suppressed activity then led to atonia. All of these findings explain why there is often an increase in the AHI in REM sleep. This additionally affects the tendency for upper airway collapse in people with anatomically narrow airways.

SUMMARY

Myofunctional therapy has been shown to have various effective treatment paths that can help with many problems. This is an important area of treatment to consider and implement in order to aid breathing and swallowing, and to promote harmonious muscle patterns and function. It is necessary to understand the effect of airway compromise on the tongue musculature, to appreciate the alterations that may occur, and the corresponding need to address them through this type of treatment. This therapy can best be provided by a trained/certified speech-language pathologist or orofacial myologist. There is a definite need for additional research to establish myofunctional therapy as an adjunctive treatment for patients with sleep related breathing disorders and those with the mouth breathing habit during the day.

REFERENCES

1. Guimaraes KC, Drager LF, Genta PR, et al. Effects of oropharyngeal exercises on patients with moderate obstructive sleep apnea syndrome. Am J Respir Crit Care Med 2009;179:962–6.

2. American Speech-Language Hearing Association. Orofacial myofunctional disorders: knowledge and skills [guidelines, knowledge, and skills]. 1993. Available at: www.asha.org/policy. Accessed August 2, 2009.

3. Marchesan I, Krakauer L. The importance of respiratory activity in myofunctional therapy. Int J Orofacial Myology 1996;22:23–7.

4. Caine A. How voice exercises can assist in orthodontic treatment. Presented at the 3rd Barcelona Orthodontic Meeting on Multidisciplinary Treatment in Orthodontics. Catalonian Dental Association, Barcelona, Spain, March 13–15, 2003.

5. Pitta DB, Pessoa AF, Sampaio AL, et al. Oral myofunctional therapy applied in cases of severe obstructive sleep apnea syndrome. Intl Arch Otorhinolaryngology 2007;11:350–4.

6. Davidson TM. The great leap forward: the anatomic basis for the acquisition of speech and obstructive sleep apnea. Sleep Med 2003;4:185–94.

7. Takahashi S, Kuribayashi G, Takashi O, et al. Modulation of masticatory muscle activity by tongue position. Angle Orthod 2005;75:35–9.

8. Demmink-Geertman L, Schouten S. Oral myofunctional diseases and the coordination therapy Dutch

Journal for Speech Therapists: Logopedie en Fonia-trie nr. April 5, 2001.

9. Harper RM, Sauerland EK. The role of the tongue in sleep apnea. In: Sleep apnea syndromes. New York: Alan R. Liss, Inc; 1976. p. 219–34.

10. Horner RL. Control of genioglossus muscle by sleep state-dependent neuromodulators. In: Integration in respiratory control from genes to systems. New York: SpringerLink; 2008. p. 262–7.

11. Saboisky JP, Butler JE, McKenzies DK, et al. Neural drive to human genioglossus in obstructive sleep apnea. J Physiol 2007;585:135–46.

12. Fogel RB, Malhotra A, Pillar A, et al. Genioglossus activation in patients with obstructive sleep apnea versus control subjects. Mechanisms of muscle control. Am J Respir Crit Care Med 2001;164(11): 2025–30.

13. Malhotra A, White DP. Pathogenesis of obstructive sleep apnea syndrome. In: Mc Nicholas WT, Phillipson EA, editors. Breathing disorders in sleep. Toronto (Philadelphia): W.B. Saunders; 2002. p. 44–63.

14. Basner RC, Simon PM, Schwartzstein SE, et al. Breathing route influences upper airway muscle activity in awake normal adults. J Appl Phys 1989; 66:1766–71.

15. Simon PM, Landry SH, Leiter JC. Respiratory control during sleep. In: Lee-Chiong TL, Sateia MJ, Carskadon MA, editors. Sleep medicine. Philadelphia: Hanley & Belfus; 2002. p. 41–51.

16. Schwab RJ, Kuna ST, Remmers JE. Anatomy and physiology of upper airway obstruction. In: Kryger MH, Roth T, Dement WC, editors. Principles and practice of sleep medicine. 4th edition. Philadelphia: Elsevier Saunders; 2005. p. 983–1000.

17. Fogel RB, Trinder J, Malhotra A, et al. Within-breath control of genioglossal muscle activation in humans: effect of sleep-wake state. J Physiol 2003;550: 899–910.

18. Douglas NJ. Respiratory physiology: control of ventilation. In: Kryger MH, Roth T, Dement WC, editors. Principles and practice of sleep medicine. 4th edition. Philadelphia: Elsevier Saunders; 2005. p. 224–31.

19. Eckert DJ, McEvoy RD, George KE, et al. Genioglossus reflex inhibition to upper-airway negative-pressure stimuli during wakefulness and sleep in healthy males. J Physiol 2007;581:1193–205.

Introduction to a Postural Education and Exercise Program in Sleep Medicine

David G. Austin, DDS, MS

KEYWORDS
• Respiration • Posture • Muscles • Exercises
• Temporomandibular dysfunction • Pain dysfunction

The evidence is compelling that dental sleep practitioners should thoroughly examine their patients for upper quarter pain and dysfunction, such as temporomandibular disorder (TMD), fibromyalgia, forward head posture (FHP), cervical dysfunction, dysphagia, and tongue thrusting.[1–28] If upper quarter pain and dysfunction is found, it should be addressed at the initiation of or along with oral appliance (OA) therapy. Moldofsky associated sleep disordered breathing with fibromyalgia.[17,18] The literature relates fibromyalgia and TMD as closely related disorders.[13,17,18,29,30] The 2001 National Heart, Lung and Blood Institute workshop related cardiovascular and sleep-related consequences of TMDs.[19] The 2006 American Academy of Sleep Medicine (AASM) Standards of Practice Committee found that OA therapy had a median adherence of 77% during the first year of appliance wear. Dropout rates were primarily related to OA intolerance. Development of temporomandibular joint (TMJ) disorder issues, such as headache and tooth, TMJ, masticatory, neck, and shoulder pain, were common reasons for

discontinued use of OAs.[20] A referral for physical medicine should be considered.[1–3,5,14,16,26]

The direct cause of upper quarter pain and dysfunction is inherent in the functional mechanism of a mandibular advancement device. By protruding the mandible to open and stabilize the airway, the entire upper quarter is biomechanically stressed. This increased workload is often beyond the patient's adaptive capacity and leads to pain and dysfunction. This situation is especially true for patients with preexisting upper quarter dysfunction.[1–3,14,20]

FHP is a global societal problem. It increases the temporomandibular condylar load, whereas sleep-disordered breathing increases sleep bruxism activities of the masticatory complex. In addition, with FHP the head weighs several times more, resulting in neck and shoulder muscle fatigue and potentially causing greater occipital nerve entrapment that facilitates headache and shoulder, head, neck, and jaw muscle hyperactivity and pain. Pain and muscle hyperactivity lead to increased constant loading and friction upon movement of

No funding or conflicts of interest.
Private Practice, Orofacial Pain, Headache, TMJ and Sleep Disorders, 3600 Olentangy River Road, Suite B-1, Columbus, OH 43214, USA
E-mail address: drdavidgaustin@hotmail.com

Sleep Med Clin 5 (2010) 115–129
doi:10.1016/j.jsmc.2009.11.002

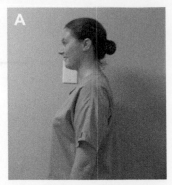
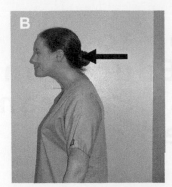
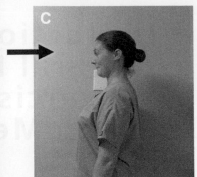

Fig. 1. Head and neck retraction "cranial glide." This stretch specifically targets the musculature of the upper neck (occipitals) and is used to assist in treating FHP. Initially, while you are learning this stretch it can be performed in front of a mirror. Stand up straight in good posture (A). With your eyes straight ahead, move your head forward (B) and backward (C) as far as possible. Do not raise or lower the head. Keep it straight. Do 3 sets of 10 each day.

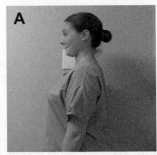
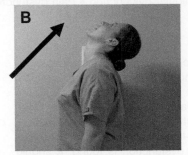

Fig. 2. Extension. This stretch targets the anterior neck musculature and assists in treating FHP. In conjunction with the head and neck retraction, begin a neck extension stretch. With the mandible relaxed, begin in the head retraction position with the teeth 5 to 10 mm apart (A), and tilt the head backward as far as possible (B). Do 3 sets of 10 each day. If you have complaints of pain with this stretch then start this stretch slowly. During the first week, begin the neck extension with 1 of 3 sets. During the second week, do the neck extension with 2 of the 3 sets. By the end of the third week, you should be doing neck extensions with all 3 sets.

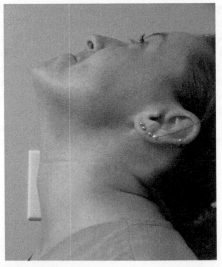
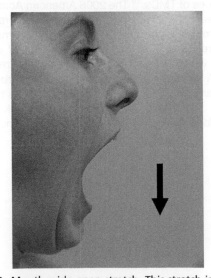

Fig. 3. Extension anterior neck stretch with jaw in protrusion. This stretch is indicated for patients with a complaint of dysphagia and/or anterior neck pain, especially the suprahyoid and infrahyoid muscles. This stretch is performed by tilting the head backward as far as possible with the mandible relaxed (mouth slightly open). When the head is fully extended, maximally protrude the mandible with a closing motion. Hold for 10 to 15 seconds. Do 3 times a day.

Fig. 4. Mouth wide-open stretch. This stretch is done for temple, cheek, teeth, TMJ, ear, or face pain. It directly lengthens the mandibular elevators, the temporalis, masseter, and medial pterygoid muscles. Stretch the mouth open as wide as possible. Hold for 10 to 20 seconds. Do as many times as needed but at least 3 times each day.

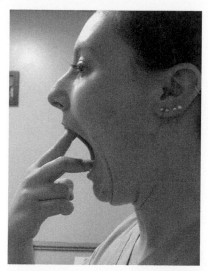

Fig. 5. Assisted opening stretch using finger pressure. This stretch is designed for mandibular hypomobility. This stretch can be held up to 30 seconds, but hold at least for 10 seconds. Do this stretch as many times as needed but at least 3 times a day.

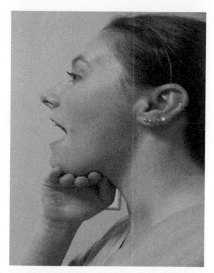

Fig. 7. Resisted opening. This exercise strengthens the mandibular depressors. The anterior digastric and the lateral pterygoid are considered the primary mandibular depressors, whereas the suprahyoid group, the geniohyoid, mylohyoid, stylohyoid, and digastric muscles can also function as accessory depressors. Do this exercise by applying light pressure against the mandible and resist opening over a count of 10 seconds. Repeat 3 to 5 times a day.

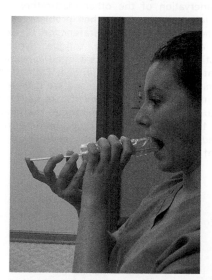

Fig. 6. Assisted opening stretch using tongue blades. This stretch is used for mandibular hypomobility. A tongue blade stretching apparatus is fabricated by stacking tongue blades to the patient's approximate mandibular opening. The tongue blades are held together loosely by a rubber band. A sandwich-sized plastic bag is placed over the tongue blades, which is then inserted between the anterior incisors. The assisted opening stretch is achieved by slowly sliding extra tongue blades into the tongue blade "stack," which thickens the stack by approximately 1.8 mm per tongue blade. This stretch is recommended for 30 seconds and can be increased up to 3 minutes with patient tolerance. Patients are instructed to apply moist heat before and/or during this stretch up to 15 minutes to relax muscles and increase stretch tolerance.

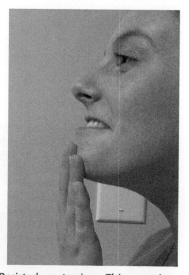

Fig. 8. Resisted protrusion. This exercise assists in strengthening mandibular protrusive movement performed by medial pterygoid and the inferior lateral pterygoid. Do this exercise by applying light pressure against the mandible and resist protrusion over a count of 10 seconds. Repeat 3 to 5 times a day.

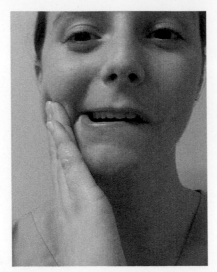

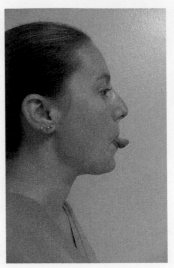

Fig. 9. Resisted lateral excursion. This exercise assists in strengthening the medial pterygoids. Do this exercise by applying light pressure against the mandible to resist lateral excursions over a count of 10 seconds. Repeat 3 to 5 times a day for each right and left lateral excursions.

Fig. 10. Tongue stretch. The tongue is often overlooked as a source of pain and dysfunction. However, the tongue is an integral part of the masticatory musculature system. It positions the bolus of food for mastication and swallowing. Considering it shares the innervation of the other masticatory elevator musculature, it also shares their problems of muscle hyperactivity and habits of parafunction. On examination, a common sign of tongue hyperactivity "thrusting or clenching" is a scalloped appearance to the lateral borders of the tongue. Patients should maximally extend the tongue and see if there is any discomfort with the movements. To perform the "tongue stretch" extend the tongue maximally for 10 to 15 seconds, then allow the tongue to relax. A relaxed tongue should have no sensation or awareness of tightness or discomfort.

the shoulder, head, neck, and jaw, which results in increased arthritic change in the upper quarter, especially C5 to C7, which becomes flexed with FHP, chronic FHP, TMD and fibromyalgia may result.[1–3,13,14,18,28]

Respiration is essentially an oxygen transportation pathway composed of an integrated series of components that are regulated by the central

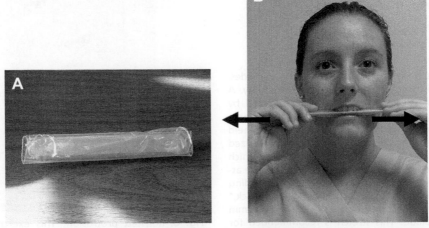

Fig. 11. Lateral excursion exercise. Place a tongue blade covered with a plastic wrap or a plastic sandwich bag (*A*) laterally between the anterior teeth. Stabilize the tongue blade with your hands while sliding your mandible side to side, performing full right and left lateral excursions (*B*). Perform 3 sets of 10 lateral excursion "warm-up" exercises each day. This exercise especially encourages articular surface health and repair through high-repetition low-force exercise, which circulates nutrient-laden synovial fluid.

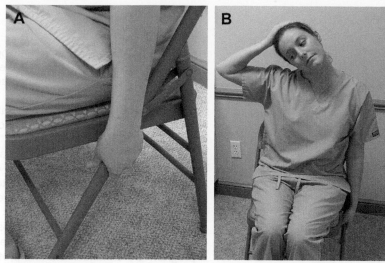

Fig. 12. Side-bending of the neck. This exercise targets the upper trapezius muscle. Begin by holding the side of your chair and sitting up straight (*A*). Slowly side-bend your head away from the side of the chair that you are holding. Place your free hand on the side of your head, and point your elbow straight out in the direction of the side-bend (*B*). Hold your head as a deadweight. Do not pull with your arm. Side-bend your head as far as possible, and hold the stretch for 10 seconds. Take a deep relaxation breath. As you exhale, let your neck and shoulder muscles relax, and the weight of your arm will gently side-bend your head. Hold the side-bend stretch for another 10 seconds; then perform the side-bend stretch for the opposite side. The side-bending stretch should be repeated at least 3 times a day.

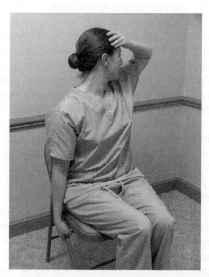

Fig. 13. Neck rotation. This exercise targets the levator scapulae muscle. Begin by holding the side of the chair and sitting up straight. Slowly turn (rotate) your head away from the side of the chair you are holding. Place your free hand on the side of your head, and point your elbow straight out in the direction you are rotating. Keep your eyes and head on the horizon. Hold your head as a deadweight. Do not pull. Turn your head as far as possible, and hold for 10 seconds. Then take a deep relaxation breath. As you exhale, let your neck and shoulder muscles relax, and the weight of your arm will gently rotate your head. Hold the rotation stretch for another 10 seconds. Then perform the rotation stretch for the opposite side. The neck rotation stretch should be repeated at least 3 times a day.

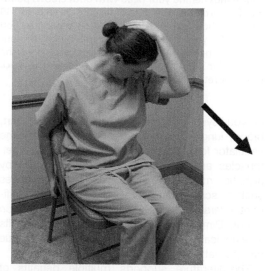

Fig. 14. 45° Neck flexion in sitting position. This stretch targets the upper and middle trapezius muscle along with posterior neck muscles, splenius capitis, splenius cervicis, and levator scapulae. Begin by holding the back corner of the chair, retracting your shoulder, and sitting up straight. Turn your head so you are looking directly at the opposite front corner of the chair, essentially a 45° angle. Place your free hand on the back of your head and point your elbow at the same 45° angle. Now, slowly lower your head forward (flexion) as far as possible at this 45° angle. Hold your head as a deadweight. Do not pull. Hold this stretch for 10 seconds, and take a relaxation deep breath. As you exhale, let your head relax, and the weight of your arm will gently pull your head forward in the 45° angle. Then hold this stretch for another 10 seconds. Repeat this stretch for the opposite side. Repeat the 45° angle stretch at least 3 times a day.

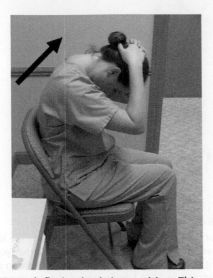

Fig. 15. Neck flexion in sitting position. This exercise targets the entire trapezius muscle along with the posterior cervical muscles. Begin by slowly lowering your head forward as far as possible (flexion). Place your hands behind your head with both elbows pointing forward. Do not pull. Hold this stretch for 10 seconds; then take a deep relaxation breath. As you exhale, let your head relax, and the weight of your arms will gently pull your head forward. Hold the stretch for another 10 seconds. Repeat the neck flexion stretch at least 3 times a day.

nervous system. These components are the heart, blood, lungs, and muscles. Muscles create the ventilator force for the exchange of gases. When muscles are inhibited by pain or restricted by arthritis, muscle weakness or fibrotic changes such as scar tissue and/or adhesions and significant overall reduction of oxygen transportation occur. Diminished oxygen transportation results in significant exercise limitation through fatigue and perpetuation of pain and dysfunction.[31–38]

The literature supports multiple benefits of a program of postural training, stretching, and exercise. Upper quarter muscular exercises, stretching, and deep breathing can potentially strengthen muscles of inspiration to increase vital capacity and expiratory airflow by reducing or eliminating tight muscle adhesions that increase the elastic recoil of the thorax and upper quarter. It is also postulated that deep breathing may increase alveolar surface area in lungs for enhanced transfer of respiratory gases. An exercise physiology principle states that lengthening a muscle by stretching increases the strength of that muscle's contraction. This principle explains the mechanism for increased vital capacity, exercise tolerance, and endurance. The medical literature provides many examples of respiratory

muscle and upper extremity training to address skeletal muscle dysfunction that created a ventilator limitation during exertion and exercise. Good posture assists respiration by reducing nerve entrapment and muscular fatigue and by creating and maintaining a mechanical advantage for respiratory muscle movement.[31–37,39–41]

Because the upper quarter plays such a vital role in respiration, the importance of a well-designed program of postural education and flexibility exercises cannot be overlooked for providing an improved ergonomic environment as well as maintenance of wellness and injury prevention. The benefits of a posture and exercise program are enhancement and protection of the airway; reduced incidence of headache, TMD, and upper quarter pain and dysfunction; and increased tolerance of and adherence to OA therapy.

POSTURAL EDUCATION AND EXERCISE PROGRAM
Reactive Exercise

Patients are instructed to maintain "body awareness" for sensations of pain and/or dysfunction. In addition, patients are taught to recognize the location of each stretching exercise, that is, "where each stretch stretches." Sensations such as pain, itching, burning, tightness, and pressure are to be considered as warning signals. Normally, a patient should feel nothing. A patient should have no sensation of discomfort and/or tightness. If patients sense that something is occurring then they should perform the stretch that "hits the spot." If the first stretch helped but did not eliminate the sensation then the stretch should be repeated. If there was no success then other stretches that affect that area should be attempted. Sometimes a combination of stretches is required to eliminate the problem. There is a learning curve, and the more the patients work with discomforting sensations, the better they will get at eliminating them.

Complainers

As patients learn their stretching exercises, they are instructed to sense the focus of each stretch, that is, "where each stretch stretches." In addition, patients are instructed to sense how each stretch feels. A normal healthy joint system should have full range of motion without pain or dysfunction. However, if the stretch produces a lot of discomfort then it should be noted as a "complainer." Patients are instructed to perform all exercises at least 3 times a day; however, "complainers" ask for special attention. Such

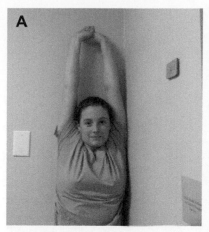 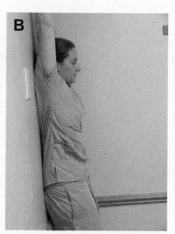 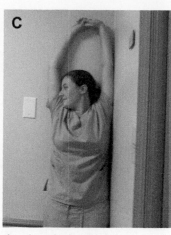

Fig. 16. Against-the-wall stretch. This stretch essentially targets the entire back, head, neck, shoulder, and scapular musculature to include important respiratory muscles, latissimus dorsi, scalene, sternocleidomastoid, intercostals, and the entire trapezius muscle with its attachments from occiput to the spinous processes C2 to T12. *Step 1*: Find an empty corner and stand up straight with your back against the wall. Take 1 step out and put your feet shoulder-width apart. Bend your knees as you lean backward against the wall pressing your entire back flat. Do not flatten your neck against the wall. Just relax the back of your head against the wall. Make sure the "corner" side of your body is against the wall. Raise your arms over your head as high as possible while keeping your arms close to the wall. Interlock your thumbs, and your fingers should touch the wall (*A*). Take a deep breath as you raise your arms, and hold this stretch for at least 10 seconds (*B*). Then exhale and relax and stretch your arms further. Repeat the stretch, and hold for another 10 seconds attempting to pull up higher with your arms and release. *Step 2*: With your arms down, rotate your head away from the corner wall and push your back flat against the wall (*C*). Then as you bring your arms up, lock your thumbs together and take a deep breath. Hold your breath and the stretch for 10 seconds. Make sure your fingers are touching the wall and as you take the deep breath, pull your arms up as high as possible. Take a deep relaxation breath. Make sure you always turn your head first, before you raise your arms up. After 10 seconds exhale and relax. Then repeat by taking another deep breath as you raise your arms as far as possible while turning your head further. Hold for another 10 seconds, and then exhale and relax. *Step 3*: Change walls so you can do the opposite side (remember, you have to turn [rotate] your head away from the wall). Repeat the directions of step 2. *Step 4*: Remain leaning against the wall. Make sure your entire back is flat against the wall and fingers are touching the wall. Repeat the directions of step 1.

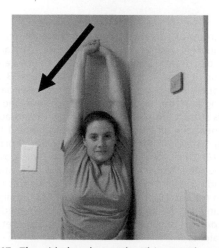

Fig. 17. The side-bend stretch. This stretch targets flank, chest, neck, and shoulder girdle muscles to include important respiratory muscles, especially latissimus dorsi and scalene. Find an empty corner as described in **Fig. 16**, step 1. Stand back flat against a wall with your feet at least shoulder-width apart, your arms raised over your head as high as possible, your thumbs interlocked, and your fingers touching the wall. Side-bend at the waist as far as you can and take a deep breath. Hold the stretch for at least 10 seconds. Repeat 3 times a day.

stretches should be done regularly at least once an hour. Stretching helps create and maintain muscle relaxation and pain reduction through increased flexibility, pliability, and extensibility. Without stretching and rest, pain causes muscle hyperactivity and increased loading of the injured joint system. Patients are instructed that they can eliminate extra stretching for complainers when they stop complaining.

Learning Good Posture for Reading

Reading with good posture is achieved by using a custom-fitted chair and headrest and sitting against the wall. A card table, adjustable music stand, or TV dinner tray table is used in this technique. While sitting against the wall, the patients are instructed to pull the table up to them. With the reading material held by the bookholder on music stand and properly aligned, reading should be easier, without any desire to bring the head forward. This position may be achieved by adjusting the book holder or music stand to eye level and focal length. With the patients' head, neck, and lumbar areas in good posture, they should be able to read as long as desired without feeling pain or fatigue.

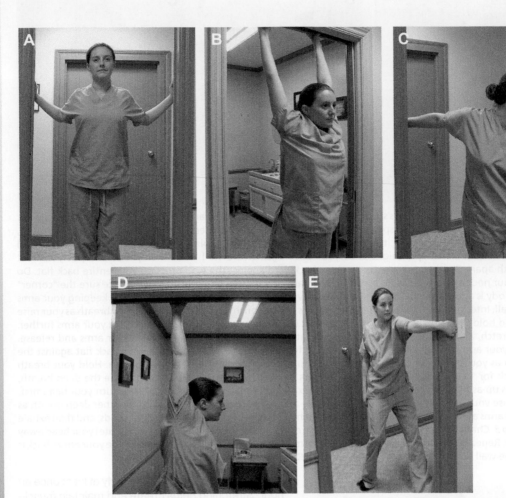

Fig. 18. Shoulder stretching exercises using a doorframe. This group of stretches focuses on the neck, scapular, shoulder, and chest musculature to help treat FHP, rounded shoulders, and muscles of respiration. (*A*) Standing in a doorway, place your hands chest high and flat against the doorframe. Lean forward as far as you can and take a deep breath. Hold the stretch and the deep breath for at least 10 seconds. Repeat at least 3 times a day. Variations of this stretch can also be performed with your hands placed higher or lower, essentially at any angle in the doorframe as in (*B*). With your hands flat against the doorframe, lean forward and take a deep breath and hold for 10 seconds. Other variations of this stretch are performed by using 1 hand against the doorframe placed at different angles as in (*C*) and (*D*). Repeat the directions for (*A*) but use only 1 hand; then repeat using the other hand. Another variation is placing 1 hand on the opposite side of the doorframe and leaning back as far as you can, such as in stretching exercise (*E*). Once you have leaned back as far as possible, take a deep breath and hold for 10 seconds; then repeat with the other hand. Another variation is performed by placing both hands on top of the doorframe while slowly bending your knees and leaning forward as in (*B*). Other variations are produced by turning the head as shown in (*C*) and (*D*), by twisting or turning the hip and low back, or by changing leg positions as shown in (*C*), (*D*), and (*E*). All stretches should be performed with a deep breath and should be held for at least 10 seconds. The patient is instructed to try the various stretching positions and focus on sore and tight musculature, the "complainers."

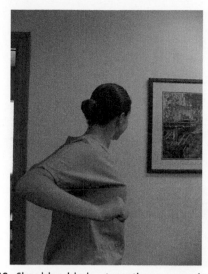

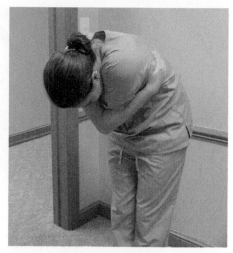

Fig. 19. Shoulder blade strengthener exercise. This exercise is intended to help correct FHP and round shoulders by strengthening overstretched and weakened muscles of the neck and shoulder. This stretch especially targets scapular muscles to include rhomboids and upper and middle trapezius. Retract arms and shoulders as far back as possible (try to touch shoulder blades). As you pull back (retract) your shoulders, take a deep breath. Hold for 3 seconds, and then relax by exhaling and returning your arms and shoulders forward for 1 to 2 seconds. Do the exercise in sets of 10 and repeat 3 times a day.

Fig. 21. "Hug yourself stretch" for shoulder blade pain. This stretch targets the rhomboid and the upper and middle trapezius muscles. Pull your shoulders forward as far as possible while wrapping your arms around you. Bend forward pulling shoulders forward, and then breathe deep and hold for up to 10 seconds. Do the exercise at least 3 times a day.

STRETCHING PROTOCOL FOR REDUCTION OF PAIN OR DYSFUNCTION

The patient is instructed to do the following:

1. Learn the location affected by each stretch, that is, "where each stretch stretches."
2. Be "body aware" for sensations. It is normal to feel absolutely nothing; no aberrant sensations

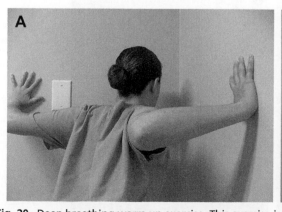

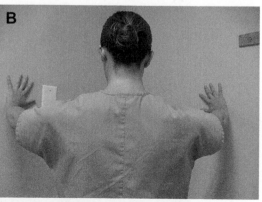

Fig. 20. Deep breathing warm up exercise. This exercise is intended to warm up and strengthen muscles of respiration and assist in eliminating muscular restrictions of respiration. In addition, this exercise assists in increasing the elastic recoil of expiration and lessens the resistive load of inspiration. This results in increased exchange of gases and increased stamina during exercise. This is especially important to the elderly. In the corner, place your hands flat against the wall. Feet should be approximately 2 ft away from corner. Keeping your head and back straight, lean into the corner as if doing a standing erect "push-up." Take a deep breath as you lean forward (*A*). Do not bump your head against the wall. Then push back as if doing a push-up and exhale (*B*). Repeat at least 5 times. This is a great exercise to do in the shower.

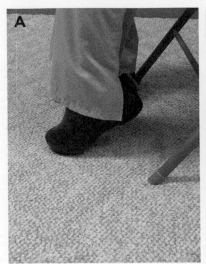
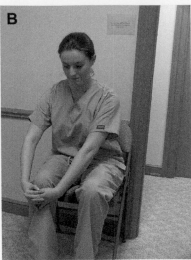

Fig. 22. Knee pull-shoulder blade exercise. This stretch targets the rhomboid and upper and middle trapezius muscles. Sit in a chair with 1 heel raised and toe touching the floor (*A*). Pull your shoulders forward as far as possible with your arms straight out (*B*). Wrap your hands around your raised knee. Lower your raised knee toward the floor while pulling backward with your upper back. When you feel the stretch across your shoulder blades, take a deep breath and hold for 10 seconds. Do this exercise at least 3 times a day.

of discomfort, tightness, burning, itch, or numb-tingling are to be tolerated.

3. If a sensation is noted, perform the stretch for that area.
4. If the sensation has partially diminished, wait a minute and repeat the original stretch.
5. If the sensation seems unaffected, perform other stretches in the region, taking note of their effect.

Sometimes it takes a combination of stretches to control a painful sensation. Good posture in sitting, use of moist heat packs and/or contrast of hot and cold packs to the region, and deep relaxation breathing may be helpful. There is a learning curve, and as patients work on their pain and dysfunction, they become empowered, gain confidence, and discover what works for

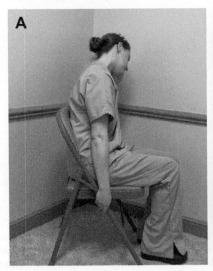
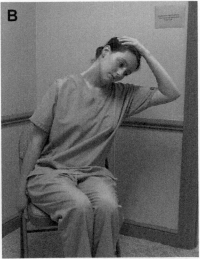

Fig. 23. The scalene stretch, part I. This stretch targets the anterior and middle scalene muscles. Sit up straight, using your right hand, grab a hold of the side bottom of your chair. Lean to the left as far as possible, stretching your right shoulder and neck (*A*), turn your head left as far as possible and tilt your head back (*B*). Hold this stretch for 10 seconds; then take a deep relaxation breath, exhale and allow the head to fall limp. Then continue to stretch for 10 more seconds. Repeat on the opposite side. Do 1 set 3 times a day.

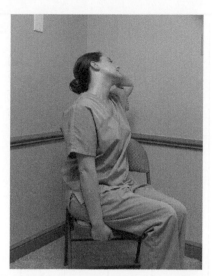

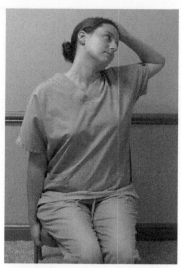

Fig. 24. The scalene stretch, part II. This stretch targets the middle and posterior scalene muscles. Sit up straight, with your right hand grab a hold of the front of your chair, turn your body approximately 45° to the left side, and tilt your head to the left side as far as possible. Hold this stretch for 10 seconds, take a deep relaxation breath, exhale, allow the head to fall limp, and then continue the stretch for 10 more seconds. Repeat on the opposite side. Do 1 set 3 times a day. After the first week of stretches, you may use your hand as a deadweight by placing it on top of your head.

them. Detailed descriptions of the recommended exercises are provided in **Figs. 1–25.**

In addition, the patient is instructed to be aware of the cause-and-effect relationships. In 1982, the author missed 8 full days of work because of migraine headache (all patients were canceled). They were all Mondays in the summer after a weekend of bending over, weeding, gardening, and trimming.

Table 1 demonstrates the symptom areas and the exercises in clinical practice in its entirety that need to be followed for pain management and to optimally improve respiration.

OTHER TECHNIQUES FOR LEARNING GOOD POSTURE

The author recommends a custom-fitted chair **(Fig. 26)** for watching TV. He also recommends going to the library and selecting movie DVDs. While you are sitting against the wall, if anything feels uncomfortable, fix it by readjusting the support layers.

While learning good posture, leave the neck support rolled towel unattached to the wall. If you start to slouch or slump forward, the towel

Fig. 25. Sternocleidomastoid stretch. This stretch targets the sternocleidomastoid muscle. Begin by holding the side of the chair and sitting up straight. Then rotate your head away from the side of the chair you are holding and place your free hand on the side of your head and point your elbow straight out in the direction you are rotating. As you rotate, keep your eyes and your head on the horizon and have your mandible relaxed (teeth apart). Upon full rotation, extend your head posteriorly as far as possible. Hold this stretch for 10 seconds, and take a deep relaxation breath. As you exhale, relax your neck and shoulder muscles. Hold the stretch for another 10 seconds. Then perform the sternocleidomastoid stretch for the opposite side. The sternocleidomastoid stretch should be repeated at least 3 times a day. *How to sit in good posture*: When sitting in good posture against the wall you should have your feet flat on the floor for a good foundation of support. You should wiggle your bottom and lower back in lumbar support area until comfortable support is achieved. Next you must address the question of what is to be done with your neck and shoulders. The answer is, let them relax against the wall. Do not force them against the wall, just let them relax. Your arms should fall loose with your hands and forearms resting on your thighs. Roll your shoulders a few times and take a deep relaxation breath, and let your shoulders relax and drop.

will fall forward and instantly alert you to bad posture. This instant feedback will assist you in learning good posture. Reposition the rolled towel for comfort and continue watching TV. The author recommends at least a few hours of TV or a movie a night. The author acquired good posture sitting in approximately 2 weeks. Once good posture while sitting becomes a habit, the rolled towel can be attached to the wall with Velcro. In addition, once good posture while sitting is a habit, a new

Table 1
Stretching protocol and guide

Symptomatic Area	Trigger Point Location	Stretch
TMJ	Deep masseter Temporalis Medial pterygoid Digastric	3, 4, 5, 8
Ear	Deep masseter Lateral pterygoid Sternocleidomastoid	4, 25 3, 4, 5, 8, 11, 12
Jaw	Superficial masseter Trapezius Digastric Medial pterygoid	4, 25
Cheek, teeth	Sternocleidomastoid Superficial masseter Entire temporalis	4, 25
Chin, face	Sternocleidomastoid	4, 8, 11
Gingiva	Superficial masseter Medial pterygoid	4, 12, 14, 15, 16, 25
Supraorbital	Sternocleidomastoid Temporalis Trapezius Occipital	14, 16, 25
Forehead	Sternocleidomastoid Splenius capitis Occipital	4, 12, 13, 14
Temple	Temporalis Trapezius Splenius capitis	3, 14, 25
Postauricular	Digastric Sternocleidomastoid Deep masseter	13, 14, 16, 25
Vertex	Splenius capitis Semispinalis capitis	

Symptom location	Muscles	References
Occipital	Trapezius, Levator scapulae, Semispinalis capitis	11, 13, 14, 16
Retro-orbital	Temporalis, Trapezius	4, 11, 13, 14
Maxillary teeth	Temporalis occipital	4, 14, 16
Maxillary molars	Temporalis occipital	4, 14, 16
Mandibular molars	Trapezius, Sternocleidomastoid	4, 11, 25
Mandibular incisors	Superficial masseter, Anterior digastric	3, 4
Throat	Sternocleidomastoid, Hyoids/anterior neck, Medial pterygoid	3, 4, 11, 23, 25
Mouth, tongue, and hard palate	Medial pterygoid, Digastric	4, 3, 11, 16
Maxillary sinus	Lateral pterygoid, Occipital	4, 14, 16
Anterior neck	Sternocleidomastoid, Anterior neck musculature	3, 23, 25
Blurred vision, Ptosis, Lacrimation	Sternocleidomastoid (sternal division), Anterior temporalis	4, 14, 16, 25
Dizziness, Tinnitus, Ear stuffiness	Deep masseter, Medial pterygoid	4, 14, 16
Salivation (excessive)	Medial pterygoid	4, 11
Sore throat	Medial pterygoid, Sternocleidomastoid, Hyoids/anterior neck musculature	3, 4, 11, 23, 25

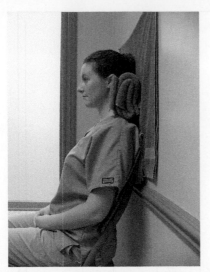

Fig. 26. Create a custom-fitted chair. Select a comfortably fitting padded folding chair that when sitting allows your feet to comfortably rest on the floor. Select a wall preferably across from a TV, so when you sit you will be looking directly at the TV. Thumbtack a bath towel lengthwise to the wall. Place the folding chair against the towel-covered wall. Then create a custom headrest using layers of cloth, such as old washcloths. Cut the washcloths in half. Then incrementally attach them to the wall behind your head with Velcro until the proper thickness is achieved. The proper thickness is where the weight of your head feels the least uncomfortable. The sensation of neck and shoulder musculature should be neutral. Roll up different towels until you find one that feels very comfortable when placed against the wall behind your neck. The custom neck support should not push your head forward. The back of your head should be resting comfortably against the wall with the arch of your neck filled in with the towel. The comfortable neck towel is then taped so that it does not unroll. Using layers of cloth incrementally attach them with Velcro to your folding chair's lumbar support area. As each layer is added, sense the feeling of support in your lower back. The proper thickness is achieved when your lower back feels maximally comfortable and well supported without strain, pressure, and/or discomfort.

habit of good posture while standing should be realized. The proprioception of the head and neck recognizes improper feet and/or hip positioning and encourages you to self-correct improper posture.

POSTURE RELATED TO SLEEP

Sleep posture is indeed a personal preference. However, anatomically correct posture significantly enhances ease of respiration, which is directly affected by biomechanical principles. Patients are taught the technique of altering sleep position to maximize ease of respiration. Through the use of pillows and layers of cloth, the head, neck, shoulder, leg, and low back positions are custom fitted to provide comfortable support to maximize respiration.

REFERENCES

1. Kraus SL. Cervical spine influences on the craniomandibular region. In: Kraus SL, editor. TMJ disorders: management of the craniomandibular complex. 2nd edition. New York: Churchill Livingstone; 1994. p. 325–412.
2. Manheimer JS, Dunn J. Cervical spine: evaluation and relation to temporomandibular disorders. In: Kaplan AS, Assael LA, editors. Temporomandibular disorders: diagnosis and management. Philadelphia: Saunders; 1991. p. 50–94.
3. American Academy of Orofacial Pain. Orofacial pain: guidelines for assessment, classification, and management. Chicago: Quintessence; 2008.
4. Attanasio R. An overview of bruxism and its management. Dent Clin North Am 1997;41:229–41.
5. Bailey DR. Oral evaluation and upper airway anatomy associated with snoring and obstructive sleep apnea. Dent Clin North Am 2001;45: 715–32.
6. Bailey DR. Sleep disorders: overview and relationship to orofacial pain. Dent Clin North Am 1997;41: 189–209.
7. Paiva T, Batista A, Martins P, et al. The relationship between headaches and sleep disturbances. Headache 1995;35:590–6.
8. Sahota RK, Dexter J. Sleep and headache syndromes: a clinical review. Headache 1990;30: 80–4.
9. Schiffman E, Heley D, Baker C, et al. Diagnostic criteria for screening headache patients for temporomandibular disorders. Headache 1995; 35:121–4.
10. Ulfberg J, Carter N, Talback M, et al. Headache, snoring and sleep apnea. J Neurol 1996;243:621–5.
11. Riley JL, Benson MB, Gremillion HA, et al. Sleep disturbance in orofacial pain patients: pain-related or emotional distress? Cranio 2001;19:106–13.
12. Kanli A, Dural S, Demirel F. Sleep disorders in chronic orofacial pain patients. Pain Clin 2004;16: 293–8.
13. Friction JR, Kroening RJ, Hathvaway KM. TMJ and craniofacial pain: diagnosis and management. St. Louis (MO): Ishiyaku Euro America Inc; 1988. p. 1–10, 39–52.
14. Austin DG. Special considerations in orofacial pain and headache. Dent Clin North Am 1997;41:325–39.

15. Austin DG, Cubillos L. Special considerations in oro-facial pain and craniomandibular disorders. Dent Clin North Am 1991;35:224–7.

16. Austin DG, Pertes RA. Examination of the TMD patient. In: Pertes RA, Gross S, editors. Clinical management of temporomandibular disorders and orofacial pain. Chicago: Quintessence; 1995. p. 123–60.

17. Moldofsky H. Sleep, neuroimmune and neuroendo-crine functions in fibromyalgia and chronic fatigue syndrome. Adv Neuroimmunol 1995;5:39–56.

18. Moldofsky H, Scarisbrick P, England R, et al. Musculoskeletal symptoms and non REM sleep disturbance in patients with fibrositis syndrome and healthy subjects. Psychosom Med 1975;34:341–51.

19. National Heart, Lung and Blood Institute (NHLBI). Cardiovascular and sleep related consequences of temporomandibular disorders, NHBI Workshop Final Report, 2001.

20. Kushida CA, Morgenthaler TI, Littner MR, et al. Practice parameters for treatment of snoring and obstructive sleep apnea with oral appliances: an update for 2005. Sleep 2006;29(2):240–3.

21. Burch JG. History and clinical examination. In: Laskin DM, Greenfield W, Gale EN, et al, editors. The President's conference on the examination. Diagnosis and management of temporomandibular disorders. Chicago: American Dental Association; 1983. p. 51–6.

22. Huggare JA, Raustia MA. Head posture and cervi-covertebral and craniofacial morphology in patients with craniomandibular dysfunction. J Craniomandib-ular Pract 1992;10:173–7.

23. Kritsineli M, Shim YS. Malocclusion, body posture and temporomandibular disorder in children with primary and mixed dentition. J Clin Pediatr Dent 1992;16(2):86–93.

24. Wallace C, Klineberg IJ. Management of cranioman-dibular disorders. Part II: clinical assessment of patients with craniocervical dysfunction. JOP 1994; 8(1):42–54.

25. Kaplan AS. Examination and diagnosis. In: Kaplan AS, Assael LA, editors. Temporomandibular disorders: diagnosis and treatment. Philadelphia: Saunders; 1991. p. 284–311.

26. Travell JG, Simons DG. Myofascial pain and dysfunc-tion: the trigger point manual. Baltimore (MD): Williams and Wilkins; 1983. p. 45–102, 183–201, 305–20.

27. Wallace C, Klineberg IJ. Management of cranioman-dibular disorders. Part I: a craniocervical dysfunc-tion index. JOP 1993;7(1):83–8.

28. Dunn J. Physical therapy. In: Kaplas AS, Assael LA, editors. Temporomandibular disorders: diagnosis and treatment. Philadelphia: Saunders; 1991. p. 455–500.

29. Moldofsky H. The contribution of sleep-wake physi-ology to fibromyalgia. In: Friction JR, Awad EA, editors. Advances in pain research and therapy, My-ofascial pain and fibromyalgia, vol. 17. New York: Raven; 1990. p. 227–40.

30. Wallace DJ, Clauw DJ. Fibromyalgia & other central pain syndromes. 9th edition. Philadelphia: Lippincott Williams & Wilkins; 2005.

31. Marchland E, Decramer M. Respiratory muscle func-tion and drive in chronic obstructive pulmonary disease. Clin Chest Med 2000;21:679–92.

32. Petty TL. Simple office spirometry. Clin Chest Med 2001;22:845–59.

33. Teixeira-Salmela LF, Parreira VF, Britto RR, et al. Respiratory pressures and thoracoabdominal motion in community dwelling chronic stroke survivors. Arch Phys Med Rehabil 2005;86:1974–8.

34. Chiara T, Martin D, Davenport PW, et al. Expiratory muscle strength training in persons with multiple sclerosis having mild to moderate disability; effect on maximal expiratory pressure, pulmonary function and maximal voluntary cough. Arch Phys Med Reha-bil 2006;87:468–73.

35. Budweiser S, Mourt LM, Jörres RA, et al. Respiratory muscle training in restrictive thoracic disease: a randomized controlled trial. Arch Phys Med Reha-bil 2006;87:1559–65.

36. Bourjeily G, Rochester CL. Exercise training in chronic obstructive pulmonary disease. Clin Chest Med 2000;21:763–81.

37. Wagner PD. Why doesn't exercise grow the lungs when other factors do? Exerc Sport Sci Rev 2005; 33(1):3–8.

38. Spring H, Illi U, Kunz HR, et al, editors. Stretching and strengthening exercises. New York: Thieme Medical Publishers; 1991. p. 2–11, 21–3, 81–97, 111–41.

39. Nici L. Mechanisms and measures of exercise toler-ance in chronic obstructive pulmonary disease. Clin Chest Med 2000;21:693–704.

40. Flaminiano LE, Celli BR. Respiratory muscle testing. Clin Chest Med 2001;22:661–77.

41. Stickland MK, Lovering AT. Exercise induced in-trapulmonary arteriovenous shunting and pulmo-nary gas exchange. Exerc Sport Sci Rev 2006; 34:99–106.

Orofacial Pain and Sleep

Robert L. Merrill, DDS, MS

KEYWORDS

- Orofacial pain • Chronic pain • Sleep disorders
- Sleep • Neuropathic pain • Temporomandibular disorders

Pain is defined by the International Association for the Study of Pain (IASP) as "…an unpleasant sensory and emotional experience associated with actual or potential tissue damage, or described in terms of such damage."[1] Acute pain is short term and although the impact on sleep may be significant, it does not have a long-standing influence. Chronic pain, however, can have a long-standing and negative impact on sleep. The IASP defines chronic pain as "pain without apparent biologic function that has persisted beyond the normal tissue healing time" (usually taken to be 3 months).[1] Chronic pain includes such disorders as arthritis, neuropathic pain, and sometimes headache. Melzack[2,3] in 1993 described a pain neuromatrix that involved all regions of the brain, helping to explain the emotional and cognitive response to the pain. Nofzinger and Derbyshire[4] described the "significant overlaps between the neuromatrix of pain and that of sleep."

The interrelationship between pain and sleep is complex and that relationship may be overlooked by clinicians treating only orofacial pain or only treating sleep disorders. Pain and sleep seem to represent opposing forces. Pain is a conscious process and in going to sleep, awareness of the surrounding environment decreases and the neural networks related to wakefulness become less active.[4] Nevertheless, pain can intrude into the unconsciousness of sleep, bringing pain into consciousness, thereby disturbing sleep.

Melzack and Wall[5] in 1965 proposed a pain modulating system called the "gate control theory of pain." This system has been modified over the years as the understanding of ascending and descending modulation has increased. Nevertheless, the basic tenets of the system have been more clearly elucidated through ongoing research. The authors described a process wherein nociception, coming from the periphery, is modulated in the substantia gelatinosa of the dorsal horn or trigeminal subnucleus caudalis. Second-order neurons in the substantia gelatinosa form part of an action system, transferring the pain signals to the somatosensory cortex. The action system stimulates a response to the pain, characterized by heightened arousal, readiness to engage in adaptive behaviors, or escape.[4] This action system functions in the awake and alert brain but is assumed to be suppressed in the sleeping brain. Brain activity decreases as sleep stages transition to non–rapid eye movement (NREM) and then increases in rapid eye movement (REM) sleep.[6] In general, imaging studies for both pain and sleep show an extensive overlap of areas that are deactivated in sleep transition but are activated by pain.

Chronic pain disorders are characterized by nonnociceptive pain, although some categories of pain have acute nociceptive components (eg, arthritis). The 1996 National Sleep Foundation: Gallup Poll on Adult Public's Experiences with Nighttime Pain found that 56 million Americans complained of chronic pain interfering with falling asleep or causing them to awaken during the night. Pain the next day was linked to getting less than 6 hours or more than 9 hours of sleep the previous night.[7] The question arises, however, whether it is caused by sleep deprivation or disturbed sleep continuity. Smith and colleagues[8] found that sleep continuity disturbance and not simple sleep restriction caused increased spontaneous pain. Furthermore, the number of awakenings that occur during the night may also

Orofacial Pain and Dental Sleep Medicine Center, UCLA School of Dentistry, Room 13-089C, 10833 Le Conte Avenue, Los Angeles, CA 90095–1668, USA
E-mail address: rmerril@ucla.edu

Sleep Med Clin 5 (2010) 131–144
doi:10.1016/j.jsmc.2009.10.008

influence subsequent pain. In the study by Smith and colleagues,[8] patients who were awakened frequently during the night reportedly had more spontaneous pain the next day than patients who were only sleep deprived.

A 1991 General Social Survey in Canada found that 44% of people with pain had difficulty getting to and staying asleep but only 19% who did not have pain had the same problem. The odds ratio of relative risk for the association of insomnia and pain increases with severity of pain.[9] A survey of Australians found that chronic pain was the strongest predictor of sleep disturbance.[10] A survey for chronic pain and insomnia in five European countries reported that 40.2% of respondents with insomnia reported chronic pain.[11] As Choinière and coworkers[12] point out, however, most of the studies rely on self-report instruments and not on objective measures obtained during sleep studies. Choinière and cowokers[12] summarize the relationship between sleep and pain as follows (**Box 1**).

The nature of the interaction between pain and sleep is threefold: (1) pain may disturb normal sleep patterns, (2) disturbed sleep may lead to pain, and (3) the two conditions may exacerbate each other. Descriptions of pain disorders in the literature and various pain classification systems often include disordered sleep as a side effect of pain.[13] Linton and Shane[14] described a survey undertaken to look at the relationship between pain and sleep, and found that 50% of respondents reported having sleep problems. They also found that 58% of the respondents reporting a pain problem also had a sleep problem, but 70% of respondents reporting a sleep problem also had a pain problem. Their findings also suggested that the participants who reported both pain and sleep problems had greater psychiatric morbidity in the form of anxiety or depression than the other two groups.

Pain levels can be exacerbated, not only by poor sleep, but also by psychologic issues that often accompany the pain condition (eg, depression and anxiety). Patients who have chronic pain often have associated anxiety or depression that negatively impacts the pain and treatment response. If the comorbid psychiatric problems are ignored, the patient does not respond optimally to the treatment of their pain. Conversely, if both the pain disorder and the comorbid problems are addressed concomitantly, the treatment outcome can be optimized.[15]

Healthy pain-free individuals who were sleep deprived at a modest level with REM sleep interrupted showed that the loss of 4 hours of sleep and specific REM sleep loss caused hyperalgesia

---

Box 1
Relationship between sleep and pain

1. The prevalence of sleep disturbances in patients who suffer from chronic pain is higher than in the general population, but there are pain conditions in which sleep dysfunctions seem to be more common (eg, rheumatoid arthritis).
2. Although the percentages of chronic pain patients who complain of poor sleep quality varies widely among studies (from 50%–89%), it seems reasonable to state that most patients with chronic pain report sleep problems.
3. The most frequent subjective sleep complaints in chronic pain patients are insomnia (difficulty falling asleep or staying asleep, or waking up too early); nonrefreshing sleep; and excessive daytime sleepiness or fatigue.
4. The most common objective-quantitative sleep abnormalities in chronic pain patients include sleep fragmentation, decreased sleep efficiency, and reduced slow wave sleep. Various other disturbances in sleep macrostructure (eg, REM sleep abnormalities) or microstructure (eg, alpha-delta intrusions during NREM sleep) have also been observed in some patient groups. Some objective sleep abnormalities are also specific to certain pain conditions (eg, types of headache).
5. Alpha-delta intrusions during NREM sleep are not specific to fibromyalgia. They have been observed in various other types of pain conditions and sleep disorders, and even in normal subjects.
6. A relatively important number of chronic pain patients have primary sleep disorders other than insomnia, most notably sleep apnea, restless leg syndrome, or periodic leg movements during sleep.

---

the following day.[16] Hyperalgesia is defined by the IASP as "an increased response to a stimulus which is normally painful."[1] The significance of this study relates to increased pain levels if the patient has poor sleep. An implication is that medications that decrease sleep or interrupt REM sleep may increase pain. Sleep deprivation studies in which the subjects' sleep is disturbed during stage N3,4 (slow wave sleep [SWS]) had increased muscle tenderness and reduced pain threshold the next day, but other studies have reported a negative relationship between SWS disturbances and pain.[17] Increased muscle tenderness to palpation is described in pain terms as "hyperalgesia."

Bastuji and colleagues,[18] in a polysomnography (PSG)-pain study, reported that giving a painful stimulus during sleep caused brain-evoked potentials to be recorded in all stages of sleep and that the painful stimuli during stage N2 sleep were followed by K complexes. They further found that the brain was not as responsive to sound as pain during stages N3,4 and REM sleep, implying that sound intrusions are different from pain intrusions. Electrical pain stimulation during different NREM and REM sleep stages found muscle reflex latencies increased in N2 and increased even further in N3,4 and REM sleep.[19] Lavigne and colleagues[20] reported that thermal stimuli of 46°C produced moderate levels of cortical arousal during all stages of sleep but was greater in N2 sleep (**Fig. 1**).

The pain-gating mechanism is also thought to mitigate non–life-threatening pain signals that could intrude on sleep and cause arousals.[21] The likely area where this modulation occurs is in the reticular activating system, a poorly defined network of neurons extending from the medulla to the mesencephalon.[4] In terms of sleep and wakefulness, brainstem arousal nuclei in the reticular activating system are the main nuclei for initiating and maintaining wakefulness. These nuclei are the locus ceruleus, the dorsal raphe nuclei,

and the pedunculopontine tegmentum and are associated with specific neurotransmitters that alert the brain (**Fig. 2**). The primary role of the reticular activating system is to maintain alertness and attention.[19,22] Soja[22] has suggested that sensory inhibition during REM sleep is driven by postsynaptic hyperpolarization in the dorsospinocerebellar and the spinoreticular tracts and that γ-aminobutyric acid (GABA) tonically mediates sensory activity in these tracts.[23,24] Presynaptic inhibitory mechanisms may also help filter and modulate sensory activity and ascending sensory signals can be filtered through mechanisms in the thalamus to protect sleep.

The brainstem arousal nuclei are part of the mesopontine reticular activating system. These nuclei modulate release of specific neurotransmitters involved in wakefulness and pain modulation. The locus ceruleus is associated with norepinephrine, the dorsal raphe nuclei are associated with serotonin, and the pedunculopontine tegmentum is associated with acetylcholine. All three of these nuclei, acting together, initiate and maintain wakefulness. Medications that block or increase release of any of the three modify wakefulness or enhance SWS or REM sleep. The neurotransmitters in this system are also involved in pain and mood modulation. Serotonergic medications, such as the

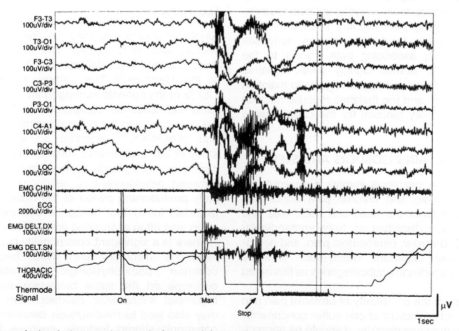

Fig. 1. Thermal stimulation causing cortical arousal during sleep. This figure is from Lavigne's study using thermal stimulation during sleep stage 2 to determine cortical response. As can be seen, the electroencephalogram leads recorded cortical activation, and electromyogram of chin and deltoid muscle in the area of the stimulation. (*From* Lavigne G, Zucconi M, Castronovo C, et al. Sleep arousal response to experimental thermal stimulation during sleep in human subjects free of pain and sleep problems. Pain 2000;84:287; with permission.)

2 KEY SLEEP-WAKE CENTERS
BAN (MESOPONTINE RETICULAR ACTIVATING SYSTEM)

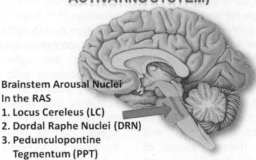

Brainstem Arousal Nuclei
In the RAS
1. Locus Cereleus (LC)
2. Dordal Raphe Nuclei (DRN)
3. Pedunculopontine
   Tegmentum (PPT)

Fig. 2. The brainstem arousal nuclei in the mesopontine reticular activating system (RAS). The area of the brainstem arousal nuclei and the neurotransmitters associated with the brainstem arousal nuclei subnuclei that are also active in pain modulation.

tricyclic antidepressants, have a positive effect not only on depression but also modulate headache, musculoskeletal, and neuropathic pain. The tricyclic antidepressants work through the serotonin and norepinephrine systems by an active reuptake system and actions on presynaptic and postsynaptic receptors. Neurotransmitter reuptake inhibition is not the main mechanism of action. It has been clinically observed that the selective serotonin reuptake inhibitors do not have as great an effect on pain as do the tricyclic antidepressants.

The ascending pain circuitry passes into the thalamus where third-order neuron synapses occur, relaying ascending pain signals to the somatosensory cortex. During sleep, thalamic nuclei filter the ascending pain signals to maintain the sleep state and the thalamic reticular nucleus plays a regulatory function for the cortex during SWS.

OROFACIAL PAIN DISORDERS AND SLEEP

Orofacial pain problems involve both acute or nociceptive pain and chronic pain conditions. The pain involves the head and neck area and includes such disorders as temporomandibular joint (TMJ) disorder, neuropathic pain, and neurovascular pain disorders. Within each of these general categories are subcategories as illustrated in **Fig. 3.**

Because of the complexity of orofacial pain and the fact that an individual can suffer concurrently with more than one disorder, it should be appreciated that the impact of these conditions on sleep can be very significant. In addition, because of the rich innervation of the head region and the proximity to the brain, the pain may be sensed

as more severe and create more distress than similar pain in another part of the body. A cross-sectional population-based study of 4000 individuals found that patients with orofacial pain had a relative risk factor of 3.7 for a high level of sleep disturbance.[25] Furthermore, there are orofacial pain conditions that are not seen in other areas of the body that have their own characteristics, impacting on sleep or being impacted by sleep.

Headache

Nighttime headaches may be associated with snoring and sleep apnea. The comorbidity of headache and orofacial pain has been reported in the literature.[26] The authors reported that 72.7% of the patients coming to an orofacial pain clinic had headache, compared with 32% of individuals coming to the general dental clinic. Paiva and coworkers,[27] reporting an epidemiologic study of 288 consecutive subjects in a headache clinic who were grouped based on a relationship between development of headache during the early prewakening period of the night and sleep disorder, found that headache occurring during sleep was often associated with a sleep disorder.

There is a significant commonality between the headache disorders and TMD because of common pathophysiologic pathways that converge on the same brainstem area in the trigeminal subnucleus caudalis. This situation may also lead to misdiagnosis because of some commonly shared features, such as throbbing temporal and cervical pain and tender masticatory and cervical muscles. These patients usually report sleep disturbances associated with their pain.

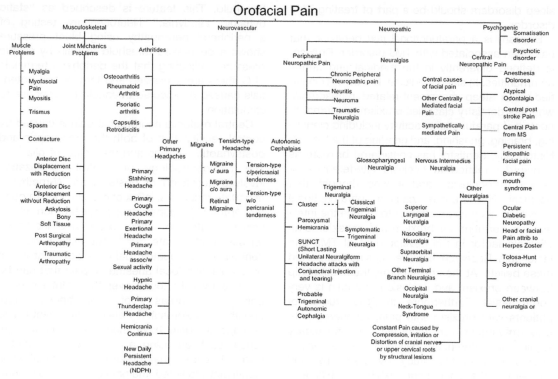

Fig. 3. General schema of pain disorders seen in the orofacial region.

TMJ Disorders

The three main categories of TMJ disorder are (1) mechanical problems of the TMJs, (2) pain problems involving the muscles, and (3) the arthritides. As in other areas of the body, pain involving the masticatory system can have a significant impact on sleep and getting restful sleep can mitigate the pain. The pain of the masticatory muscles and TMJs can be exacerbated by sleep position. This problem impacts sleep conditions, such as obstructive sleep apnea (OSA), where often the apnea is exacerbated while sleeping in a supine position and is reduced when side-sleeping. Sleeping supine usually does not put pressure on the masticatory system and usually does not aggravate pain, whereas sleeping on the side often puts pressure on the TMJ and jaw muscles, aggravating the pain.

In those individuals susceptible to TMJ disk derangements, supine sleeping may cause disk dislocation when the jaw muscles relax, allowing the jaw to move posteriorly and the disk to slip forward and dislocate. Often these patients report that when they arise in the morning and attempt to open their mouths, the jaw is locked. This may be a temporary condition not requiring treatment, but may be a more persistent condition requiring focused treatment by a dentist skilled in TMJ disorder.

Pain in the TMJ is a common complaint in TMJ disorder clinics. The pain may be caused by microtrauma, macrotrauma, or arthritis. One of the key features of pain in the TMJ is pain with pressure applied over the joint or to the jaw. Sleeping on the side often exacerbates the jaw pain from the pressure of the bed or pillow and this may disturb sleep. In addition, the TMJ is as susceptible to arthritis as other joints in the body. Moffitt and coworkers[10] found that arthritis was the most significant factor contributing to pain, and patients with TMJ arthritis are not an exception to this observation.

TMJ disorders are multifactorial and include muscle pain disorders, mechanical problems of the TMJ, and arthritis. The pain associated with these problems is caused by inflammation of the joints and muscles. Jaw function usually aggravates the problem so patients who clench or grind their teeth during the night may experience sleep-interrupting pain. Patients presenting with TMJ disorder often report poor sleep associated with their pain.[28] Smith and colleagues[29] found that patients with orofacial pain and specifically masticatory muscle pain were more likely to have a sleep disorder. Edwards and colleagues[30] reported TMJ pain may be related to sleep fragmentation that negatively impacts the pain modulating system, suggesting that evaluating and treating comorbid sleep disorders should be a part of treating TMJ disorder.

Bruxism is a parafunctional jaw behavior that has been associated with TMJ disorder. Bruxism is defined differently in the medical and dental communities. In sleep medicine, bruxism is classified as a sleep movement-related parasomnia, whereas dentistry classifies bruxism as diurnal or nocturnal parafunctional activity including clenching, bracing, gnashing, and grinding of the teeth.[31] Historically, dentistry has considered bruxism as a disorder related to occlusal interferences or dental malocclusion and it was thought that occlusal interferences caused parafunctional activity at night as an attempt to reduce the interference. Furthermore, bruxism was considered an etiologic factor in the development of TMJ and facial pain. Research, however, has not supported these beliefs. At the present time, the relationship between bruxism and occlusion and pain is very controversial. Furthermore, in PSG studies of patients with bruxism with pain, compared with bruxism without pain, there were no statistically significant differences between the groups.[32] Interestingly, in the study by Camparis and Siqueira,[32] the pain group exhibited 20% less bruxism than in the nonpain group, possibly indicating an inhibitory reflex in the masticatory muscles in the presence of pain.

Neuropathic Pain

Orofacial neuropathic pains involve the trigeminal sensory system. Neuropathic pain is described as "pain arising as a direct consequence of a lesion or disease affecting the somatosensory system."[33] It is important to differentiate between neuropathic pain of peripheral and central nervous systems because the characteristics and pathophysiology of these conditions are different and successful treatment of the neuropathy depends on the correct diagnosis. A case in point is the diagnosis of atypical facial pain that was given primarily to middle-aged postmenopausal women because of lack of understanding of the possible conditions that could cause the facial pain. There is now a better understanding of the conditions that can be missed in making the diagnosis. Many of these pain problems are neuropathic pain of both peripheral and central origin.[34–39] The pathophysiology of peripheral neuropathic pain involves sensitization of peripheral nociceptors by peripherally released neurotransmitters after trauma to the sensory nerves.[40] The ongoing release of the neurotransmitters mediates the chronic sensitization of the small diameter unmyelinated nociceptors, resulting in lowered pain

threshold. This feature is described as "static dynamic allodynia." Neurosensory testing of a peripheral neuropathy using blunt pressure shows a decreased threshold to pain by simple pressure, indicating that the peripheral terminals of C fibers are sensitized and form action potentials caused by lowered threshold of response to stimulation.

Central orofacial neuropathic pain is caused by central sensitization of both the presynaptic and postsynaptic neurons and the adjacent glia.[40–42] The pathophysiology of central sensitization involves activation of postsynaptic N-methyl-D-aspartate receptors, influx of calcium ions through the N-methyl-D-aspartate–associated ion channels, formation of nitric oxide, and increased release of glutamate.[40,43,44] The clinical signs of centralized neuropathic pain are pain that is not blockable with local anesthetic; pain that can be induced by light touch over the painful site; or pain in areas of numbness (eg, anesthesia dolorosa).[33] Patients with centralized neuropathic pain have increased pain to light touch, such as using a cotton wisp or cotton swab. Because the threshold to stimulation is significantly lowered, the painful site is easily stimulated during the night as the patient moves in bed, resulting in sleep disturbance. Centralized neuropathic pain may be caused by sympathetic mediation. The clinical manifestation in the orofacial region is similar to centralized neuropathic pain without sympathetic mediation, although some early papers on this variation found a difference in thermographically determined temperature in the facial region involved in the sympathetic mediation.[45,46]

Both peripheral and central orofacial neuropathic pains are described as diurnal but fluctuating over a 24-hour period. Patients may indicate that the pain does not awaken them but if they do awaken during the night, they are usually aware of the pain. Most of these patients report some degree of sleep onset and maintenance difficulties. In contrast, patients with trigeminal neuralgia usually indicate that they do not have pain during the night but note its recurrence shortly after arising in the morning. In addition, they do not usually report sleep difficulties.[35,47,48] Trigeminal neuralgia, however, typically occurs in individuals from 40 to 65 years of age. This age also tends to have increased likelihood of having sleep-disordered breathing.

Trigeminal neuralgia typically is not active during sleep. Although individuals have severe bouts of the lancinating pain during the day, the condition generally becomes quiet during sleep. The mechanism for this phenomenon is unclear, and the mechanism for trigeminal neuralgia remains unclear. If the patient awakens during the night, they do not usually have the bouts of pain but the pain returns within minutes of arousing in the morning.[49] In contrast, peripheral and centralized trigeminal neuropathies seem to remain active during sleep, although sufferers often indicate that they are able to sleep and are not aware of the pain; they usually experience it if they awaken or move during the night.

The presence of the trigeminal neuropathies, with the exception of trigeminal neuralgia, are associated with diurnal or 24-hour pain of moderate intensity. Although they may not report that the pain wakens them during the night, they consistently report difficulty with sleep, either delayed sleep onset, insomnia, or problems maintaining sleep. In addition, these patients have increased likelihood of having depression and anxiety that can also impact on their sleep.

Burning Mouth Syndrome

Burning mouth syndrome remains a puzzling disorder. The pathophysiology is not understood but the clinical presentation is consistent. The pain is described as a bilateral moderate burning sensation involving the lips, palate, gingiva, or tongue. The pain is not blockable and may become more intense with application of topical anesthetic. This pain is also described as diurnal and the patient usually has accompanying sleep difficulty. The condition is most commonly seen in perimenopausal and postmenopausal women in whom one is more likely to see sleep disorders, such as insomnia, and psychiatric disorders, such as depression or anxiety.

THE IMPACT OF PAIN ON SLEEP STAGES

Anyone who has had significant pain, whether from a chronic pain condition or from trauma or surgery, knows how pain can interfere with restful sleep. What is not apparent, however, is how the pain can alter the normal sleep architecture. These

changes are observed in PSG studies and are discussed next.

Alpha Waves

In general, the frequency of electroencephalogram (EEG) activity recorded in PSG studies slowly decreases. Alpha wave and mixed wave recordings (8–13 Hz) are characteristic of the awake subject and in subjects transitioning to other sleep stages or following arousal.[50] Alpha activity usually appears when the patient is asked to close their eyes. As sleep onset occurs progressing to N1 stage sleep, less than 50% of an epoch contains alpha waves and activity decreases, being replaced by theta wave activity in the range of 4 to 8 Hz. N1 stage sleep represents 3% to 8% of total sleep time.[51] Perlis and coworkers[52] have suggested that other factors may increase alpha activity in SWS, such as hyperarousals.

N2 Stage Sleep

A further decrease in frequency is seen in N2 stage sleep with predominantly theta wave activity but sleep spindles (12–14 Hz) lasting approximately 0.5 seconds and K complexes begin to appear, defining N2 sleep (**Fig. 4**).

Sleep Spindles and K Complexes

K complexes are characterized by higher amplitude fast negative wave deflections that are followed by slower positive higher amplitude slow wave deflections. They are generated spontaneously and may occur in response to outside disturbances and represent a partial arousal response. In addition, delta waves characteristic of stage N3 may also appear in the pattern of theta wave in N2 sleep. N2 sleep represents approximately 50% of the total sleep time.[51]

Although K complexes are noted in transient arousal activity in normal sleep, when PSG studies are done with patients who have chronic pain, increased K complexes are observed. These large amplitude EEG waves often accompany short

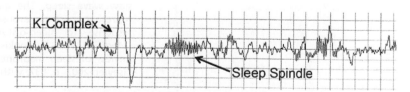

Fig. 4. An example of a K complex and sleep spindle intrusion in N2 sleep pattern. This figure shows the typical pattern of sleep spindles and K complexes that appear in PSG recordings in response to afferent nociceptive activity coming from below the thalamus. These phenomena serve to filter ascending nociceptive activity from intruding into the cortex and cause arousals. (*Modified from* Barkoukis TJ, Avidan A. Review of sleep medicine. Philadelphia: Elsevier, 2007. p. 537; with permission.)

bursts of alpha EEG activity. Similar to alpha intrusions, it has been postulated that K complexes are an indication of the brain's attempt to change from the sleep state to arousal. PSGs of fibromyalgia patients show increased numbers of the intrusive K complexes during their sleep and are associated with complaints of nonrestorative sleep, fatigue, and pain.[53]

In contrast to alpha wave and K complex intrusions, sleep spindles are brief periods (0.5–2 seconds) of EEG activity in the frequency range of 10 to 12 Hz that are thought to be sleep-promoting phenomena. The spindles increase in the presence of pain and represent an attempt to filter the intrusiveness of pain in the sleep pattern. Sleep spindles are generated in the reticular nucleus of the thalamus and function as a gating mechanism to inhibit ascending activity, such as noxious signals from below the thalamus reaching the cortex and causing arousal.

N3 Stage Sleep

N3 stage sleep, also called "slow wave sleep," is associated with slow delta wave frequencies (0.5–2 Hz) that help to identify this stage. Generally, N3 takes 15% to 20% of a total sleep time. In addition, electromyogram recorded muscle activity is less in N3 sleep than in wakefulness or in N1 sleep. A phenomenon observed in PSG studies of pain patients is intrusion of alpha waves (8–13 Hz) into the SWS (see **Fig. 4**). Alpha wave activity is characteristic of wakefulness and represents arousal activity when intruding into SWS. When these intrusions occur, they are at the expense of SWS, causing an upward shift in the sleep cycle pattern and decreasing total sleep time. In terms of pain, the net result of this, as illustrated in the study by Roehrs and coworkers,[16] can be an increase in hyperalgesia (**Fig. 5**).

THE IMPACT OF SLEEP ON OROFACIAL PAIN

Moldofsky and coworkers[54] studied two groups of young, healthy, nonathletic volunteers who were subjected to selective sleep stage deprivation. Six subjects were deprived of N3,4 sleep and seven subjects of REM sleep. The N3,4-deprived group reported more musculoskeletal symptoms during the deprivation condition than did the REM-deprived group. The N3,4-deprived group also showed a significant increase in muscle tenderness between the baseline and deprivation conditions and an altered pattern of overnight change in muscle tenderness in response to deprivation. The REM-deprived group did not show either of these changes. Although the sample size is small, this study suggests that loss of N3,4 sleep can result in lower pain thresholds in muscles.

Fragmented sleep continuity has also been found to increase musculoskeletal pain. Drewes and coworkers[55] conducted a longitudinal study of clinical and sleep parameters in patients with rheumatoid arthritis and showed a relationship between pain, morning stiffness, and sleep architecture. Macfarlane and coworkers[56,57] found that poor sleep was a predictor for persistence of orofacial pain (ie, the poorer the sleep, the more likely it was that the patient would have persistent orofacial pain). It has been observed that treating an underlying OSA or upper airway resistance syndrome in chronic pain disorders, such as fibromyalgia, results in a decrease in severity of the pain.[58]

Heavy snoring, independent of OSA, is also a risk factor for headache. The headache is usually mild to moderate; diffuse; and not associated with other symptoms, such as nausea, phonophobia, or photophobia. These headaches tend to resolve within 30 to 60 minutes after arising. The headache is classified as a tension-type headache. In a study of 206 individuals assessing the prevalence of

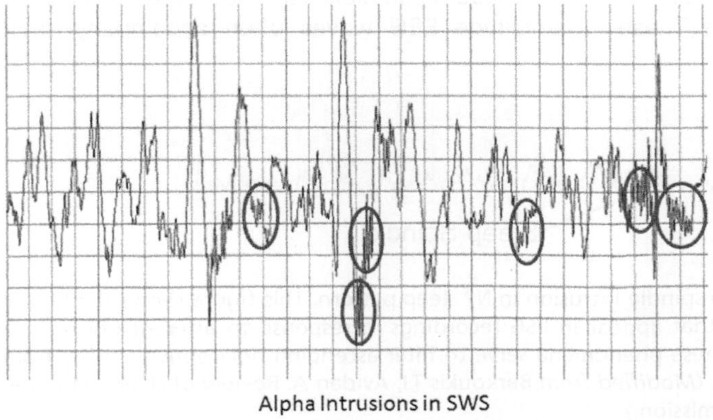

Alpha Intrusions in SWS

Fig. 5. Alpha intrusions into slow wave sleep (SWS). This figure shows alpha wave intrusions circled in the pattern of slow wave sleep. The alpha intrusions represent cortical arousal activity in response to sleep-disturbing signals. (*Modified from* Barkoukis TJ, Avidan A. Review of sleep medicine. Philadelphia: Elsevier, 2007. p. 537; with permission.)

snoring with chronic daily headache, compared with a control group of 507, it was found that habitual snoring was more common in the chronic daily headache group (24% of chronic daily headache snored vs 14% of controls).[59]

Patients with insomnia experience enhanced spontaneous pain and hyperalgesia.[60] A common feature of OSA or upper airway resistance syndrome is morning headache, and treating the OSA with continuous positive airway pressure reduces the headache. The frequency, depending on the study, ranges between 36% and 58%.[61,62] The intensity of the headache is variable and the pain is described as aching to throbbing. Of all the headache disorders, tension-type headache has the strongest association with OSA. Goder and coworkers[63] found that morning headache was not linked to mean O_2 saturation but to the number of awakenings and decreased total sleep time.

Insomnia has been linked with tension-type headache. This link is strongest in women and stress is one of the strongest factors in the linkage. The postulated mechanism for this association is through stress-increased autonomic activation of the hypothalamic-pituitary-adrenal axis that induces release of cortisol from the adrenal gland.[64] Cortisol acts in the hypothalamus to stimulate arousal mechanisms leading to wakefulness. Increased stress has been linked to onset of tension-type headache and migraine.

THE OVERLAP IN NEUROBIOLOGY OF SLEEP AND PAIN
Neurotransmitters of Sleep and Wakefulness

The main center for wakefulness is the brainstem arousal nuclei, comprised of several nuclei that function together to initiate and maintain wakefulness. There are two types of wakefulness: excited wakefulness and quiet wakefulness. The neurotransmitters for each of these states are different. The neurotransmitters of excited wakefulness are norepinephrine, acetylcholine, serotonin, and dopamine. In addition to the action of these wakeful state neurotransmitters, cortisol also functions as a neurotransmitter involved in hyperarousal through activity in the hypothalamic-pituitary-adrenal axis. The neurotransmitter for quiet wakefulness is histamine, which is released in the tuberomammillary nucleus in the hypothalamus (Fig. 6, Table 1).

The most important neurotransmitter of sleep is GABA. GABA is an inhibitor neurotransmitter that functions as a sleep-inducing neurotransmitter through the suprachiasmatic nucleus to the

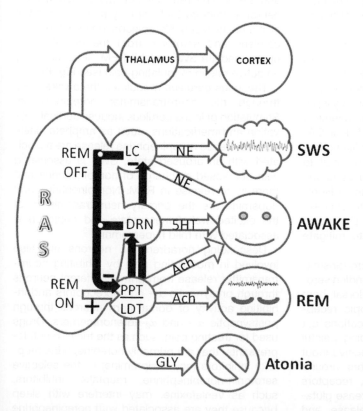

Fig. 6. Reticular activating system neurotransmitters of sleep and pain. The reticular activating system (RAS) oversees the wakefulness state through activity of four subnuclei: (1) the locus ceruleus (LC), which releases norepinephrine; (2) the dorsal raphe nuclei (DRN), which release serotonin (5HT); (3) the pedunculopontine (PPT); and (4) the laterodorsal tegmentum (LDT), which are associated with acetylcholine (Ach). The PPT-LDT neurons are active not only in wakefulness but also in REM sleep and are thought to be the REM on-switch. Lesions in the PPT-LDT area do not affect wakefulness but lead to loss of REM sleep. SWS is modulated through LC and DRN by decreasing the release of NE. Wakefulness is achieved through the combined activity of the PPT, LC, and DRN nuclei releasing Ach, norepinephrine, and serotonin, respectively. The primary neurotransmitter of REM is Ach. SWS is achieved through suppression of the wakefulness neurotransmitters NE and 5HT and release of Ach. (Data from Webster HH, Jones BE. Neurotoxic lesions of the dorsolateral pontomesencephalic tegmentum-cholinergic cell area in the cat. II. Effects upon sleep-waking states. Brain Res 1988;458(2):285–302.)

Table 1
Neurotransmitters of wakefulness and sleep

	Excited Wakefulness	Quiet Wakefulness	REM Sleep	Slow Wave Sleep
ACH	++	−	+++	−
NE	+++	−	−	+
5HT	+++	−	−	+
DA	+++	−	++	+
Orex	+++	+++	−	−
Hist	+	++	−	−
GABA	−	−	+++	+++

Abbreviations: 5HT, serotonin; Ach, actylcholine; DA, dopamine; GABA, γ-aminobutyric acid; Hist, histamine; NE, norepinephrine; Orex, orexin (hypocretin); REM, rapid eye movement.

ventrolateropreoptic nucleus to induce sleepiness. The neurotransmitters of wakefulness and sleep are shown in **Table 1**, with their impact on the stages of wakefulness and sleep.

The important neurotransmitters for pain modulation are serotonin, norepinephrine, histamine, GABA, and acetylcholine. GABA is an inhibitory neurotransmitter and functions on the GABA-A receptors. These receptors are associated with chloride ion channels. When GABA binds to the receptor, the ion channel opens allowing chloride to enter the neurons, causing hyperpolarization of the neuron and blocking propagation of action potentials. Medications that increase GABA activity or act on the GABA-associated neurons tend to cause sleepiness or sedation, as GABA does in the sleep side of the sleep-wake cycle. In addition, GABA release in the thalamus mediates the thalamic sensory filter to filter out sensory input coming to the thalamus from spinal and trigeminal ascending transmission. If there is deficient GABAergic neurotransmission at night, the filter effect is reduced allowing ascending sensory input to pass through the thalamic filter, impacting the cortex and causing hyperarousal. Using GABAergic medications helps to restore the effectiveness of the filter and enhance sleepiness. Enhancing GABAergic neurotransmission helps to mitigate pain and enhance sleep.

Serotonin is also one of the main neurotransmitters involved in pain modulation. Descending serotonergic neurons inhibit activity of dorsal horn neurons through $5HT_{1B/1D}$ metabotropic receptors. Serotonin or serotonergic medications act on these receptors to inhibit ascending painful activity of dorsal horn neurons that receive input from muscles, joints, and nociceptors around blood vessels. Post synaptic $5HT_{2A}$ receptors excite cortical pyramidal neurons, increase glutamate release, decrease dopamine release, and

are involved in sleep and hallucinations. Blocking the $5HT_{2A}$ receptor by an antagonist, such as trazodone or mirtazapine, helps to restore sleep and reduce anxiety that may disturb sleep. The $5HT_{2C}$ receptors regulate dopamine and norepinephrine release, playing a role in obesity, mood, and cognition. $5HT_3$ receptors regulate inhibitory interneurons in the brain, mediating vomiting by activity on the vagal nerve. $5HT_6$ receptors regulate release of neurotrophic factors and $5HT_7$ receptors may be involved in circadian rhythms, mood, and sleep. The reticular activating system uses neurotransmitters that not only mediate pain but also mediate sleep. Norepinephrine from the locus ceruleus and serotonin from the dorsal raphe nuclei mediate SWS, inhibit REM sleep, and play an active role in modulating pain (see **Fig. 6**).

The locus ceruleus modulates the awake state through the neurotransmitter norepinephrine. Stimulation of locus ceruleus induces cortical activation and medications, such as amphetamines, which increase norepinephrine release are associated with an aroused state. SWS is associated with decreased discharge of norepinephrine and there is no release in REM. Norepinephrine and dopamine are the primary neurotransmitters of the excited wakefulness state and depletion is associated with mild hypersomnia.[65]

Descending noradrenergic neurons are also involved in modulating pain by inhibiting neurotransmitter release from primary afferent neurons through presynaptic α_2- adrenoreceptors and inhibiting activity of dorsal horn neurons through postsynaptic α_1- and α_2-adrenoreceptors. Drugs used for treating pain, such as the tricyclic antidepressants, that are primarily norepinephrine reuptake inhibitors (eg, desipramine) or the selective serotonin-norepinephrine reuptake inhibitors, such as venlafaxine, may interfere with sleep because they are associated with norepinephrine reuptake inhibition. Patients taking noradrenergic tricyclic antidepressants may experience agitation and difficulty initiating sleep. Drugs that increase availability of both serotonin and norepinephrine can enhance sleep (see **Fig. 6**). The typical tricyclic antidepressants used for pain and sleep are amitriptyline and nortriptyline. These drugs can help pain and increase SWS possibly through blockade of the postsynaptic $5HT_{2A}$ and $5HT_{2C}$ receptors and blockade of H1 histamine and α_1- adrenergic receptors (see **Table 1**).

The main hypothalamic subnuclei involved in sleep-wakefulness and pain are the ventrolateral preoptic nucleus, which modulates sleep through GABA and functions as the off switch for wakefulness; the tuberomammilary nucleus, which uses histamine as the on-switch for arousal; and the lateral hypothalamic nucleus with orexin (**Fig. 7**).

GABA is also one of the main inhibitory neurotransmitters that play a role in pain modulation through GABA-A and GABA-B receptors. In addition, GABA is linked to anxiety and most anxiolytic drugs act on GABA receptors. The $GABA_A$ receptor plays an important role in benzodiazepines anxiolysis and different subtypes of the receptor have been identified, each performing a different function. Although phasic inhibition is primarily associated with anxiolytic action, tonic inhibition might eventually play a role in the development of novel anxiolytics. The thinking is that dysregulation of inhibitory tone may cause abnormal neural excitability, which may be involved in various anxiety disorders. Current understanding suggests that the benzodiazepine-type drugs target benzodiazepine-sensitive GABA-A receptors to enhance phasic

postsynaptic inhibition. This increases the inhibitory presence of GABA, particularly in the amygdala and the cortico-striatal-thalamic-cortical loop in the prefrontal cortex, where overly active output neurons would otherwise cause fear and worry. Anxiety increases pain levels and pain can be modulated through anxiolytic activity on GABA-A receptors.

It has been suggested that orexin may also be involved in pain signaling. Ozcan and colleagues[66] reported that orexin activates intracellular calcium signaling through a protein kinase C–dependent pathway that may be involved in pain modulation. Holland and Goadsby,[67] in a study involving orexin-A and orexin-B, reported that orexin-B had no effect on trigeminal firing but orexin-A played a key inhibitory role in trigeminal A fiber responses to electrical stimulation. Additionally, orexin-A acting on OX-1 receptors inhibited dural vasodilatation, which may be involved in the mechanism of neurogenic inflammation and headache.[68,69]

SUMMARY

The relationship between orofacial pain and sleep disorders is well documented in the literature. The orofacial pain specialist is well advised to evaluate their pain patients for sleep disorders that are comorbid with orofacial pain. As indicated, the interrelationship between sleep disorders and pain is complex and a two-way street. The central effects of sleep disorders on pain modulating circuitry may account for much of the association, indicating that sleep disorders should be considered in the orofacial pain population. Medications that can modulate sleep may also modulate pain where

Hypothalamic Control of Sleep-wake System

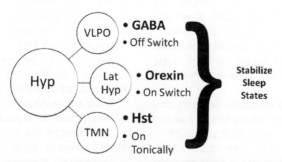

Fig. 7. Hypothalamic neurotransmitter control of sleep-wake system. This figure shows the relationship between the hypothalamic nuclei that control the sleep wake system. γ-Aminobutyric acid (GABA) is an inhibitory neurotransmitter and is the off-switch to turn the brain off for sleep. Histamine (Hst) is part of the on-switch to cause arousal. In addition, orexin functions to maintain wakefulness as part of the on-switch. (*Data from* Stahl S. Diagnosis and treatment of sleep wake disorders. Carlsbad (CA); Neuroscience Education Institute; 2007.)

there is an overlap between the pain and sleep circuitry in which they act.

REFERENCES

1. Merskey HB, Bogduk N, editors. Classification of chronic pain: descriptions of chronic pain syndromes and definitions of pain terms. 2nd edition. Seattle (WA): IASP Press; 1994. p. 209–13.
2. Melzack R. From the gate to the neuromatrix. Pain 1999;(Suppl 6):S121–6.
3. Melzack R. Labat lecture: phantom limbs. Reg Anesth 1989;14(5):208–11.
4. Nofzinger EAD, Derbyshire S. Pain imaging in relation to sleep. In: Lavigne GS, Barry JS, Choiniere M, et al, editors. Sleep and pain. Seattle (WA): IASP; 2007. p. 153–74.
5. Melzack R, Wall PD. Pain mechanisms: a new theory. Science 1965;150:971–9.
6. Meyer JS, Hayman LA, Amano T, et al. Mapping local blood flow of human brain by CT scanning during stable xenon inhalation. Stroke 1981;12(4):426–36.
7. Edwards RR, Almeida DM, Klick B, et al. Duration of sleep contributes to next-day pain report in the general population. Pain 2008;137(1):202–7.
8. Smith MT, Edwards RR, McCann UD, et al. The effects of sleep deprivation on pain inhibition and spontaneous pain in women. Sleep 2007;30(4):494–505.
9. Sutton DA, Moldofsky H, Badley EM. Insomnia and health problems in Canadians. Sleep 2001;24(6):665–70.
10. Moffitt PF, Kalucy EC, Kalucy RS, et al. Sleep difficulties, pain and other correlates. J Intern Med 1991;230(3):245–9.
11. Ohayon MM. Relationship between chronic painful physical condition and insomnia. J Psychiatr Res 2005;39(2):151–9.
12. Choiniere M, Racine M, Raymond-Shaw I. Epidemiology of pain and sleep disturbances and their reciprocal interrelationships. In: Lavigne G, Sessle B, Choiniere M, et al, editors. Sleep and pain. Seattle (WA): IASP Press; 2007. p. 267–84.
13. Menefee LA, Cohen MJ, Anderson WR, et al. Sleep disturbance and nonmalignant chronic pain: a comprehensive review of the literature. Pain Med 2000;1(2):156–72.
14. Linton SJM, Shane BJ. Pain and sleep disorders: clinical consequences and maintaining factors. Pain and sleep. Seattle (WA): IASP Press; 2007. p. 417–37.
15. Argoff CE. The coexistence of neuropathic pain, sleep, and psychiatric disorders: a novel treatment approach. Clin J Pain 2007;23(1):15–22.
16. Roehrs T, Hyde M, Blaisdell B, et al. Sleep loss and REM sleep loss are hyperalgesic. Sleep 2006;29(2):145–51.
17. Moldofsky H, Scarisbrick P. Induction of neurasthenic musculoskeletal pain syndrome by selective sleep stage deprivation. Psychosom Med 1976;38(1):35–44.
18. Bastuji H, Perchet C, Legrain V, et al. Laser evoked responses to painful stimulation persist during sleep and predict subsequent arousals. Pain 2008;137(3):589–99.
19. Sandrini G, Milanov I, Rossi B, et al. Effects of sleep on spinal nociceptive reflexes in humans. Sleep 2001;24(1):13–7.
20. Lavigne G, Zucconi M, Castronovo C, et al. Sleep arousal response to experimental thermal stimulation during sleep in human subjects free of pain and sleep problems. Pain 2000;84(2–3):283–90.
21. Lavigne G, Okura K, Smith MT. Pain perception-nociception during sleep. In: Basbaum AI, Bushnell MC, editors. Science of pain. New York: Elsevier; 2009. p. 783–94.
22. Soja PJ. Modulation of prethalamic sensory inflow during sleep versus wakefulness. In: Lavigne G, Sessle B, Choiniere M, et al, editors. Sleep and pain. Seattle (WA): IASP; 2007. p. 45–76.
23. Soja PJ, Pang W, Taepavarapruk N, et al. On the reduction of spontaneous and glutamate-driven spinocerebellar and spinoreticular tract neuronal activity during active sleep. Neuroscience 2001;104(1):199–206.
24. Merrill RL. Intraoral neuropathy. Curr Pain Headache Rep 2004;8(5):341–6.
25. Macfarlane TVW. Association between orofacial pain and other symptoms: a population-based study. Oral Biosci Med 2004;1(1):45–54.
26. Mitrirattanakul S, Merrill RL. Headache impact in patients with orofacial pain. J Am Dent Assoc 2006;137(9):1267–74.
27. Paiva T, Farinha A, Martins A, et al. Chronic headaches and sleep disorders. Arch Intern Med 1997;157(15):1701–5.
28. Yatani H, Studts J, Cordova M, et al. Comparison of sleep quality and clinical and psychologic characteristics in patients with temporomandibular disorders. J Orofac Pain 2002;16(3):221–8.
29. Smith MT, Wickwire EM, Grace EG, et al. Sleep disorders and their association with laboratory pain sensitivity in temporomandibular joint disorder. Sleep 2009;32(6):779–90.
30. Edwards RR, Grace E, Peterson S, et al. Sleep continuity and architecture: associations with pain-inhibitory processes in patients with temporomandibular joint disorder. Eur J Pain 2009;23.
31. De Leeuw R, editor. Orofacial pain: guidelines for assessment, diagnosis, and management. 4th edition. Hanover Park (IL): Quintessence Books; 2008. p. 136.
32. Camparis CM, Siqueira JT. Sleep bruxism: clinical aspects and characteristics in patients with and without chronic orofacial pain. Oral Surg Oral

Med Oral Pathol Oral Radiol Endod 2006;101(2): 188–93.

33. Baron R. Neuropathic pain: clinical. In: Basbaum AIB, Catherine M, editors. Science of pain. New York: Elsevier; 2009. p. 865–900.

34. Merrill RL. Differential diagnosis of orofacial pain. In: Laskin DMG, Charles S, Hylander WL, editors. Temporomandibular disorders: an evidence-based approach to diagnosis and treatment. Chicago: Quintessence Publishing Co Inc; 2006. p. 299–317.

35. Merrill RL, Graff-Radford SB. Trigeminal neuralgia: how to rule out the wrong treatment. J Am Dent Assoc 1992;123(2):63‑8.

36. Padilla M, Clark GT, Merrill RL. Topical medications for orofacial neuropathic pain: a review. J Am Dent Assoc 2000;131(2):184–95.

37. Murphy E, Merrill RL. Non-odontogenic toothache. J Ir Dent Assoc 2001;47(2):46–58.

38. Graff-Radford SB, Solberg WK. Atypical odontalgia. CDA J 1986;14(12):27–32.

39. Graff-Radford SB, Solberg WK. Atypical odontalgia. J Craniomandib Disord 1992;6(4):260–5.

40. Sessle B. What is pain, and why and how do we experience pain. In: Lavigne G, Sessle BJ, Choiniere M, et al, editors. Sleep and pain. Seattle (WA): IASP Press; 2007. p. 23–43.

41. Watkins LR, Hutchinson MR, Milligan ED, et al. "Listening" and "talking" to neurons: implications of immune activation for pain control and increasing the efficacy of opioids. Brain Res Rev 2007;56(1):148–69.

42. Watkins LR, Milligan ED, Maier SF. Spinal cord glia: new players in pain. Pain 2001;93(3):201–5.

43. Butera JA. Current and emerging targets to treat neuropathic pain. J Med Chem 2007;50(11):2543–6.

44. Miyoshi K, Narita M, Takatsu M, et al. mGlu5 receptor and protein kinase C implicated in the development and induction of neuropathic pain following chronic ethanol consumption. Eur J Pharmacol 2007;562(3):208–11.

45. Gratt BM, Sickels EA, Graff-Radford SB, et al. Electronic thermography in diagnosis of atypical odontalgia: a pilot study. Oral Surg Oral Med Oral Pathol 1989;68:472–81.

46. Graff-Radford SB, Ketelaer M-C, Gratt BM, et al. Thermographic assessment of neuropathic facial pain. J Orofac Pain 1995;9(2):138–45.

47. Fromm GH. Pathophysiology of trigeminal neuralgia. In: Fromm GH, Sessle BJ, editors. Trigeminal neuralgia, current concepts regarding pathogenesis and treatment. Boston: Butterworth-Heinemann; 1991. p. 105–30.

48. Dubner R. Neuropathic pain: new understanding leads to new treatments. J Pain 1993;2(1):8–11.

49. Merrill RL. Central mechanisms of orofacial pain. Dent Clin North Am 2007;51(1):45–59, v.

50. Rama A, Cho SC, Kushida CA. Normal human sleep. In: Lee-Chiong T, editor. Sleep medicine essentials. Hoboken (NJ): Wiley-Blackwell; 2009. p. 1–4.

51. Smith MT, Buenaver LF. Electroencephalographic correlates of pain and sleep interactions in humans. In: Lavigne G, Sessle BJ, Choiniere M, et al, editors. Sleep and pain. Seattle (WA): IASP Press; 2007. p. 189–212.

52. Perlis ML, Giles DE, Bootzin RR, et al. Alpha sleep and information processing, perception of sleep, pain, and arousability in fibromyalgia. Int J Neurosci 1997;89(3–4):265–80.

53. Dauvilliers Sleep YC. Pain interactions in medical disorders: the examples of fibromyalgia and headache. In: Lavigne G, Sessle B, Choiniere M, et al, editors. Sleep and pain. Seattle (WA): IASP Press; 2007. p. 285–309.

54. Moldofsky H, Scarisbrick P, England R, et al. Musculoskeletal symptoms and non-REM sleep disturbance in patients with fibrositis syndrome and healthy subjects. Psychosom Med 1975;37(4):341–51.

55. Drewes AM, Nielsen KD, Hansen B, et al. A longitudinal study of clinical symptoms and sleep parameters in rheumatoid arthritis. Rheumatology (Oxford) 2000;39(11):1287–9.

56. Macfarlane TV, Blinkhorn AS, Davies RM, et al. Predictors of outcome for orofacial pain in the general population: a four-year follow-up study. J Dent Res 2004;83(9):712–7.

57. Macfarlane TV, Gray RJM, Kincey J, et al. Factors associated with the temporomandibular disorder, pain dysfunction syndrome (PDS): Manchester case-control study. Oral Dis 2001;7(6):321–30.

58. Gold AR, Dipalo F, Gold MS, et al. Inspiratory airflow dynamics during sleep in women with fibromyalgia. Sleep 2004;27(3):459–66.

59. Scher AI, Lipton RB, Stewart WF. Habitual snoring as a risk factor for chronic daily headache. Neurology 2003;60(8):1366–8.

60. Haack M, Santangello G, Scott-Sutherland J, et al. Patients with primary insomnia experience more spontanous pain and hyperalgesia. Paper presented at: Sleep 2009, 23 Annual Meeting of the Associated Professional Sleep Societies, LLC2009. Seattle, Washington, June 6–11, 2009.

61. Guilleminault C, Eldridge FL, Tilkian A, et al. Sleep apnea syndrome due to upper airway obstruction: a review of 25 cases. Arch Intern Med 1977; 137(3):296–300.

62. Boutros NN. Headache in sleep apnea. Tex Med 1989;85(4):34–5.

63. Goder R, Friege L, Fritzer G, et al. Morning headaches in patients with sleep disorders: a systematic polysomnographic study. Sleep Med 2003;4(5):385–91.

64. Ong JC, Stepanski EJ, Gramling SE. Pain coping strategies for tension-type headache: possible implications for insomnia? J Clin Sleep Med 2009;5(1):52–6.

65. King CD, Jewett RE. The effects of -methyltyrosine on sleep and brain norepinephrine in cats. J Pharmacol Exp Ther 1971;177(1):188–95.

66. Ozcan M, Ayar A, Serhatlioglu I, et al. Orexins activates protein kinase C-mediated Ca(2+) signaling

in isolated rat primary sensory neurons. Physiol Res 2009. [Epub ahead of print].

67. Holland P, Goadsby PJ. The hypothalamic orexinergic system: pain and primary headaches. Headache 2007;47(6):951–62.

68. Holland PR, Akerman S, Goadsby PJ. Modulation of nociceptive dural input to the trigeminal nucleus caudalis via activation of the orexin 1 receptor in the rat. Eur J Neurosci 2006;24(10):2825–33.

69. Holland PR, Akerman S, Goadsby PJ. Orexin 1 receptor activation attenuates neurogenic dural vasodilation in an animal model of trigeminovascular nociception. J Pharmacol Exp Ther 2005;315(3): 1380–5.

Sleep and Headache

Steven B. Graff-Radford, DDS[a,b,*],
Antonia Teruel, DDS, MS, PhD[c], Satish K.S. Kumar, MDSc[c]

KEYWORDS

- Sleep disorders • Headaches • Migraine
- Cluster headache • Obstructive sleep apnea

The relationship between headache and sleep is diverse and complex. It has been studied and explained in many ways at the epidemiologic, clinical, anatomic, and pathophysiologic levels.[1–4] The prevalence of sleep dysregulation and sleep disorders is significantly higher in individuals with primary headaches, such as migraine and cluster headache.[5,6] In addition, research has shown that in patients with sleep disorders, nonspecific morning headaches, chronic daily headaches, and chronic awakening headaches (headaches awakening patients from sleep) are present in higher prevalence than the general population.[7] These sleep disorders may include sleep-disordered breathing, insomnia, circadian rhythm disorders, and parasomnia, among others.[8] In several studies, obstructive sleep apnea (OSA) has been associated with morning and awakening headaches, and with migraine and cluster headaches. Variations in sleep duration, as well as in sleep schedule, have been reported to be common triggers for headaches, and sleeping itself relieves headaches.[9] Patients with headaches and sleep disturbances also have psychiatric comorbidities, such as anxiety and depression.[8,10,11] Management of sleep disorders, regulation of sleep, and management of associated psychiatric comorbidities, such as anxiety or depression, may improve or resolve associated headache.[12,13] Although there is no definable cause-and-effect relationship between sleep and headache, sleep disorders pose a significant clinical implication in the management of patients with headaches.[1–3]

CLASSIFICATION

Several investigators who have studied the complex relationship between sleep and headache have attempted to explain the interactions between sleep and headache by classifying them in groups. Paiva and colleagues[14] identified four groups:

Headaches that are symptoms of a primary sleep disturbance

Sleep disturbances that are symptoms of a primary headache disorder

Sleep disturbance and headaches that are symptoms of an unrelated medical disorder

Sleep disorders and headaches that are both manifestations of a similar underlying pathogenesis.

Dodick and colleagues[4] in 2003 identified three groups:

Headaches as a result of sleep disruption

Headaches as a cause of sleep disruption

Headaches as a sleep-related disorder.

EPIDEMIOLOGIC AND CLINICAL EVIDENCE: SLEEP AND HEADACHE ASSOCIATION

Several studies in the general population as well as in the clinical population have shown an association between sleep disorders or sleep dysregulation and various headaches, including primary

a The Program for Headache and Orofacial Pain, The Pain Center, Cedars Sinai Medical Center, 444 South San Vicente # 1101, Los Angeles, CA 90048, USA
b UCLA School of Dentistry, Los Angeles, CA 90024, USA
c University of Southern California School of Dentistry, 925 West 34th Street, Room # 4333, Los Angeles, CA 90089, USA
* Corresponding author. The Program for Headache and Orofacial Pain, The Pain Center, Cedars Sinai Medical Center, 444 S San Vicente # 1101, Los Angeles, CA 90048.
E-mail address: graffs@cshs.org (S.B. Graff-Radford).

Sleep Med Clin 5 (2010) 145–152
doi:10.1016/j.jsmc.2009.09.002
1556-407X/10/$ – see front matter © 2010 Elsevier Inc. All rights reserved.

headache, secondary headache, and nonspecific morning/awakening headaches. The following sections outline selected studies that have documented this relationship. The limitation of some studies in defining the headaches, their chronicity, and presence of comorbid factors, such as anxiety and depression, has been reported.[4]

Sleep Disorders and Dysregulation

Sleep disturbances have been reported to trigger headaches and sleeping itself relieves headaches. Severe sleep problems have been shown to predict new headache in patients headache-free at baseline. Absence of sleep problems predicted recovery during 1-year follow-up in patients with recent headache at baseline.[15] The general association between sleep and headache is also seen in specific sleep disorders.

Obstructive sleep apnea

OSA is the most common sleep-related breathing disorder.[16,17] There is increased risk in patients with OSA for developing cardiovascular diseases, such as hypertension, coronary artery disease, arrhythmias, heart failure, and stroke, as well as metabolic syndrome, including type 2 diabetes. OSA also impairs cognition and predisposes depression. Significant morbidity and mortality from these associated conditions have been reported.[16,17] OSA has also been associated with headaches in numerous publications.[18–21]

The International Classification of Headache Disorders II (ICHD-II) has established a separate class of secondary headaches termed 10.1.3–Sleep apnea headache under the broader classification of 10–Headache attributed to disorders of homeostasis and 10.1–Headache attributed to hypoxia or hypercapnia.[22] Although the strength of the association between OSA and headaches in epidemiologic studies merits a separate classification, Rains and Poceta[2] emphasize the need to validate these criteria and point out the deficiencies, particularly the exclusion of other sleep-related breathing disorders, such as upper airway resistance syndrome (UARS).

Snoring, commonly seen in chronic daily headache patients,[23] is within the spectrum of obstructive sleep-related breathing disorders, including UARS and OSA.[1,24–27] Awakening headaches have been shown to be significantly associated with patients with OSA when compared with patients with periodic limb-movement disorder. These headaches are brief, and their occurrence and severity increase with increasing OSA severity. Fluctuations in nighttime oxygen saturation with hypercapnia, increased intracranial pressure, vasodilatation, and impaired sleep quality

have all been implicated pathogenically in the relationship of OSA and headache.[21]

Treatment of OSA with continuous positive airway pressure (CPAP) or uvulopalatopharyngoplasty has shown to improve awakening headaches in OSA patients. Interestingly, patients in the same cohort with primary headache disorders, such as migraine and tension-type headache (TTH), showed minimal improvement with OSA treatment.[19]

In children with headaches, polysomnographic studies have revealed that severe and chronic migraine were associated with sleep disturbances. Compared with other children, children with headaches have shorter sleep time, longer sleep latency, and shorter rapid eye movement (REM) and slow-wave sleep. In addition, sleep-disordered breathing was seen more commonly in children with migraine and nonspecific headaches. Interestingly, TTH was not associated with sleep-disordered breathing, but was noted to be associated with sleep bruxism.[28]

Mitsikostas and colleagues[18] conducted polysomnography on 72 patients with chronic and refractory headaches that occurred during sleep or in whom sleep was accompanied by snoring. Twenty-one cases (29.2%) had OSA. Their headaches were classified, and the majority were medication overuse headache (9) and cluster headache (6). Results with treatment were mixed. Five (23.8%) had a greater than 50% reduction in headache days. Fourteen (66.6%) had increased headache frequency requiring medication management. In the remaining 2 cases (9.5%), headache frequency did not change. Neau and colleagues[20] noted in 68% (36 of 53 cases) with headache and OSA a similar finding with regards to treatment of OSA reducing headache burden. They showed improvement in headache symptoms after sleep apnea treatment.

Although managing OSA in healthy patients does not completely resolve the headache, favorable results often occur in most headache populations. These data warrant evaluating sleep and headache with polysomnography and managing the underlying OSA and UARS when discovered.

Insomnia

Insomnia is the most common sleep disorder seen in headache patients, both in adults and in children.[9,12,29–33] Chronic morning headache may indicate a major depressive disorder.[5] Kelman and Rains,[29] in a study of 1283 migraineurs, found that over 50% had difficulty initiating and maintaining sleep at least occasionally. Over one third reported that they experienced this difficulty frequently. The investigators also reported insomnialike symptoms in migraineurs were at least threefold greater than the incidence in the general population.[29] Ong and colleagues[9] studied self-report data from patients with TTH and control patients with minimal pain. The TTH patients reported more sleep problems and stress as a headache trigger, while going to sleep was used as a pain-coping measure. With these findings, they hypothesized that the sleep-seeking behavior itself might be a mediating factor in the development of insomnia among TTH patients.

Dyssomnias and parasomnias

In a large epidemiologic study done in Europe, circadian rhythm disorder (as defined in the *Diagnostic and Statistical Manual of Mental Disorders, Fourth Edition* [*DSM-IV*]) was found to be significantly associated with chronic morning headache patients compared with other subjects.[5]

Restless leg syndrome (RLS) was shown to occur in significantly higher frequency in a cohort of 200 headache patients (22.4% vs 8.3%) than in control subjects (n = 120). About 60% of RLS patients (n = 27) were affected by migraine without aura and 30% (n = 13) were affected by a combination of two headache types. In addition, headache patients with RLS reported sleep disturbances more frequently compared with those without RLS (50.0% vs 32.7%).[34] In a study involving 584 children, sleep disorders were more common in the 300 children with headache than in the control group with 284 children. Parasomnia symptoms included sleep talking (48.3% in the headache group vs 38.7% in the control group), bruxism (23.3% in the headache group vs 16.5% in the control group), leg movement (20.3% in the headache group vs 18.0% in the control group), and nightmares (16.7% in the headache group vs 7.4% in the control group).[6]

A case-control study investigating excessive daytime sleepiness in 100 patients with episodic migraine found that excessive daytime sleepiness was more frequent in migraineurs than in controls and that excessive daytime sleepiness was noted to correlate with migraine disability, sleep problems, and anxiety.[35] In children with migraine, a high frequency of somnambulism (sleep walking) has been reported.[36] In another study done with a sample of 100 patients (54 women and 46 men) with proven narcolepsy, migraine prevalence was noted in 44.4% of women and in 28.3% of men, about 40% of the total narcoleptic study population.[37] Parasomnias have also been reported in children with migraines[38] and in a group of 4 children with nocturnal cluster headaches who responded to indomethacin.[39]

Headaches

Nonspecific, chronic morning headaches and awakening headaches; primary headache disorders, such as migraine, TTH, and cluster headache; and secondary headache disorders, such as hypnic headaches, have been associated with sleep disturbances and sleep disorders.

Chronic morning headaches and awakening headaches

In a large European epidemiologic study, investigators reported chronic morning headache prevalence as 7.6% (n = 1442). The data were gathered through a telephone questionnaire evaluation done involving 18,980 individuals (15 years or older) across five European countries. Several factors were found to be significantly associated with chronic morning headache, including comorbid anxiety and depressive disorders (28.5% vs 5.5%), major depressive disorder alone (21.3% vs 5.5%), dyssomnia not otherwise specified (17.1% vs 6.9%), insomnia disorder (14.4% vs 6.9%), circadian rhythm disorder (20.0% vs 7.5%), and sleep-related breathing disorder (15.2% vs 7.5%).[5] A prospective longitudinal study done over a 3-year period in 1698 migraineurs (3582 migraine attacks) found that nearly half of all attacks occurred between 4 AM and 9 AM, indicating that migraine occurred predominantly in REM sleep.[40] Morning headaches in patients with sleep disorders have been proposed to have anatomically identical central origin regulating sleep and pain.[41] Awakening headaches have been shown to be common among patients with migraine (n = 1283), with 71% reporting at least occasional headaches awakening them from sleep.[29]

Migraine

Several studies in adult and child migraineurs have shown sleep dysregulation and sleep disorders are related to headache.[29,38,40,42,43] Migraine has also been shown to occur during sleep, predominantly in REM sleep, and sleeping itself has been palliative for migraineurs.[29,31] Thus, the relationship between migraine and sleep is complex and hypotheses on common or overlapping pathophysiology of migraine and other sleep-related headaches with sleep disorders have been suggested.[4,44]

In a study done with 1283 migraineurs (84% female, 16% male), over half of migraineurs reported difficulty initiating and maintaining sleep at least occasionally. Sleep disturbances triggered the onset of migraines in 50% of patients; 85% of patients "chose to" and 75% were "forced to" sleep or rest because of headache. Patients who slept an average of 6 hours per night experienced more frequent and severe headaches and headaches on awakening than patients who slept longer. Patients with chronic migraine slept shorter during nights (6 hours) and experienced more sleeping difficulties compared with patients with episodic migraine.[29]

In a prospective study involving 68 female migraine patients with recorded 1869 migraine attacks, the relationship between insomnia and migraine was recorded. The migraine attacks were designated as insomnia-related if the patients reported difficulties in falling asleep and/or maintaining sleep the night before the reported attack or the night of the attack. Of the 1869 migraine attacks, 533 (29%) were considered insomnia-related and occurred mainly in the morning hours. A key observation is that patients experienced insomnia before the onset of migraine attacks (79% of attacks).[31]

In a recent controlled family study, a significant association between migraine and the number of sleep problems, as well as several specific sleep symptoms among migraineurs and their adult relatives, was reported. Interestingly, these associations between sleep problems and migraine persisted after controlling for usual comorbidities of both lifetime and current anxiety and mood disorders.[30]

A case-control study determining the comorbidity of RLS and migraine with patients with migraine (n = 411) and an equal number of sex- and age-matched control subjects, reported that RLS frequency was significantly higher in migraine patients than in control subjects (17.3% vs 5.6%, $P<.001$; odds ratio 3.5 [95% CI, 2.2–5.8]).[45]

There is evidence as discussed that regulation of sleep may improve migraine.[13] Children with migraine who not only have sleep disturbances but also have behavioral problems may be helped in overcoming behavioral problems related to sleep and migraine.[42] Thus, clinical evaluation and management of sleep problems are critical in migraineurs.

Tension-type headache
Ong and colleagues[9] studied self-report data from patients with TTH and from control patients with minimal pain. A significant proportion of TTH patients reported sleep problems. Many also reported stress as a trigger of headaches. Meanwhile, TTH patients, like migraine patients, used sleep as a palliative measure. In a study involving 2226 school children (6–13 years old), the overall prevalence of headache was 31% with higher prevalence of TTH (5.5%) than migraine (1.7%). However, abnormal sleep pattern was noted to be significantly associated with migraine, but not in TTH.[43] Sleeping problems have been shown to be a poor prognostic indicator in episodic TTH[46] and thus sleep regulation is essential in management of episodic TTH.

Cluster headache
Cluster headache presents with attacks of severe, strictly unilateral pain in orbital, supraorbital, or temporal sites, or in any combination of these sites. It typically lasts 15 to 180 minutes. The attacks are typically associated with ipsilateral autonomic features, such as conjunctival injection and lacrimation.[22] Cluster headaches occur during specific sleep stages (REM phase) and patients often wake up from sleep.[47,48] The circadian rhythm of cluster headache has led to the findings of critical role played by hypothalamus in cluster headache.[49–51] Sleep disorders have been associated with cluster headache, including OSA, insomnia, and narcolepsy.[47,52–54] There have been reports that management of OSA may improve cluster headache symptoms and, in fact, the high incidence of OSA seen in cluster headache population have led clinicians to consider sleep evaluation and appropriate management with CPAP or an oral appliance.[53] Successful treatment of the sleep apnea does not usually translate to decreasing cluster headache. It is postulated that there are two coexisting conditions causing the headache and apnea.[49]

Chronic paroxysmal hemicrania, another form of trigeminal autonomic cephalalgia, has been shown to be associated with sleep disturbances[7] and to occur in REM phase of sleep.[55]

Hypnic headache
Hypnic headache occurs exclusively during sleep and has been shown to arise both from non-REM[56,57] and REM sleep,[58,59] with majority of cases recorded arising from REM sleep, in particular, the first REM stage. Snoring was noted in patients with hypnic headache. However, a sleep disorder is uncommon and only few reports have associated hypnic headaches with OSA and oxygen desaturation.[60,61] Caffeine before sleep often prevents hypnic headache.

PATHOPHYSIOLOGY

Dodick and colleagues[4] have reviewed in detail the underlying pathophysiology of sleep disorders and headache, as well as associated psychiatric comorbidities. They have reviewed in particular the role of hypothalamus, serotonin, and melatonin in sleep, headache, and mood.

As explained, hypothalamic involvement has been shown in primary headache disorders, including migraine; in trigeminal autonomic cephalalgias, including cluster headaches; and in hypnic headaches.[44,58,62] Blood investigations in chronic migraine patients (338 blood samples from 17 chronic migraine patients) have shown alterations in hormones related to hypothalamus, including decreased nocturnal prolactin peak and increased cortisol concentrations. Also, lower melatonin concentration in patients with chronic migraine with insomnia was observed.[62] These findings have potential clinical implications in evaluation and management.[63] In another study, the chances of having RLS in migraine patients were found to be more than five times higher in the presence of dopaminergic premonitory symptoms, which could support a role for dopamine involvement in the pathogenesis of both disorders.[64] Sabayan and colleagues[65] proposed a joint origin for RLS and migraine based on (1) the observations of the same genetic origin for migraine without aura and RLS in a single Italian family on chromosome 14q2, where the gene coding survival motor neuron-interacting protein 1 is believed to play a role in both diseases; (2) correlation of both RLS and migraine with the chronic pain syndrome fibromyalgia; and (3) the cortical excitability alteration.

CLINICAL AND MANAGEMENT IMPLICATIONS

Research has revealed and will continue to reveal specific patterns and connections related to sleep and headache. These revelations will improve clinical assessment and management. For instance, screening for and treating sleep disorders and implementing sleep-regulation strategies will help clinicians prevent headache, especially in high-risk individuals. Managing sleep disorders may resolve or improve headaches.[7,12,29,66]

A recent randomized, placebo-controlled study done in 43 women with transformed migraine assessed the impact that behavioral sleep modification had on headache. Patients either received behavioral sleep instructions or placebo behavioral instructions in addition to usual medical care. The patients were followed at 6-week intervals. At the first follow-up, all patients received behavioral sleep modification. Subjects recorded their headache symptoms in standard headache diaries. Patients who received behavioral sleep modification in the first 6 weeks reported statistically significant reduction in headache frequency and headache intensity compared with the placebo behavioral group. Also, those patients who received behavioral sleep modification were more likely to revert to episodic migraine, while none of the patients from placebo group reverted to episodic migraine. Interestingly, at the final visit, 48.5% of those who had received behavioral sleep modification instructions had reverted to episodic migraine.[13]

OSA carries a high morbidity and mortality because of consequent cardiovascular sequelae and metabolic syndrome.[16,17] In addition, a recent literature review has shown that sleep-disordered breathing may cause permanent brain changes, including gray- and white-matter loss, alteration in autonomic and motor regulation, and damage to higher cognitive functions, and that these changes can start early in the progression of sleep disorders.[67] Hence, early diagnosis of disorders, especially OSA, is essential and, because such disorders are common in headache populations, screening for OSA is prudent.[1,2]

A Cochrane systematic review has concluded that CPAP is effective in patients with moderate and severe OSA. Although CPAP is more effective than oral appliances, patients seem to prefer oral appliances in managing OSA, probably because an oral appliance is easier to use.[68] Mandibular advancement with 50% of protrusive capacity with an oral appliance has shown to be beneficial in management of mild to moderate sleep apnea.[69,70] Hence, dentists involved in the management of OSA with oral appliances can help in screening headache patients for a possible underlying sleep disorder, such as UARS and OSA. Dentists can also help in management of OSA by appropriate construction of oral appliances on the physician's recommendation. Also, dentists can play a critical role in managing sleep bruxism, which is often associated with TTH, with oral appliance therapy along with other multidisciplinary treatment approaches, such as stress management, biofeedback, physical therapy, and pharmacologic treatment of headaches.[71]

SUMMARY

Sleep, shown to be associated with headaches in diverse and complex ways, has been palliative in many headaches. Sleep regulation and management of sleep disorders via multiple modalities, including CPAP, oral appliances, medications, surgery, behavioral sleep regulation, and psychological and cognitive behavioral management, will help not only in resolving the direct consequences of poor sleeping habits and sleep disorders (eg, cardiovascular diseases and metabolic syndrome in the case of OSA), but also in resolving or improving associated comorbidities, such as headaches and mood disorders. Hence, a thorough evaluation of patients with headaches and/or sleep disturbances is necessary for effective management. Dentists can play a critical role in management of these comorbid disorders of sleep and headaches.

REFERENCES

1. Rains JC, Poceta JS, Penzien DB. Sleep and headaches. Curr Neurol Neurosci Rep 2008;8(2):167–75.
2. Rains JC, Poceta JS. Headache and sleep disorders: review and clinical implications for headache management. Headache 2006;46(9):1344–63.
3. Jennum P, Jensen R. Sleep and headache. Sleep Med Rev 2002;6(6):471–9.
4. Dodick DW, Eross EJ, Parish JM, et al. Clinical, anatomical, and physiologic relationship between sleep and headache. Headache 2003;43(3):282–92.
5. Ohayon MM. Prevalence and risk factors of morning headaches in the general population. Arch Intern Med 2004;164(1):97–102.
6. Zarowski M, Mlodzikowska-Albrecht J, Steinborn B. The sleep habits and sleep disorders in children with headache. Adv Med Sci 2007;52(Suppl 1): 194–6.
7. Paiva T, Farinha A, Martins A, et al. Chronic headaches and sleep disorders. Arch Intern Med 1997; 157(15):1701–5.
8. Bruni O, Russo PM, Ferri R, et al. Relationships between headache and sleep in a non-clinical population of children and adolescents. Sleep Med 2008;9(5):542–8.
9. Ong JC, Stepanski EJ, Gramling SE. Pain coping strategies for tension-type headache: possible implications for insomnia? J Clin Sleep Med 2009;5(1): 52–6.
10. Blay SL, Andreoli SB, Gastal FL. Chronic painful physical conditions, disturbed sleep and psychiatric morbidity: results from an elderly survey. Ann Clin Psychiatry 2007;19(3):169–74.
11. Lake AE 3rd, Rains JC, Penzien DB, et al. Headache and psychiatric comorbidity: historical context, clinical implications, and research relevance. Headache 2005;45(5):493–506.
12. Rains JC. Optimizing circadian cycles and behavioral insomnia treatment in migraine. Curr Pain Headache Rep 2008;12(3):213–9.
13. Calhoun AH, Ford S. Behavioral sleep modification may revert transformed migraine to episodic migraine. Headache 2007;47(8):1178–83.
14. Paiva T, Batista A, Martins P, et al. The relationship between headaches and sleep disturbances. Headache 1995;35(10):590–6.
15. Boardman HF, Thomas E, Millson DS, et al. The natural history of headache: predictors of onset and recovery. Cephalalgia 2006;26(9):1080–8.
16. Rakel RE. Clinical and societal consequences of obstructive sleep apnea and excessive daytime sleepiness. Postgrad Med 2009;121(1):86–95.
17. Bradley TD, Floras JS. Obstructive sleep apnoea and its cardiovascular consequences. Lancet 2009;373(9657):82–93.
18. Mitsikostas DD, Vikelis M, Viskos A. Refractory chronic headache associated with obstructive sleep apnoea syndrome. Cephalalgia 2008;28(2):139–43.
19. Loh NK, Dinner DS, Foldvary N, et al. Do patients with obstructive sleep apnea wake up with headaches? Arch Intern Med 1999;159(15):1765–8.
20. Neau JP, Paquereau J, Bailbe M, et al. Relationship between sleep apnoea syndrome, snoring and headaches. Cephalalgia 2002;22(5):333–9.
21. Provini F, Vetrugno R, Lugaresi E, et al. Sleep-related breathing disorders and headache. Neurol Sci 2006; 27(Suppl 2):S149–52.
22. The international classification of headache disorders: 2nd edition. Cephalalgia 2004;24(Suppl 1): 9–160.
23. Scher AI, Lipton RB, Stewart WF. Habitual snoring as a risk factor for chronic daily headache. Neurology 2003;60(8):1366–8.
24. Stoohs RA, Knaack L, Blum HC, et al. Differences in clinical features of upper airway resistance syndrome, primary snoring, and obstructive sleep apnea/hypopnea syndrome. Sleep Med 2008;9(2): 121–8.
25. Gold AR, Gold MS, Harris KW, et al. Hypersomnolence, insomnia and the pathophysiology of upper airway resistance syndrome. Sleep Med 2008;9(6): 675–83.
26. Gold AR, Dipalo F, Gold MS, et al. The symptoms and signs of upper airway resistance syndrome: a link to the functional somatic syndromes. Chest 2003;123(1):87–95.
27. Guilleminault C, Kirisoglu C, Poyares D, et al. Upper airway resistance syndrome: a long-term outcome study. J Psychiatr Res 2006;40(3):273–9.
28. Vendrame M, Kaleyias J, Valencia I, et al. Polysomnographic findings in children with headaches. Pediatr Neurol 2008;39(1):6–11.
29. Kelman L, Rains JC. Headache and sleep: examination of sleep patterns and complaints in a large clinical sample of migraineurs. Headache 2005;45(7): 904–10.
30. Vgontzas A, Cui L, Merikangas KR. Are sleep difficulties associated with migraine attributable to anxiety and depression? Headache 2008;48(10):1451–9.
31. Alstadhaug K, Salvesen R, Bekkelund S. Insomnia and circadian variation of attacks in episodic migraine. Headache 2007;47(8):1184–8.
32. Luc ME, Gupta A, Birnberg JM, et al. Characterization of symptoms of sleep disorders in children with headache. Pediatr Neurol 2006;34(1):7–12.
33. Alberti A, Mazzotta G, Gallinella E, et al. Headache characteristics in obstructive sleep apnea syndrome and insomnia. Acta Neurol Scand 2005;111(5): 309–16.

34. d'Onofrio F, Bussone G, Cologno D, et al. Restless legs syndrome and primary headaches: a clinical study. Neurol Sci 2008;29(Suppl 1):S169–72.

35. Barbanti P, Fabbrini G, Aurilia C, et al. A case-control study on excessive daytime sleepiness in episodic migraine. Cephalalgia 2007;27(10): 1115–9.

36. Barabas G, Ferrari M, Matthews WS. Childhood migraine and somnambulism. Neurology 1983; 33(7):948–9.

37. Dahmen N, Kasten M, Wieczorek S, et al. Increased frequency of migraine in narcoleptic patients: a confirmatory study. Cephalalgia 2003;23(1):14–9.

38. Isik U, Ersu RH, Ay P, et al. Prevalence of headache and its association with sleep disorders in children. Pediatr Neurol 2007;36(3):146–51.

39. Isik U, D'Cruz OF. Cluster headaches simulating parasomnias. Pediatr Neurol 2002;27(3):227–9.

40. Fox AW, Davis RL. Migraine chronobiology. Headache 1998;38(6):436–41.

41. Goder R, Friege L, Fritzer G, et al. Morning headaches in patients with sleep disorders: a systematic polysomnographic study. Sleep Med 2003;4(5): 385–91.

42. Heng K, Wirrell E. Sleep disturbance in children with migraine. J Child Neurol 2006;21(9):761–6.

43. Ayatollahi SM, Khosravi A. Prevalence of migraine and tension-type headache in primary-school children in Shiraz. East Mediterr Health J 2006;12(6): 809–17.

44. Cortelli P, Pierangeli G. Hypothalamus and headaches. Neurol Sci 2007;28(Suppl 2):S198–202.

45. Rhode AM, Hosing VG, Happe S, et al. Comorbidity of migraine and restless legs syndrome—a case-control study. Cephalalgia 2007;27(11):1255–60.

46. Lyngberg AC, Rasmussen BK, Jorgensen T, et al. Prognosis of migraine and tension-type headache: a population-based follow-up study. Neurology 2005;65(4):580–5.

47. Nobre ME, Leal AJ, Filho PM. Investigation into sleep disturbance of patients suffering from cluster headache. Cephalalgia 2005;25(7):488–92.

48. Nobre ME, Filho PF, Dominici M. Cluster headache associated with sleep apnoea. Cephalalgia 2003; 23(4):276–9.

49. Graff-Radford SB, Teruel A. Cluster headache and obstructive sleep apnea: Are they related disorders? Curr Pain Headache Rep 2009;13(2):160–3.

50. Holle D, Obermann M, Katsarava Z. The electrophysiology of cluster headache. Curr Pain Headache Rep 2009;13(2):155–9.

51. Brittain JS, Green AL, Jenkinson N, et al. Local field potentials reveal a distinctive neural signature of cluster headache in the hypothalamus. Cephalalgia 2009;29(11):1165–73.

52. Weintraub JR. Cluster headaches and sleep disorders. Curr Pain Headache Rep 2003;7(2):150–6.

53. Graff-Radford SB, Newman A. Obstructive sleep apnea and cluster headache. Headache 2004; 44(6):607–10.

54. Chervin RD, Zallek SN, Lin X, et al. Sleep disordered breathing in patients with cluster headache. Neurology 2000;54(12):2302–6.

55. Kayed K, Godtlibsen OB, Sjaastad O. Chronic paroxysmal hemicrania IV: "REM sleep locked" nocturnal headache attacks. Sleep 1978;1(1):91–5.

56. Dolso P, Merlino G, Fratticci L, et al. Non-REM hypnic headache: a circadian disorder? A clinical and polysomnographic study. Cephalalgia 2007; 27(1):83–6.

57. Manni R, Sances G, Terzaghi M, et al. Hypnic headache: PSG evidence of both REM- and NREM-related attacks. Neurology 2004;62(8):1411–3.

58. Dodick DW. Polysomnography in hypnic headache syndrome. Headache 2000;40(9):748–52.

59. Pinessi L, Rainero I, Cicolin A, et al. Hypnic headache syndrome: association of the attacks with REM sleep. Cephalalgia 2003;23(2):150–4.

60. Evers S, Goadsby PJ. Hypnic headache: clinical features, pathophysiology, and treatment. Neurology 2003;60(6):905–9.

61. Evers S, Rahmann A, Schwaag S, et al. Hypnic headache—the first German cases including polysomnography. Cephalalgia 2003;23(1):20–3.

62. Peres MF, Sanchez del Rio M, Seabra ML, et al. Hypothalamic involvement in chronic migraine. J Neurol Neurosurg Psychiatry 2001;71(6):747–51.

63. Nagtegaal JE, Smits MG, Swart AC, et al. Melatonin-responsive headache in delayed sleep phase syndrome: preliminary observations. Headache 1998;38(4):303–7.

64. Cologno D, Cicarelli G, Petretta V, et al. High prevalence of dopaminergic premonitory symptoms in migraine patients with restless legs syndrome: a pathogenetic link? Neurol Sci 2008;29(Suppl 1): S166–8.

65. Sabayan B, Bagheri M, Borhani Haghighi A. Possible joint origin of restless leg syndrome (RLS) and migraine. Med Hypotheses 2007; 69(1):64–6.

66. Rains JC. Chronic headache and potentially modifiable risk factors: screening and behavioral management of sleep disorders. Headache 2008;48(1): 32–9.

67. Simmons MS, Clark GT. The potentially harmful medical consequences of untreated sleep-disordered breathing: the evidence supporting brain damage. J Am Dent Assoc 2009;140(5):536–42.

68. Giles TL, Lasserson TJ, Smith BH, et al. Continuous positive airways pressure for obstructive sleep apnoea in adults. Cochrane Database Syst Rev 2006;3:CD001106.

69. Tegelberg A, Walker-Engstrom ML, Vestling O, et al. Two different degrees of mandibular advancement

with a dental appliance in treatment of patients with mild to moderate obstructive sleep apnea. Acta Odontol Scand 2003;61(6):356–62.

70. Hammond RJ, Gotsopoulos H, Shen G, et al. A follow-up study of dental and skeletal changes associated with mandibular advancement splint use in obstructive sleep apnea. Am J Orthod Dentofacial Orthop 2007;132(6):806–14.

71. Biondi DM. Headaches and their relationship to sleep. Dent Clin North Am 2001;45(4):685–700.

Surgical Therapy for Sleep Breathing Disorders

Michael Friedman, MD[a,b,c],*,
Meghan N. Wilson, MD[b,c]

KEYWORDS

- Obstructive sleep apnea
- Surgical treatment of obstructive sleep apnea
- Minimally invasive surgery • Sleep-disordered breathing

Current thinking in surgical treatment of obstructive sleep apnea/hypopnea syndrome (OSAHS) has evolved since uvulopalatopharyngoplasty (UPPP) was first introduced by Fujita in 1981.[1] The major change has been the recognition that UPPP, or some modification of UPPP as an isolated procedure, is not the standard but is appropriate only for a select group of patients with disease limited to the palate and tonsils. Multilevel surgical treatment is accepted as the standard for most patients.

Surgery involves either resection of tissue, reconstruction of tissue or both. Although techniques for removal may be standard, reconstructive procedures are as varied as patients' anatomy and symptomatology. Innovation is based on the need to achieve an ideal result, and just as there is no limit to perfection, there is no limit to innovation.

Recent thinking has created many more innovations. The three common anatomic areas assumed to obstruct the airway in OSAHS are the nose, the palate, and the retrolingual area. Because patients vary greatly in anatomy, it is clearly logical that different types of reconstruction may be required for each location. Standard corrective procedures need to be individualized based on patients' needs; in many cases nonstandard techniques are needed to meet these goals. Once the sites of obstruction have been identified in patients, the corrective means for each anatomic site can be planned, which may include surgical and nonsurgical procedures. Often palatal and retrolingual obstruction can be corrected or improved with a mandibular advancement device. This article highlights just a few of the standard and innovative techniques used to address each area of obstruction.

NASAL VALVE REPAIR

Difficulty breathing through the nose is a frequent complaint of otolaryngology patients. Although obstruction caused by septal deviation and turbinate hypertrophy are routinely examined for, nasal valve obstruction is frequently overlooked. In a study by Elwany and Thabet[2] of 500 subjects who had chronic nasal obstruction, 13% had an incompetent nasal valve as the cause of nasal obstruction. Because patients who have OSAHS have increased respiratory effort, it is likely that nasal valve collapse is more common in this group of patients. Many have had turbinate reduction and correction of their deviated septum but continue to have nocturnal nasal obstruction.

The anterior nostril may be narrowed by incompetence at the internal nasal valve, the external nasal valve, or both. There are several causes of

---

There are no financial relationships to disclose.
ᵃ Department of Otolaryngology, Section of Sleep Surgery, Rush University Medical Center, Chicago, IL, USA
ᵇ Department of Otolaryngology, Advocate Illinois Masonic Medical Center, Chicago, IL, USA
ᶜ Advanced Center for Specialty Care, 3000 North Halsted Street, Suite 400, Chicago, IL 60657, USA
* Corresponding author. Advanced Center for Specialty Care, 3000 North Halsted Street, Suite 400, Chicago, IL 60657.
E-mail address: hednnek@aol.com (M. Friedman).

Sleep Med Clin 5 (2010) 153–162
doi:10.1016/j.jsmc.2009.10.006

an incompetent nasal valve including congenital weakness of the nasal sidewalls, aging, reduction rhinoplasty, and trauma; reduction rhinoplasty accounts for the majority of cases.[2,3] Decreased airflow through the nostril may contribute to snoring and OSAHS.

Corrective procedures aim to increase the minimum cross-sectional area of the nasal valve through strengthening support structures including the nasal septum, nasal sidewalls, or columella using grafts of septal or conchal cartilage or anchored sutures. Some techniques are done endoscopically, but open procedures often allow better visualization and more precise graft placement. Many approaches to correct the nasal valve have been described as follows. Internal valve repair can be accomplished with spreader grafts,[4] cartilage overlay grafts,[5] or splay conchal grafts.[5] Repair of the external nasal valve may be done with lateral suspension sutures,[6,7] alar batten grafts,[8,9] or columelloplasty.[10] For patients who have OSAHS, the simplified approach of orbital suspension reported by Friedman and colleagues[6,7] is often the preferred technique.

This technique is shown in **Figs. 1–3**. The procedure can be performed under general anesthesia or local anesthesia. The nasal valve area is examined to identify the area of collapse before injection of local anesthesia to avoid distortion of tissue. The Mitek Soft Tissue Anchor system (1.3 mm

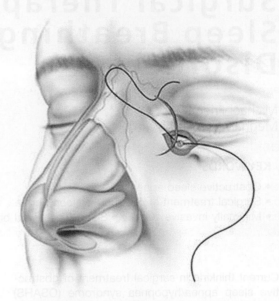

Fig. 2. The suture is inserted into a curved, tapered needle and passed into the nasal valve area, through the incised mucosa. (*From* Friedman M. Sleep apnea and snoring: surgical and non-surgical therapy. Philadelphia: Saunders; 2009; with permission.)

Micro Quick Anchor; Ethicon), which includes a drill bit, bone anchor, and attached suture, is used to anchor a suture to the orbital rim. After identifying the site of collapse and the intended site of

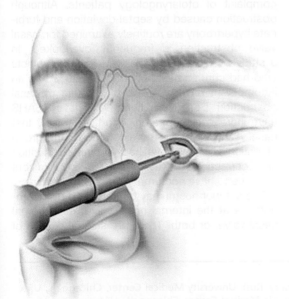

Fig. 1. A small drill hole is made in the orbital rim, in preparation for insertion of the anchoring system and suture. (*From* Friedman M. Sleep apnea and snoring: surgical and non-surgical therapy. Philadelphia: Saunders; 2009; with permission.)

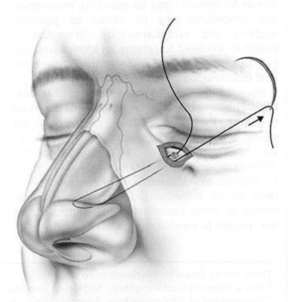

Fig. 3. The needle is then rethreaded and passed through the opening in the mucosa toward the anchor. (*From* Friedman M. Sleep apnea and snoring: surgical and non-surgical therapy. Philadelphia: Saunders; 2009; with permission.)

suspension, the needle is then rethreaded and passed from the caudal point toward the anchor. The suture is then tightened and tied with the proper amount of tension to open the valve but to avoid significant distortion of the external valve area. The orbital rim incision is closed with sterile adhesive skin closure strips.

PALATAL AND HYPOPHARYNGEAL OBSTRUCTION: CLINICAL ASSESSMENT

Determining the sites of obstruction is critical to effective treatment planning. Friedman and colleagues[11–13] introduced a simple clinical assessment to predict hypopharyngeal obstruction, which is based on a simple examination of the tongue/palate relationship as seen when patients opens their mouth. **Fig. 4** illustrates

Friedman Tongue Position (FTP) I through IV. Staging is based on a combination of FTP, tonsil size (**Fig. 5**), and body mass index (BMI). Patients who have a favorable tongue position (I or II), large tonsils (3 or 4), and a BMI less than 40 have primarily palatal/tonsil obstruction (stage I). Treatment directed at the palate and tonsils, classic UPPP, is effective in these patients (80% success).[12] Patients who have an unfavorable FTP (III or IV) and small tonsils (1 or 2) [stage III] are not likely to benefit from palate/tonsil surgery without treatment of the hypopharynx.

UVULOPALATOPHARYNGOPLASTY

Classical treatment of palatal/tonsil obstruction was UPPP introduced by Fujita.[1] It includes tonsillectomy and partial resection of the soft palate

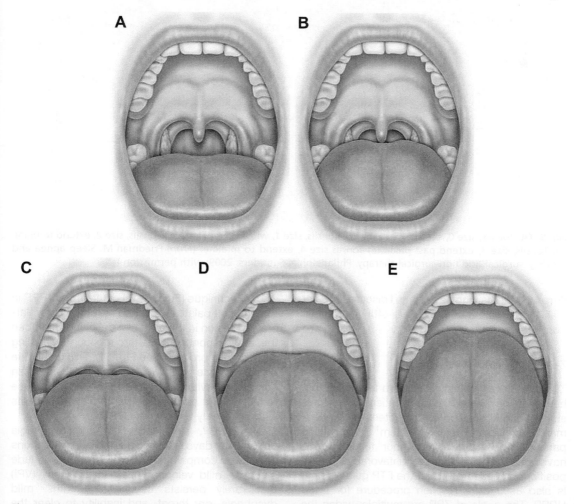

Fig. 4. (*A*) FTP I allows visualization of the entire uvula and tonsils/pillars. (*B*) FTP IIa allows visualization of most of the uvula, but the tonsils/pillars are absent. (*C*) FTP IIb allows visualization of the entire soft palate to the base of the uvula. (*D*) In FTP III some of the soft palate is visualized, but the distal structures are absent. (*E*) FTP IV allows visualization of the hard palate only. (*From* Friedman M. Sleep apnea and snoring: surgical and non-surgical therapy. Philadelphia: Saunders; 2009; with permission.)

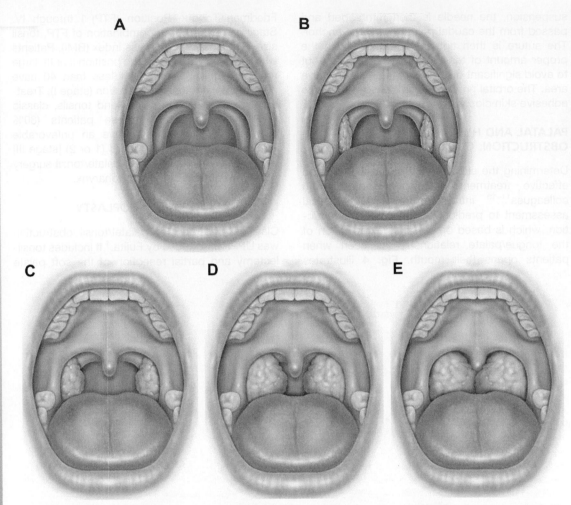

Fig. 5. (*A*) Tonsils, size 0, s/p tonsillectomy. (*B*) Tonsils, size 1, within the pillars. (*C*) Tonsils, size 2, extend to pillar. (*D*) Tonsils, size 3, extend past pillar. (*E*) Tonsils size 4, extend to midline. (*From* Friedman M. Sleep apnea and snoring: surgical and non-surgical therapy. Philadelphia: Saunders; 2009; with permission.)

(**Fig. 6**). Patients who have stage I disease (FTP I or II and tonsil size 3 or 4 and BMI <40) may benefit from this procedure.[12]

Z-PALATOPHARYNGOPLASTY

Z-palatopharyngoplasty (ZPP) is a technique that has been developed to treat patients who have stage II and III disease as characterized by Friedman's Anatomic Staging System[11–13] including patients who have had a prior tonsillectomy, have small tonsils, or have unfavorable tongue positioning measured using the FTP guidelines. It is also used as a revision procedure for failed UPPP. The goals of ZPP are multiple: widen the distance between the palate and posterior pharyngeal wall, widen the distance between the base of the tongue and the palate, and widen the lateral diameter of the pharynx.

This technique (**Figs. 7–11**) differs from UPPP in that the soft palate is split and retracted anterolaterally. Tension in the anterolateral plane will widen the airway continuously throughout the healing and scarring process (see **Fig. 11**). This technique preserves the palatal tissue. ZPP is often combined with radiofrequency tongue-base reduction and can also be performed on patients who previously underwent UPPP.

Like UPPP, significant pain and dysphagia occur in the days following surgery. Complications are also comparable to UPPP and include bleeding, mild velopharyngeal insufficiency (VPI) that rarely persists beyond 3 months, mild dysphagia, dry throat, and inability to clear the throat. The rate of VPI is slightly higher in ZPP than UPPP.[14]

Objective cure rate for stage II patients treated with ZPP and radiofrequency of the tongue base

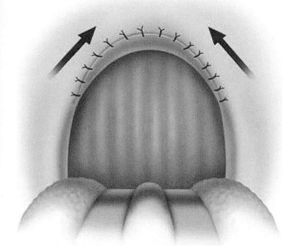

Fig. 6. In UPPP, the tonsils are removed and the soft palate is partially resected. (*From* Friedman M. Sleep apnea and snoring: surgical and non-surgical therapy. Philadelphia: Saunders; 2009; with permission.)

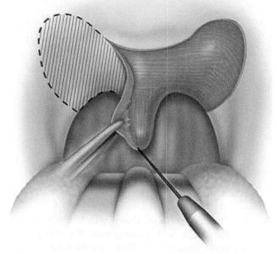

Fig. 8. The mucosa over the palatal flap is removed and the palatal musculature is exposed. (*From* Friedman M. Sleep apnea and snoring: surgical and non-surgical therapy. Philadelphia: Saunders; 2009; with permission.)

is nearly 70%.[14] This cure rate far exceeds the cure rate of approximately 39% for stage II patients undergoing classic UPPP with TBRF as an isolated procedure.[12,15]

PALATAL STIFFENING

Patients who have palatal obstruction without large tonsils may often be treated with minimally invasive palatal stiffening techniques. Often this can be combined with minimally invasive surgical or nonsurgical treatment of the nasal airway and

hypopharyngeal airway. Palatal stiffening is often combined with mandibular advancement devices to correct palatal and hypopharyngeal obstruction. The most popular palatal stiffening technique is the soft palate implant technique.

Previously described,[16] it involves the placement of three polyester pillars to stiffen the palate (**Figs. 12** and **13**). The oral cavity is prepped with chlorhexidine gluconate rinse. Implantation sites

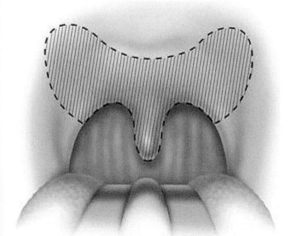

Fig. 7. Outline of the palatal flaps, marked before incision. (*From* Friedman M. Sleep apnea and snoring: surgical and non-surgical therapy. Philadelphia: Saunders; 2009; with permission.)

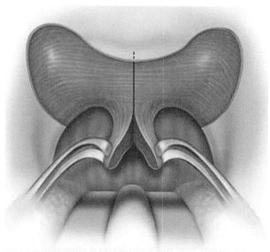

Fig. 9. The uvula and palate are split in the midline with a cold knife. (*From* Friedman M. Sleep apnea and snoring: surgical and non-surgical therapy. Philadelphia: Saunders; 2009; with permission.)

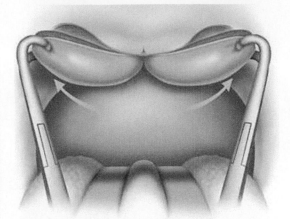

Fig. 10. The uvular flaps along with the soft palate are reflected back and laterally over the soft palate. Two-layered closure is then performed. (*From* Friedman M. Sleep apnea and snoring: surgical and non-surgical therapy. Philadelphia: Saunders; 2009; with permission.)

are marked just in front of the hard palate/soft palate junction (the midline and points 3 mm on either side of midline are marked). Approximately 0.5 mL of 1% lidocaine with adrenaline 1:100,000 is injected into each of the marked sites. The Pillar implant system includes an applicator and a polyester implant. The applicator tip is introduced into the soft palate until the third mark, taking care not to bypass the soft palate. The device is then withdrawn until the second mark can be seen and the palatal implant is delivered into the soft palate. In

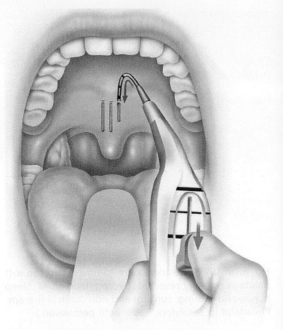

Fig. 12. One central implant is placed at the midline of the soft palate. The two lateral implants are placed as close as possible to the midline implant, approximately 2 mm apart. (*From* Friedman M. Sleep apnea and snoring: surgical and non-surgical therapy. Philadelphia: Saunders; 2009; with permission.)

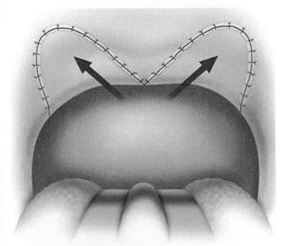

Fig. 11. After ZPP, the anterolateral direction of pull on the soft palate widens the retropharyngeal space. (*From* Friedman M. Sleep apnea and snoring: surgical and non-surgical therapy. Philadelphia: Saunders; 2009; with permission.)

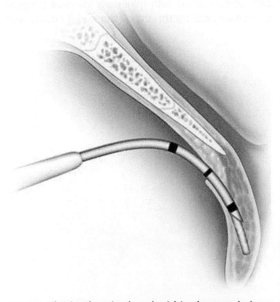

Fig. 13. The implant is placed within the muscle layer of the soft palate. (*From* Friedman M. Sleep apnea and snoring: surgical and non-surgical therapy. Philadelphia: Saunders; 2009; with permission.)

same fashion, the other two implants are applied on each side of the midline.

TRANSPALATAL ADVANCEMENT PHARYNGOPLASTY

Retropalatal airway obstruction is common and most often treated surgically by UPPP. When UPPP fails to relieve obstruction or airway narrowing is too severe to be relieved by standard UPPP, transpalatal advancement pharyngoplasty is indicated.

In transpalatal advancement pharyngoplasty, a portion of the posterior hard palate is excised, and the soft palate is advanced anteriorly, which allows enlargement of the upper pharyngeal space in an anterior-posterior and lateral direction without soft-palate tissue destruction.[16]

Possible complications, although rare, include wound breakdown, fistula formation, nasopharyngeal reflux, dysphagia, and VPI. A soft diet may be started on day one, but dentures or upper retainers may not be worn for at least 4 weeks and may require refitting by a dentist.

The studies performed on this technique show improved efficacy over UPPP success rates. Woodson and colleagues[17] found a greater decrease in the apnea-hypopnea index (AHI) in patients undergoing transpalatal advancement pharyngoplasty than UPPP and an odds ratio of success for palatal advancement over UPPP of 3.88. Because advancement pharyngoplasty does not generate as much scar tissue within the soft palate as other procedures, snoring may persist because of flutter of soft tissues. When this occurs, patients may undergo additional procedures, such as palatal implants or radiofrequency of the palate. These success rates show that transpalatal advancement pharyngoplasty can be used as an alternative treatment to aggressive UPPP.

RADIOFREQUENCY REDUCTION OF THE TONGUE BASE

One of the least invasive techniques to increase the retrolingual space is radiofrequency reduction of the tongue base. Treatment to increase retrolingual space is indicated in all patients who have Friedman anatomic stage II or III disease regardless of OSAHS severity. Radiofrequency reduction is a simple, safe procedure that provides minimal levels of reduction. It can be done under local or general anesthesia. The authors' standard techniques involve using a double probe made by Gyrus (Southborough, MA) that delivers radiofrequency energy to both sides of the midline

simultaneously. The probe is set so that each treatment site is 5 mm off the midline. The authors use five sites spaced between the circumvallate papillae and the vallecula. Each site delivers 60 J equally divided to a right and left lesion for a total of 3000 J delivered over 10 sites.

Postoperative pain is usually less than 3 on a 10-point visual analog scale (with 0 being no pain and 10 being the worst pain) and narcotics are rarely needed. Patients usually resume full diet within 4 days.

Complications include temporary or permanent hypoglossal paralysis that can occur if the probes are placed more than 2 cm lateral to the midline. Another potential complication is mucosal burns, if the probe is not seated properly. Local infections can also occur, but abscess formation is extremely rare (<0.1%). Treatment can be repeated if necessary.

MINIMALLY INVASIVE SUBMUCOSAL GLOSSECTOMY

Retrolingual airway obstruction is usually caused by many factors, one being macroglossia. Standard surgical procedures for macroglossia require removal of a wedge of the tongue base mucosa and musculature, an operation that causes significant dysphagia and odynophagia and requires prolonged recovery time.[18] Submucosal glossectomy is a minimally invasive technique designed to reduce tongue base mass without mucosal alteration. There is greatly reduced associated morbidity and pain than with conventional procedures.[18,19]

Multiple techniques have been described by the senior author,[20] Robinson and colleagues,[19] Maturo and Mair,[18] and Woodson and Fujita.[22] Although Woodson and Fujita have described a technique requiring only local anesthesia,[21] general anesthesia is required in most cases. A radiofrequency or coblator probe is positioned in the tongue base through either a percutaneous approach through the neck[19] or an intraoral approach.[18,20] Endoscopic guidance may be performed with the intraoral approach. One technique, the SMILE (submucosal minimally invasive lingual excision) procedure, was originally designed for use in children but is also applicable for adult patients.[18,20]

Possible complications include hematoma, delayed bleeding into the airway or tongue, hypoglossal nerve paralysis, and wound dehiscence in techniques that use an incision. There is no subjective alteration of swallowing or speech following the initial postoperative period.[18]

Few trials have been performed to analyze the success rates of this procedure. A 40% response rate was achieved in 15 subjects using the percutaneous approach.[19] The SMILE procedure has been successful in four reported pediatric cases.[18] In adults, the SMILE procedure had increased efficacy in decreasing the AHI over radiofrequency in a series of 96 subjects.[21] Additional studies must be performed to objectively quantify the efficacy in long-term follow-up.

TONGUE BASE STABILIZATION USING MINIMALLY INVASIVE TECHNIQUE

Because the base of the tongue is also part of the pharyngeal wall, muscle tonicity is required during sleep to prevent collapse of the tongue and obstruction of the hypopharyngeal airway. Tongue-base suspension stabilizes the airway during sleep to maintain patency. Because it is minimally invasive, morbidity is lower than conventional glossectomy and advancement procedures.

This procedure involves looping a submucosal suture through the posterior base of tongue and anchoring it to a screw placed in the lingual surface of the mandible. This suture will prevent passive collapse during sleep, but will not alter the anterior movements of the tongue required for speech and swallowing. As with most therapies for OSAHS, tongue-base stabilization may be performed as a single treatment or as part of multi-level surgical therapy.[22]

Studies to date show success rates of 20% to 57%.[22–27] Few trials have examined the efficacy and long-term results of tongue-base stabilization. Possible complications include transient VPI and limited tongue protrusion.[24,25] This procedure is potentially reversible and does not prohibit future surgery on the tongue base. Although advantages include low morbidity and preservation of normal tongue movement, additional studies, including long-term follow-up, must be performed to quantify efficacy of this procedure.

HYOID SUSPENSION

Hyoid suspension targets relief of obstruction at the hypopharyngeal airway. The hyoid complex is structurally connected to the hypopharynx, and anterior traction on the hyoid will open the retrolingual space, relieving obstruction at the tongue base. Hyoid suspension is often combined with other hypopharyngeal procedures or UPPP to achieve maximum effectiveness for the treatment of OSAHS.

Patient selection is critical; patients who have multiple levels of obstruction are not ideal candidates for hyoid suspension as single-modality treatment. Ideal patients have moderate to severe OSAHS and major obstruction at the tongue base without enlarged tonsils or other signs of retropalatal obstruction.

During this procedure, the hyoid bone is stabilized inferiorly through an attachment to the superior border of the thyroid cartilage using permanent sutures. Complications may include hematoma, bleeding into the airway, and temporary dysphagia.[25,28]

The four published studies examining hyoid suspension as a single-level therapy show success rates ranging from 17% to 78%.[28–31] Because there is no mucosal damage or tissue destruction, postoperative pain following this procedure is lower than after UPPP. Hyoid suspension is most useful as an adjunctive treatment in conjunction with UPPP and other hypopharyngeal procedures. Further trials with a larger number of patients and longer follow-up are needed to better assess the value of this procedure as a treatment for moderate to severe OSAHS.

HYOMANDIBULAR SUSPENSION AND HYOID EXPANSION FOR OBSTRUCTIVE SLEEP APNEA

Hyoid expansion with hyomandibular suspension treats patients who have severe OSAHS and hypopharyngeal obstruction.[32] This procedure decreases airway obstruction in multiple ways including anterior-superior repositioning of the tongue base, enlargement of the lateral diameter of the pharynx through division of the hyoid, and partial separation of the tongue base from the lower airway by infrahyoid myomotomy. This procedure can be done in combination with tongue-base suspension if necessary.

Potential complications, though not common, include prolonged odynophagia and dysphagia, change in speech, hematoma, airway obstruction, wound infection, and intense pain.[32] This procedure offers several advantages. It is a minor procedure and the only treatment for OSAHS that has the ability to widen the pharyngeal airway in a lateral diameter. A literature search revealed no published trials on the efficacy of this procedure. Therefore, studies using large patient populations and long-term follow-up will be necessary to obtain statistical data for the efficacy and rate of complications.

SUMMARY

The procedures outlined in this article are just a few of the standard methods and new advances in the treatment of OSAHS. Thorough examination of patients' airways is necessary for identification of areas of obstruction and creation of a successful treatment plan. Multilevel therapy has been accepted as the standard for treatment because many patients have multiple levels of airway obstruction. It is important to be aware of multiple techniques for airway reconstruction to be able to tailor therapy to meet individual patient's needs.

REFERENCES

1. Fujita S, Conway W, Zorick F, et al. Surgical correction of anatomic abnormalities in obstructive sleep apnea syndrome: uvulopalatopharyngoplasty. Otolaryngol Head Neck Surg 1981;89(6):923–34.
2. Elwany S, Thabet H. Obstruction of the nasal valve. J Laryngol Otol 1996;110:221–4.
3. Kosh MM, Jen A, Honrado C, et al. Nasal valve reconstruction: experience in 53 consecutive patients. Arch Facial Plast Surg 2004;6:167–71.
4. Sheen JH. Spreader graft: a method of reconstruction the roof of the middle nasal vault following rhinoplasty. Plast Reconstr Surg 1984;73:230–9.
5. Stucker FJ, Lian T, Karen M. Management of the keel nose and associated valve collapse. Arch Otolaryngol Head Neck Surg 2002;128:842–6.
6. Friedman M, Ibrahim H, Lee G, et al. A simplified technique for airway correction at the nasal valve area. Otolaryngol Head Neck Surg 2004;131(4): 519–24.
7. Friedman M, Ibrahim H, Syed Z. Nasal valve suspension: an improved, simplified technique for nasal valve collapse. Laryngoscope 2003;113(2):381–5.
8. Toriumi DM, Josen J, Weinberger M, et al. Use of alar batten grafts for correction of nasal valve collapse. Arch Otolaryngol Head Neck Surg 1997; 123:802–8.
9. Millman B. Alar batten grafting for management of the collapsed nasal valve. Laryngoscope 2002; 112:574–9.
10. Ghidini A, Dallari S, Marchioni D. Surgery of the nasal columella in external valve collapse. Ann Otol Rhinol Laryngol 2002;(11):701–3.
11. Friedman M, Ibrahim H, Bass L. Clinical predictors of OSA. Laryngoscope 1999;109:1901–8.
12. Friedman M, Ibrahim H, Bass L. Clinical staging for sleep-disordered breathing. Otolaryngol Head Neck Surg 2002;127:13–21.
13. Friedman M, Ibrahim H, Joseph N. Staging of obstructive sleep apnea/hypopnea syndrome: a guide to appropriate treatment. Laryngoscope 2004;114:454–9.
14. Friedman M, Ibrahim HZ, Vidyasagar R, et al. Z-palatoplasty (ZPP): a technique for patients without tonsils. Otolaryngol Head Neck Surg 2004;131: 89–100.
15. Friedman M, Ibrahim H, Lee G, et al. Combined uvulopalatopharyngoplasty and radiofrequency tongue base reduction for treatment of obstructive sleep apnea/hypopnea syndrome. Otolaryngol Head Neck Surg 2003;129:611–21.
16. Woodson TB. Retropalatal airway characteristics in uvulopalatopharyngoplasty compared with transpalatal advancement pharyngoplasty. Laryngoscope 1999;107(6):735–40.
17. Woodson TB, Robinson S, Lim H. Transpalatal advancement pharyngoplasty outcomes compared with uvulopalatopharyngoplasty. Otolaryngol Head Neck Surg 2005;133(2):211–7.
18. Maturo SC, Mair EA. Submucosal minimally invasive lingual excision (SMILE): an effective, novel surgery for pediatric tongue base reduction. Ann Otol Rhinol Laryngol 2006;115(8):624–30.
19. Robinson S, Lewis R, Norton A, et al. Ultrasound-guided radiofrequency submucosal tongue-base excision for sleep apnoea: a preliminary report. Clin Otolaryngol Allied Sci 2003;28:341–5.
20. Friedman M, Soans R, Gurpinar B, et al. Evaluation of submucosal minimally invasive lingual excision technique for treatment of obstructive sleep apnea/hypopnea syndrome. Otolaryngol Head Neck Surg 2008;139:378–84.
21. Woodson BT, Fujita S. Clinical experience with lingualplasty as part of the treatment of severe obstructive sleep apnea. Otolaryngol Head Neck Surg 2006;133:211–7.
22. Miller FR, Watson D, Malis D. Role of the tongue base suspension suture with the repose system bone screw in the multilevel surgical management of obstructive sleep apnea. Otolaryngol Head Neck Surg 2002;126:392–8.
23. Woodon BT. A tongue suspension suture for obstructive sleep apnea and snorers. Otolaryngol Head Neck Surg 2001;124:297–303.
24. DeRowe A, Gunther E, Fibbi A, et al. Tongue-base suspension with a soft tissue-to-bone anchor for obstructive sleep apnea: preliminary clinical results of a new minimally invasive technique. Otolaryngol Head Neck Surg 2000;122:100–3.
25. Terris DJ, Junda LD, Gonella MC. Minimally invasive tongue base surgery for obstructive sleep apnea. J Laryngol Otol 2002;116(9):716–21.
26. Thomas AJ, Chavoya M, Terris DJ. Preliminary findings from a prospective, randomized trial of two tongue-base surgeries for sleep-disordered breathing. Otolaryngol Head Neck Surg 2003;129: 539–46.
27. Sorrenti G, Piccin O, Latini G, et al. Tongue base suspension technique in obstructive sleep apnea: personal experience. Acta Otorhinolaryngol Ital 2003;23:274–80.
28. Bowden MT, Kezirian EJ, Utley D, et al. Outcomes of hyoid suspension for the treatment of obstructive sleep apnea. Arch Otolaryngol Head Neck Surg 2005;131:440–5.

29. Den Herder C, van Tinteren H, de Vries N. Hyoid-thyroidpexia: a surgical treatment for sleep apnea syndrome. Laryngoscope 2005;115(4): 740–5.

30. Vilaseca I, Morello A, Montserrat JM, et al. Usefulness of uvulopalatopharyngoplasty with genioglossus and hyoid advancement in the treatment of obstructive sleep apnea. Arch Otolaryngol Head Neck Surg 2002;128:435–40.

31. Neruntarat C. Hyoid myotomy with suspension under local anesthesia for obstructive sleep apnea syndrome. Eur Arch Otorhinolaryngol 2003;260: 286–90.

32. Krespi J. Hyo-mandibular suspension and hyoid expansion for obstructive sleep apnea. In: Friedman M, editor. Sleep apnea and snoring: surgical and non-surgical therapy. Philadelphia: Saunders; 2009. p. 321–5.

Obstructive Sleep Apnea and Bruxism in Children

Stephen H. Sheldon, DO[a,b,*]

KEYWORDS

- Obstructive sleep apnea • Bruxism • Children
- Temporalis muscle

Obstructive sleep apnea (OSA) is common in childhood. Current epidemiologic data have shown that snoring occurs in 7% to as much as 30% of school-aged children.[1] The most common cause of OSA in pediatric patients is hypertrophy of the tonsils or adenoids.[2] Nonetheless, various factors are involved in upper airway obstruction during sleep in children. Craniofacial structure and function of the upper airway musculature are extensively involved in airflow dynamics.[3] Conversely, obstructive upper airway disease can contribute to abnormalities in craniofacial structure and function. This article focuses on differences between upper airway function in children and adults, factors that predispose children to OSA, and treatment options. Bruxism, jaw clenching, and rhythmic mandibular thrusting have been associated with OSA in children, and the frequency and prevalence of these findings are discussed.

Sleep bruxism is defined as a stereotyped movement disorder characterized by grinding or clenching of the teeth during sleep.[4] Sound made by grinding or clenching of the teeth is often disturbing, but need not be present. Rhythmic clenching or wearing of the teeth can result in tooth damage, periodontal damage, or pain. Pain may be facial, associated with the temporomandibular joint, or associated with head pain and headaches. When the characteristic noise of bruxism is present, it is often brought to the attention of the health care practitioner by a parents or caretaker.

Bruxism may occur during both wakefulness and sleep. Bruxism during wakefulness seems to be etiologically different from sleep-related bruxism. If clenching or intermittent rhythmic movements of the muscles of mastication are present, this may be identified by the dentist or the patient may present with symptoms that are somewhat unrelated. Symptoms may include atypical facial pain or headaches, particularly in the morning. Presentation can be variable because considerable variation exists in the intensity and duration. Temporomandibular joint dysfunction may also occur and be associated with facial or head pain.

Although little is known about the clinical course of bruxism, dental damage with abnormal wear to the crowns of the teeth is common. Periodontal recession, inflammation, and alveolar resorption have been reported.

Polysomnographic findings include increased masseter and temporalis muscle activity. Although most frequent in N2 sleep, this rhythmic activity can occur in all sleep states, and in some individuals is most common during rapid eye movement (REM) sleep,[4] although not associated with dream mentation. Rhythmic movements of the muscles of mastication occur in the absence of epileptiform activity on electroencephalogram (EEG).

Reported prevalence of bruxism in children range from 7% to 88%.[5] Bruxism can occur during any stage of sleep and has been reported in non-REM (NREM) and REM sleep.[6] Many causes have been proposed and range from centrally mediated primary movement disorder to mandibular dystonia.[7] In many cases the cause is considered multifactorial.

[a] Northwestern University, Feinberg School of Medicine, Chicago, IL, USA
[b] Sleep Medicine Center, Children's Memorial Hospital, 2300 Children's Plaza, Box 43, Chicago, IL 60614, USA
* Sleep Medicine Center, Children's Memorial Hospital, 2300 Children's Plaza, Box 43, Chicago, IL 60614.
E-mail address: ssheldon@childrensmemorial.org

Sleep Med Clin 5 (2010) 163–168
doi:10.1016/j.jsmc.2009.10.004
1556-407X/10/$ – see front matter © 2010 Elsevier Inc. All rights reserved.

Because of the frequency of sleep-related bruxism in the pediatric population, the authors evaluated for the presence of bruxism noted on comprehensive polysomnography in 119 consecutive patients with possible OSA referred to the Pediatric Sleep Medicine Center of Children's Memorial Hospital.

METHODS

Patients between ages 3 and 16 years, referred to the Pediatric Sleep Medicine Center with symptoms of snoring that more than half the time could be heard in other rooms, were evaluated for the presence of bruxism. Bruxism was defined as three or more rhythmic contractions of the temporalis muscles, as measured with temporalis muscle electromyogram (EMG), occurring during NREM or REM sleep lasting more than 3 seconds, but less than 15 seconds (**Figs. 1** and **2**). Additionally, this rhythmic muscle activity was associated with electrocortical arousal or brief waking (<15 seconds) noted on EEG. For bruxism to be considered present, the frequency of the rhythmic temporalis muscle activity had to be a minimum of 75% of the arousal index for each patient. Bruxism was dichotomized into either present or absent. Patients who met the criteria for bruxism were considered "bruxism present" and those who did not were "bruxism absent."

Respiration was measured using multiple variables. Airflow was detected at the nose and mouth using standard thermistry. Additionally, nasal pressure was recorded at the nares and continuous monitoring of the end-tidal carbon dioxide ($EtCO_2$) waveform was performed. Respiratory effort was continuously monitored using inductive plethysmography of the chest and abdomen and continuous monitoring of the intercostal EMG.

Obstructive apneas and hypopneas were classified according to the American Academy of Sleep Medicine 2007 guidelines.[8] Obstructive apneas were scored when a greater than 90% decrease was present in the signal amplitude for 90% or greater of the entire respiratory event compared with pre-event baseline amplitude. A mixed apnea was scored if it met the criteria and was associated with absent inspiratory effort in the initial portion of the event, followed by resumption of inspiratory effort before the end of the event. A central apnea was scored if it was associated with absent inspiratory effort throughout the entire duration of the event and the event either lasted longer than 20 seconds, lasted at least 2 missed breaths, or was associated with an arousal, an awakening, or 3% or greater desaturation.

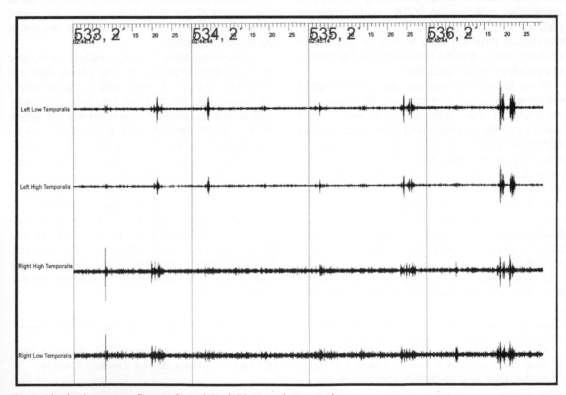

Fig. 1. Rhythmic temporalis muscle activity (120-second segment).

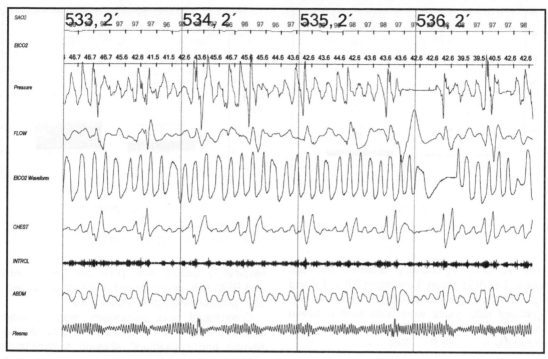

Fig. 2. Apneas and hypopneas associated with bruxism (120-second segment).

An obstructive hypopnea was scored if the event was associated with a 50% or greater decline in the amplitude of the nasal pressure for at least two respiratory efforts, the fall in nasal pressure lasted 90% or more of the entire respiratory event compared with the amplitude preceding the event, and the event was associated with an arousal, awakening, or 3% or greater oxygen desaturation.

The apnea index (AI) represented the total number of apneas per hour of sleep. The apnea–hypopnea index (AHI) represented the total apneas and hypopneas per hour of sleep, and the REM AHI represented the total number of apneas and hypopneas per hour of REM sleep.

AI, AHI, and REM AHI were then compared using nonparametric 2-tailed Mann-Whitney test for statistical significance.

RESULTS

A total of 119 patients were recorded. Ages ranged from 2 to 16 years, with a mean age of 7.0 ± 4.0 years (median, 8.5 years; mode, 3.0 years). Bruxism was identified in 70 patients (group 1). Rhythmic temporalis muscle activity was not identified or temporalis muscle activity did not meet the criteria for bruxism in 49 patients (group 0). Analysis of groups may be found in **Table 1**. Stem and leaf plots may be found in **Figs. 3–5**.

Table 1 Nonparametric Mann-Whitney tests of presence of bruxism[a]				
Index	Mann-Whitney	Wilcoxon	z Score	Significance (2-tailed)
Apnea index	12,334.5	2539.5	−2.344	.019[b]
Apnea–hypopnea index	1049.5	2274.5	−3.595	.000[b]
Rapid eye movement apnea–hypopnea index	1169.0	2394.0	−2.956	.003[b]

[a] N = 119.
[b] Significant.

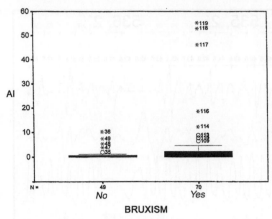

Fig. 3. Stem and Leaf Plot: Bruxism versus apnea index (AI).

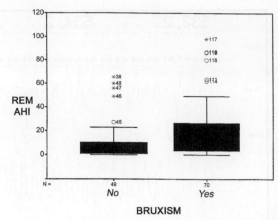

Fig. 5. Stem and Leaf Plot: Bruxism versus rapid eye movement apnea–hypopnea index.

The AI was significantly different between groups. The AI in group 0 averaged 0.8 ± 1.6 and in group 1 average 4.0 ± 10.8 (2-tailed $P = .02$). Significant differences were also seen between groups for the AHI ($z = -3.60$; $P < .001$) and the REM AHI ($z = -2.96$; $P = .003$).

DISCUSSION

OSA is common in childhood, present in approximately 1% to 3% of all school-aged children. Various factors are involved in the genesis of upper airway obstruction in children. Craniofacial structure and physiology of the upper airway musculature are extensively involved in maintenance of patency and airflow dynamics. The converse is also true: upper airway obstruction can contribute to abnormalities in craniofacial structure and oral, nasal, and pharyngeal function.

The authors showed sleep-related rhythmic temporalis muscle activity associated with arousal is significantly associated with indices of

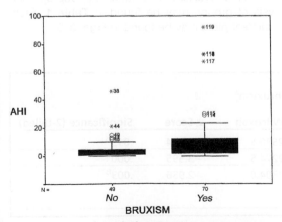

Fig. 4. Stem and Leaf Plot: Bruxism versus apnea–hypopnea index (AHI).

respiratory disturbance, particular the AI, AHI, and REM AHI, as measured using standard pediatric polysomnographic techniques.

Craniofacial pain, particularly morning headaches, are common in children who have OSA. Kampe and colleagues[9] showed a statistically significant correlation between frequent tooth clenching and headache pain.

Complex influences of normal physiologic mechanisms occur during sleep. The relationship between causes of disordered sleep and pathophysiologic mechanisms that result in the symptom complex are important to understand. Substantial improvement in nocturnal or early-morning headaches associated with OSA has been shown to occur once OSA is adequately treated.[10]

Studies have shown that bruxism occurs in all stages of sleep[11]; it can disrupt state percentages as proportions of the total sleep time. Bruxism previously showed a positive correlation with sleep-disordered breathing in children.[12]

DeFrancesco and colleagues[12] compared the incidence of bruxism before and after adenotonsillectomy in children who had sleep apnea. Almost half of the children had both clinical and reported findings of bruxism; however, 3 months after surgery, none presented with breathing problems during sleep and fewer than 12% still had symptoms of bruxism. In another study, Oksenberg and Arons[13] showed that OSA was the highest risk factor for tooth grinding during sleep.

In the authors' sample of children who had sleep-disordered breathing, rhythmic temporalis muscle activity occurred during both NREM and REM sleep. This activity was associated with arousal and is consistent with earlier physiologic data associating arousal and bruxism during sleep.[14] Other studies have also shown a correlation between habitual snoring and bruxism.[15]

Children who have migraine headaches have been shown to have a high prevalence of sleep disturbances, including snoring and bruxism. Of 118 children who had migraine headaches studied by Miller and colleagues,[16] 29% reported bruxism and 23% habitual snoring.

Associated Findings

Several conditions and symptoms may be present that indicate an increased level of risk for OSA. Dentists often recognize the presence of sleep bruxism clinically, and may need to investigate the additional findings, conditions, and symptoms that, when considered together, further increase the potential for OSA (**Box 1**).

SUMMARY

Sleep-related bruxism is a common problem in the pediatric population. Sleep bruxism seems to be associated with pediatric OSA. The authors' significant findings between objective evidence of rhythmic temporalis muscle activity and pediatric

OSA, as measured using the AI, AHI, and REM AHI, support this correlation. Further investigations are needed to assess the correlation among OSA, rhythmic temporalis muscle activity, and headaches in children. Additional studies will need to look into the underlying mechanisms and potential for temporalis muscle pain as the underlying cause of morning headaches associated with sleep-disordered breathing in children.

Box 1
Associated findings that further indicate the risk for obstructive sleep apnea
Attention Deficit Disorder/Attention Deficit–Hyperactivity Disorder
Cognitive changes
Hypersomnia
Snoring
Enlarged tonsils
Long, narrow face
Dental crossbite
Asthma
Enuresis
Obesity
Somnambulism
Restless leg syndrome symptoms
Narrow maxilla
Tongue thrusting
Behavioral Disorders
Hyperactivity
Nasal airway obstruction
Restless/disturbed sleep
Poor school performance
Allergic shiners
Scalloped tongue

REFERENCES

1. Marcus CL. Sleep disordered breathing in children. Am J Respir Crit Care Med 2001;164:16–30.
2. Ali NJ, Pitson D, Stardling JR. Sleep disordered breathing: effect of adenotonsillectomy on behaviour and psychological functioning. Eur J Pediatr 1996;155:56–62.
3. Ionescu CM, Segers P, DeKeyser R. Mechanical properties of the respiratory system derived from morphologic insight. IEEE Trans Biomed Eng 2009;56: 949–59.
4. American Academy of Sleep Medicine. International classification of sleep disorders. Diagnostic and coding manual. 2nd edition. Westchester (IL): American Academy of Sleep Medicine; 2005.
5. Attanasio R. Nocturnal bruxism and its clinical management. Dent Clin North Am 1991;45:245.
6. Tosun T, Karabuda C, Cuhadaroglu C. Evaluation of sleep bruxism by polysomnographic analysis in patients with dental implants. Int J Oral Maxillofac Implants 2003;18:286–92.
7. Clark GT, Koyano K, Browne PA. Oral motor disorders in humans. J Calif Dent Assoc 1993; 21:19.
8. Iber C, Ancoli-Israel S, Chesson A, et al. The AASM manual for the scoring of sleep and associated events: rules, terminology and technical specifications. 1st edition. Westchester (IL): American Academy of Sleep Medicine; 2007.
9. Kampe T, Tagdae T, Bader G, et al. Reported symptoms and clinical findings in a group of subjects with long-standing bruxing behaviour. J Oral Rehabil 1997;24: 581–7.
10. Biondi DM. Headaches and their relationship to sleep. Dent Clin North Am 2001;45:685–700.
11. Boutros NN, Montgomery MT, Nishioka G, et al. The effects of severe bruxism on sleep architecture: a preliminary report. Clin Electroencephalogr 1993; 24:59–62.
12. DiFrancesco RC, Junqueira PA, Trezza PM, et al. Improvement of bruxism after T&A surgery. Int J Pediatr Otorhinolaryngol 2004;68:441–5.
13. Oksenberg A, Arons E. Sleep bruxism related to obstructive sleep apnea: the effect of continuous positive airway pressure. Sleep Med 2002;3:513–5.

14. Kato T, Thie NM, Huynh N, et al. Topical review: sleep bruxism and the role of peripheral sensory influences. J Orofac Pain 2003;17:191–213.

15. Ng DK, Kwok KL, Poon G, et al. Habitual snoring and sleep bruxism in a paediatric outpatient population in Hong Kong. Singapore Med J 2002;43:554–6.

16. Miller VA, Palerms TM, Powers SW, et al. Migraine headaches and sleep disturbances in children. Headache 2003;43:362–8.

A Glossary of Dental Terminology for the Sleep Medicine Clinician

Dennis R. Bailey, DDS[a,b,*], Teofilo Lee-Chiong Jr, MD[c]

Angle classification: Classification of occlusion or malocclusion based on the relationship between the teeth in the maxilla and mandible. Divided into Class I, Class II, and Class III. The most commonly used opposing teeth used to make this determination are the canines (cuspids) and the first molars.

> Class I: The most ideal relationship between the maxilla and mandibular teeth.
>
> Class II: From a dental perspective, the mandibular teeth are positioned posterior to the maxillary teeth and the mandible is considered retrognathic.
>
> Class III: The mandibular teeth are advanced forward of the maxillary teeth. Appears to be an anterior crossbite. The mandible is considered prognathic.

Bite: see Occlusion

Bite splint: see Night guard

Bruxism: The act of the teeth being pressed together and actively moving the mandible such that the teeth wear against one another.

Bruxism appliance: see Night guard

Buccal: The cheek-side of a tooth, most often the posterior teeth (premolars and molars).

Calculus: Tartar. A hard, calcified substance that will develop on the teeth and is often related to periodontal (gum) disease. It frequently has a white-to-gray color with a chalky appearance, and can form on oral appliances.

Capsule (of the temporomandibular joint [TMJ]): The fibrous tissue that covers the TMJ on its lateral surface.

Capsulitis: Inflammation of the TMJ capsule often associated with joint pain, tenderness on palpation, or pain of the TMJ with function.

Cary (plural, caries): Tooth decay or cavity. The active destruction of a tooth starting in the enamel and progressing into the underlying dentin of the tooth causing the breakdown of a portion of the crown.

Cavity: The end result of the carious process (decay) that destroys the integrity of the enamel and progresses into the underlying dentin leaving a void in the tooth.

Cephalometric: Lateral head plate. Used to evaluate the skeletal structures of the head and neck most often as it relates to growth and development or for planning orthodontic treatment.

Cleaning: see Prophylaxis, Scaling

Clenching: The act of pressing the teeth tightly together. May be intermittent or sustained.

Contact: The side-to-side relationship of the teeth. Open contact: The teeth are not sufficiently contacting; associated with food becoming lodged between the teeth or little-to-no resistance when flossing between the teeth.

Crenation: The imprints of the teeth on the lateral border of the tongue and occasionally at the anterior aspect of the tongue, often associated with clenching of the teeth.

Crossbite: The maxillary teeth contact the mandibular teeth such that the maxillary teeth are inside (to the tongue or palatal side) relative to the mandibular teeth. Buccal crossbite: The maxillary teeth are not in occlusion with the mandibular teeth and totally positioned over them buccally (to the cheek or lip side).

[a] Orofacial Pain and Dental Sleep Medicine, Dental Sleep Medicine Mini-Residency, UCLA School of Dentistry, Los Angeles, CA, USA
[b] 7901 East Belleview Avenue, Suite 200, Englewood, CO 80111, USA
[c] Division of Sleep Medicine, Department of Medicine, National Jewish Health, 1400 Jackson Street, Denver, CO 60206, USA
* Corresponding author. 7901 East Belleview Avenue, Suite 200, Englewood, CO 80111.
E-mail address: rmc4e@aol.com (D.R. Bailey).

Sleep Med Clin 5 (2010) 169–171
doi:10.1016/j.jsmc.2009.09.006
1556-407X/10/$ – see front matter © 2010 Published by Elsevier Inc.

Crown: (a) The aspect of the tooth that is visible in the mouth and is above the gingivae. (b) The restoration that covers the tooth as a means of rebuilding or restoring the tooth. It is fabricated with all metal, partially covered with porcelain for esthetics, or all porcelain. The part that restores the tooth may be referred to as a cap.

Cusp: The high point on a posterior tooth. In chewing, it acts like the pestle part of the mortar and pestle.

Deep bite: The maxillary and mandibular anterior teeth have 50% or more vertical overlap when the teeth are in full occlusion.

Dental appliance: see Oral appliance. Nonpreferred, but often encountered, term for a device that is utilized to manage sleep-related breathing disorders.

Dental arch: The mandible or maxilla. The visualization of the teeth in horseshoe form over their boney base.

Denture: Plate, full prosthesis. (a) Full denture: Replaces all of the teeth in either the maxilla or the mandible. (b) Partial denture: Replaces those teeth that are missing in the maxilla or the mandible; often supported by the remaining teeth.

Disc (of the TMJ): The fibrocartilage structure (biconcave) interposed between the mandibular condyle and the glenoid fossa that allows for smooth joint movement.

Disc displacement: The TMJ disc is out of position and may cause limited mandibular movement or be associated with joint sounds (eg, clicking or popping).

Distal: The side of the tooth away from the midline.

Edentulous: (a) Fully edentulous: The absence of all of the teeth in the maxilla and/or or mandible. (b) Partially edentulous: The absence of some of the teeth in the maxilla mandible.

Facial: The surface of the tooth facing the lip, mainly the incisors and cuspids (canines).

Filling: see Restoration

Fixed bridge (prosthesis): A series of crowns joined as one unit that replaces one or more teeth.

Fossa: The depression or concave portion of the molars and premolars. In chewing, it acts as the mortar part of the mortar and pestle.

Frenum (Frenulum): Structure that restrains certain movements of the tongue, cheeks, or lips. Usually a thin band of tissue at the base of the tongue (lingual frenum), at the midline of the lips (labial frenum), and in the cheek area in the area of the premolars (buccal frenum).

Gingiva (plural, gingivae): Gum. The soft tissue surrounding the teeth.

Gingivitis: Active inflammation of the soft tissue that can include swelling, pain, bleeding; associated with the presence of plaque or calculus.

Gum disease: see Periodontal disease

Incisal: The biting edge of the incisors (anterior teeth).

Interincisal distance: The distance between the incisal edges of the maxillary and mandibular incisors. Most often encountered as the measurement related to the degree of bite opening when fabricating an oral appliance.

Implants: A device or fixture that is placed into the bone to eventually allow for the replacement of a tooth or teeth. Most allow bone to integrate into them (osseous integration). A number of them may be used in a single arch to support a denture.

Lingual: The tongue side (eg, the lingual of the tooth).

Malocclusion: The teeth do not fit together in an acceptable or near-normal fashion. Indicates that the bite is "off."

Mandibular advancement device (MAD): see Oral appliance

Mandibular repositioning device (MRD): see Oral appliance

Mandibular repositioning appliance (MRA): see Oral appliance

Mesial: The side of the tooth facing the midline.

Night guard: Bite splint, occlusal guard, bruxism appliance. An intraoral appliance used at night that is worn over the maxillary or mandibular teeth mostly to protect the teeth against harmful habits such as clenching or bruxism.

Occlusal guard: see Night guard

Occlusion: Bite. The assessment of how the teeth come together when the patient is asked to bite. The full interdigitation of the teeth. It is delineated as Class I, II, III, or by Angle classification.

Open bite: The teeth are in full occlusion and some of the maxillary and mandibular teeth are not in contact or do not relate properly. (a) Anterior open bite: When the posterior teeth are in contact there is a space that is visible between the front teeth. The front teeth do not overlap properly. (b) Posterior open bite: A space between the posterior teeth when the teeth are together.

Oral appliance: Dental appliance (in sleep), MRA, MAD, or MRD. An appliance worn in the mouth during sleep to reposition the mandible as a means of managing sleep apnea and snoring.

Orofacial pain: Pain in the facial, oral, TMJ, and/or head area. Encompasses TMJ disorders, headache, trigeminal neuropathies, and intraoral pain such as burning mouth or burning tongue syndrome.

Overbite: The amount of vertical overlap of the incisors of the teeth when viewed from the front. May be expressed in percent of overlap or by number of millimeters. Generally considered a deep bite when there is greater than 50% overlap.

Overjet: The distance between the incisal edges of the maxillary and mandibular incisor teeth on a horizontal plane. The farther the mandibular incisors are behind the maxillary incisors, the more the mandible is thought to be retrognathic.

Partial denture: see Dentures

Periodontal disease: Gum disease. Active inflammation of the gingivae. May involve the loss of bone that surrounds and supports the teeth.

Periodontal pocketing: The depth of the sulcus found between the gingivae that surround the teeth and the tooth itself. Measured in millimeters. Should normally be 2 to 3 mm deep. With active disease, the increased depth of the pocket indicates the presence of periodontal disease.

Periodontitis: Pyorrhea. Gum disease. Periodontal disease. Inflammatory disease of the periodontal structures that includes the gingivae and the supporting bone; often associated with bone loss around the teeth.

Periodontosis: Degenerative disease of the periodontal structures that is not associated with inflammation.

Plaque: A soft material that is found on the teeth that easily removed by flossing and brushing. If not removed periodically, it may develop into calculus.

Pocketing: Gingival sulcus. See Periodontal pocketing

Prognathic (Prognathism): An exaggerated forward position of the mandible or maxilla; usually the relationship of the mandible to the maxilla. Class III when the mandible appears to be forward of the maxilla.

Prophylaxis: Cleaning. Scaling. A process where the calculus and plaque are removed from the teeth to improve the health of the soft tissues. Also, polishing of the teeth.

Restoration: Filling, crown, or cap. This is the repair or rebuilding of the crown portion of a tooth that is deemed necessary by virtue of caries (decay) or if a tooth is broken, fractured, or sustains trauma.

Retrodiscitis (of the TMJ): Tenderness or pain associated with the posterior aspect of the TMJ between the condyle and posterior aspect of the fossae.

Retrognathia (Retrognathism): The posterior positioning of the maxilla or mandible; the mandible as it appears in relationship to the mandible. Class II when the mandible appears to be posterior to the maxilla.

Scaling: The process of removing hard deposits (calculus) from the teeth and the upper part of the root structures. It also involves the removal of diseased tissue from the sulcus around the tooth to improve gingival health.

Scalloping (of the tongue): see Crenation

Taking a bite: A process to determine the relationship between the maxillary and mandibular teeth to assess the occlusion and in sleep to determine the position of the mandible for the fabrication of an oral appliance.

Temporomandibular Joint (TMJ): Jaw joint. The joint that articulates the mandible with the maxilla and provides for movement of the mandible.

TMJ/TMD: TMJ and TMD (temporomandibular dysfunction). Abbreviation for dysfunction as it relates to the joints. Thought to involve numerous symptoms such as joint sounds, joint pain, headache, facial pain, otalgia, and neck pain.

Torus (plural, tori): Boney area at the lingual aspect of the mandible approximate to the bicuspids (premolars) and first molars, or a boney prominence in the palate at the midline. Nonpathologic; usually appears in early adulthood and stops growing between the ages of 30 to 40.

Underbite: Inaccurate term for the mandible appearing prognathic or forward of the maxilla (Class III).

Wear facets: Small areas indicative of wear in the area of the cusps or incisal edges of the teeth; associated with a malocclusion or with parafunction (clenching or bruxing).

Index

Note: Page numbers of article titles are in **boldface** type.

A

Adults, orthodontic treatment approaches to sleep-disordered breathing, 83–84

Airway, analysis of, with computed tomography, cone beam (CBCT), **59–70**

    airway, 68–69

    anatomic accuracy, 60

    degenerative joint disease, 63–68

    facial growth and the airway, 60–62

    image analysis and, 59–60

anatomy of, overview of, **45–57**

evaluation of, in oral and nasal airway screening by the dentist, 4

Ambulatory monitoring, in sleep bruxism evaluation, 13–14

Ambulatory testing, for adult obstructive sleep apnea by the dentist, **99–108**

    case presentation, 99–100

    classification of methods for diagnosis, 100

    comparison of portable monitor with polysomnography, 102–103

    criteria to support use of, 107–108

    definitions of obstructive sleep apnea by portable monitoring, 104–105

    evidence to date, 106–107

    proper study design to validate a portable home sleep testing monitor, 101

    sleep staging, 103–104

    supervision of, 100

    technical considerations, 105–106

Amitryptiline, for sleep bruxism, 26

Anatomy, airway, overview of, **45–57**

    nasal airway, in screening by the dentist, 4

    upper airway, and neurologic basis of sleep breathing disorders, 34–39

Apnea. *See* Obstructive sleep apnea syndrome.

Appliances, oral. *See* Oral appliances.

Awakening headaches, sleep and, 147

B

Behavioral therapy, for sleep bruxism, 22–23

Benzodiazepines, for sleep bruxism, 26

Bi-maxillary transverse distraction osteogenesis, for obstructive sleep apnea therapy, 87

Botulinum toxin type A, for sleep bruxism, 27

Breathing disorders, sleep-related, 1–171

ambulatory testing for adult obstructive sleep apnea by the dentist, **99–108**

anatomy of airway, **45–57**

cone beam computed tomography (CBCT)

    analysis in, **59–70**

    airway, 68–69

    anatomic accuracy, 60

    degenerative joint disease, 63–68

    facial growth and the airway, 60–62

    image analysis and, 59–60

    mandibular growth, 62–63

neurologic basis of, **37–44**

    histopathologic correlates, 41–42

    impaired cortical processing, 40–41

    motor deficits, 41

    reversal of neurologic lesions with treatment, 42

    sensory dysfunction, 39–40

    upper airway anatomy, 34–39

obstructive sleep apnea and bruxism in children, **163–168**

oral and nasal airway screening by the dentist, **1–8**

    clinical recognition of a patient at risk, 2

    detailed evaluation, 2–6

    nasal airway evaluation, 6–7

oral appliance therapy for, **91–98**

    adverse effects, 95–96

    effectiveness, 93–95

    indications for, 96–97

    mechanism of action, 91–92

    medical devices, 93

    selection of, 93

    types of, 92–93

orofacial myology and myofunctional therapy, **109–113**

    common signs of myofunctional disorder, 109

    head and neck growth and development, 109–110

    tongue muscle physiology, 110–111

orthodontic considerations related to, **71–89**

    cephalometric evaluation, 74–75

    clinical examination and study model evaluation, 72–74

    growth and development, 75–80

    in adults, 83–84

    in pediatric patients, 80–83

doi:10.1016/S1556-407X(10)00022-6
1556-407X/10/$ – see front matter © 2010 Elsevier Inc. All rights reserved.

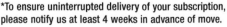

Printed and bound by CPI Group (UK) Ltd, Croydon, CR0 4YY
03/11/2024
01040554-0020

Printed and bound by CPI Group (UK) Ltd, Croydon, CR0 4YY

03/10/2024

01040353-0020